Pediatric Acupuncture

With love for my daughters Alyssa and Alexandra,
and my aging Mother

For Churchill Livingstone:

Publishing Manager, Health Professions: Inta Ozols
Project Manager: Gail Wright
Designer: Judith Wright

PEDIATRIC ACUPUNCTURE

May Loo MD

*Assistant Clinical Professor, Department of Pediatrics and Department of
Pediatric Anesthesiology, Stanford Medical Center, Palo Alto, CA;
Director, Neurodevelopmental Program, Department of Pediatrics,
Santa Clara County Valley Medical Center, San Jose, CA, USA*

Foreword by

John Spencer PhD ABPN

*Silver Spring, MD; Formerly, Director of Extramural Programs of Research,
The Office of Medicine, NIH, Bethesda, MD and Associate Dean and
Director of the Doctorate Program in Clinical Psychology, Regent University,
Virginia Beach, VA, USA*

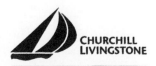

CHURCHILL
LIVINGSTONE

CHURCHILL LIVINGSTONE
An imprint of Elsevier Limited

First published 2002
    Reprinted 2005

ISBN 0 443 07032 6

British Library Cataloguing in Publication Data
A catalogue record for this book is available from the British Library

Library of Congress Cataloguing in Publication Data
A catalogue record for this book is available from the Library of Congress

Note
Medical knowledge is constantly changing. As new information becomes
available, changes in treatment, procedures, equipment and the use of drugs
become necessary. The authors and the publishers have taken care to ensure
that the information given in this text is accurate and up to date. However,
readers are strongly advised to confirm that the information, especially with
regard to drug usage, complies with the latest legislation and standards of
practice.

                                                                    The Publisher

ELSEVIER **your source for books,
journals and multimedia
in the health sciences**
www.elsevierhealth.com

Working together to grow
libraries in developing countries
www.elsevier.com | www.bookaid.org | www.sabre.org

ELSEVIER   BOOK AID   Sabre Foundation
           International

Transferred to digital print 2007
Printed and bound by CPI Antony Rowe, Eastbourne

The
publisher's
policy is to use
**paper manufactured
from sustainable forests**

Contents

Foreword

As conventional medicine moves into the 21st century, consumers can expect a variety of changes that will both improve and move healthcare to an exciting and new plateau. Sophisticated technologies exist for evaluating brain (dys)function during specified behavioral tasking. Synthetically produced medications are being tested in a range of areas, from keeping arterial shunts open to enhancing neuronal synaptic capabilities and potentially reversing dementia. Along with these changes, however, also comes another kind of medicine that has its origins dating back thousands of years. It encompasses a multitude of techniques that have come under various descriptions including "holistic, alternative, complementary, naturopathic or botanical medicine". Many therapies, which are part of these larger categories: a) are increasingly utilized by patients both in the USA and abroad; b) are being reimbursed by insurance companies; c) are the subject of much discussions by governments throughout the world interested in providing optimal healthcare to their constituents. One such therapy technique, *medical acupuncture*, is the feature of this book. The patient population discussed and reviewed—children—presents a unique opportunity to begin to better understand at a clinical and more importantly an integrative level, ways for healthcare and medicine to provide for a more balanced, thorough and potentially efficacious treatment opportunity.

Historically acupuncture has been used for many medical conditions. Until recently it was less important to understand how or why it worked than it was to report on its usefulness, including patient "satisfaction". With the advent of modern medicine pushing for a more focused scientific-evidence base, a challenge has gone out to all therapies, both conventional and non-conventional, essentially to prove that they deliver what they say they can—efficacious outcomes—along with an eye toward cost and safety issues. Although it has been difficult understanding how sticking a needle in the skin (and potentially activating and driving a so-called energy force of "Qi" to balance dysfunctional systems) might relate to Western healthcare, pre-clinical research is currently demonstrating that this stimulation is in fact activating specific brain pathways and centers that have their connections with the autonomic and peripheral nervous system(s)—areas directly relevant and tied to much of medical physiology. Thus, acupuncture is simply more than just folklore or a "placebo acting event"; several respected research conferences at NIH have lent scientific credibility to and suggested acupuncture's usefulness in treating specific medical disorders such as nausea and pain. Noteworthy though, there will always be a recognizable and ongoing debate between Western scientists who demand that any clinical procedure be proven through a large number of patients enrolled in clinical trials and those Eastern clinicians who stress the larger importance of tailoring treatment(s) to the individual. Both groups need to listen to and learn from each other. Medical programs such as the one at the University of Arizona now formally teach many of the same principles of integration that are reviewed in this book. Conventional medicine is aware that accommodation is not enough. With evidence now accumulating that acupuncture as well as other "alternative or complementary" techniques can be "proven" to be medically helpful and safe, allopathic physicians and healthcare providers are going to be required to understand its basic principles if for no other reason than to make sensible referrals. Today's consumer is much more health-driven and expects a degree of sophistication on the part of their provider that all tools are readily made available to maximize the delivery of good and complete healthcare. But beyond sophistication also lies a second important goal of providing for a more ethnically focused medicine, sensitive to all patients' healthcare concerns and needs.

Against this backdrop *Pediatric Acupuncture* by May Loo MD has just the right balance of descriptors of conventional and Chinese medicine. All chapters are well organized and easy to follow. Chapter 7 on "Pediatric acupuncture modalities and treatment protocols" is especially important because it accurately details information about acupuncture needles, and associated techniques of electric stimulators, magnets, and lasers along with the current position of the Food and Drug Administration toward usage. Also, the section on dietary management eloquently describes the important bridge between health and prevention as viewed from two different cultures. Providers should consider carefully the usefulness of much of this material for integrative potential in their own practices. There is presented throughout the book the important distinction between Western and Chinese medicine components and the ways they should be viewed in the context of the total medical–diagnostic–treatment continuum. The tables and figures clearly illustrate easy-to-follow information, linking target organs and acupuncture points so that the healthcare provider has easy-to-visualize pictures of sometimes difficult textual descriptions.

Who says that "East is East and West is West and never the twain shall meet"? This book provides a resounding "No." Rather, conventional and Chinese medicine can and should when clinically necessary use each other's strengths. One example of co-integration and utilization of acupuncture with allopathic medicine could be the example of reducing dosage of medication (to avoid or reduce unwanted side-effects in certain patients) or the tapering down of medication dosage and its eventual replacement with acupuncture for continuation of lasting treatment benefit, cost, and safety. Or, in some patients, simply using acupuncture as appropriate, standard care. The seminal goal still remains to maximize treatment benefit.

Pediatric Acupuncture should be in the library and used by any dedicated physician or healthcare provider interested in giving the best and the most complete quality of care to patients. It will be a relevant addition to any medical practice as well as to students learning more about a "new" and "old" but important component of healthcare—integrative medicine. I highly recommend this book for such purposes.

John Spencer

Acknowledgements

With thanks to my many teachers, East and West, who have imparted their knowledge and wisdom; to Gail Wright and Inta Ozols for their patience and support; and to my sister Margaret for her help with the innumerable references. Thanks to my family for their love, which sustained me throughout the writing of the manuscript.

1 Introduction

Look, it cannot be seen, it is beyond form.
Listen, it cannot be heard, it is beyond sound.
Grasp, it cannot be held, it is intangible. . .
It is called indefinable, and beyond imagination.
Stand before it and there is no beginning.
Follow it and there is no end.
Stay with the ancient Tao, move with the present.
Knowing the ancient beginning is the essence of Tao.

Tao Te Ching—Lao Tsu

Chinese pediatrics is an ancient healing art that was mentioned as early as the first century BC in the *Nei Jing* (*The Inner Classics*). The roots of Western pediatrics were planted in the writings of Plato and Aristotle, but it was not until the twentieth century that pediatrics became a major subspecialty. Chinese treatment of children continues to follow the teachings of Traditional Chinese Medicine (TCM), based on the Taoist view of man as a being of nature that follows the laws of nature. The child, as the adult, is an individual, whole entity consisting of energetic, physical, emotional, and spiritual beings. So many of those beings have no solid form, cannot be seen or heard with even the most sophisticated technological instruments. Western pediatrics, together with Western medicine, has made phenomenal scientific strides and uncovered massive information on the bioanatomic and biochemical aspects of children. This knowledge engendered a more segmental view of the child, as pediatrics branches into over a dozen subspecialties, each focusing on one physical aspect of the child.

This book is based on more than 25 years' experience in working with children. Having been trained both as a Western pediatrician and as a Chinese medical practitioner, I have been able to appreciate the immense value each school of healing has to offer. Although neither discipline has a complete picture of children, their approaches complement each other. The purpose of this book is to integrate Western knowledge and modern technology with ancient Chinese wisdom for a more comprehensive understanding of the pediatric population. Up-to-date evidence-based information is interpreted in the light of ancient concepts. Having had post-doctoral training in developmental pediatrics, I have also proposed an original theory of childhood development, integrating the teachings of Freud and Piaget with the Five Elements.

This book is intended for pediatric practitioners with training in either or both TCM and Western pediatrics. The Chinese acupuncturist can benefit from learning Western factual information about children. The Western pediatrician can benefit from viewing children from another perspective, especially in conditions that are baffling to Western science. The MD acupuncturist can see for the first time the integration of two major schools of pediatric healing. In order to accommodate the diversity of readers, this book reviews the basic physiology and pathophysiology of both Western and Chinese pediatrics. In addition, I have learned in teaching MD and DO acupuncturists around the country, that many of the basic concepts in Chinese medicine are difficult for the Western, scientific mind to comprehend. Therefore, some of the chapters are written in simple, easy to understand, less technical language; sometimes using simple metaphors to help illustrate important concepts. In order to avoid the confusion of the same terminology for the various organs, the Chinese organs will be capitalized. Illustrations of the meridians are included in the appendix. The reader is encouraged to read more basic textbooks for background information, and for description and location of acupuncture points.

When we "follow the ancient Tao, move with the present," we expand our pediatric knowledge and pave the way to raising healthier and happier children.

The Chinese medicine background information discussed throughout the book is a composite of material obtained from the author's education and experiences, and from the "General and Chinese Medicine Texts and References" list in the bibliography on p. 346.

2 History of Pediatrics: East and West

The treatment of children has undergone evolutionary changes in both Chinese and Western medicine. Chinese pediatrics dates back several thousand years, and has preserved many basic principles throughout the ages. By comparison, Western pediatrics is a relatively new field, but has rapidly become complex and segmentalized with numerous subspecialties.

Pediatrics massage, Tui Na, was mentioned in the *Nei Jing*,[1] the classical acupuncture textbook that dates to the first century BC. However, children were generally considered as adults until the Han Dynasty in the late 200 AD, when medical textbooks began to include separate chapters on treatment of children. In the twelfth century Song Dynasty, 1031–1113 AD, the famous child specialist, Qian Yi, wrote the first pediatric textbook that recognized children as unique beings with distinctive physiology and pathophysiology of diseases that merit different diagnoses and treatment from adults.

During the Ming Dynasty in the fourteenth to the seventeenth centuries, pediatrics flourished with formulation of specific herbal and acupuncture protocols for children, and introduction of preventive measures. In 1534, Wang Luan's *You Ke Lei Cui* (*A Collection of Pediatric Cases*) was a comprehensive text that described the pulse, treatment principles, acupuncture protocols, and herbal formulas for individual pediatric diseases. The distinguished imperial physician, Xue Liang-Wu wrote *Bao Ying Cuo Yao* (*Essentials for the Care & Protection of Infants*) in 1556, which stressed the importance of adjusting the dosage of herbal formulas for children according to their age and size. One of the most famous Ming Dynasty pediatricians, Wan Mi-zhai, introduced preventive pediatric measures, such as exposing children to sunlight and fresh air, protecting them from being frightened, avoiding overfeeding them or giving them too much medication.

During the last dynasty, the Qing Dynasty (1644–1911), many famous pediatric textbooks were written. Some of them are still being used as references today: *You Ke Liang Fang* (*Fine Formulas in Pediatrics*) and *Dou Zhen Liang Fang* (*Fine Formulas for Poxes & Rashes*).

The twentieth century witnessed the publication of hundreds of pediatric textbooks and the establishment of Pediatric Departments in TCM hospitals. In 1999 and 2000, I was invited to lecture at the Xinhua Hospital in Shanghai and the University Hospital in Beijing. I also had the opportunity to tour other TCM pediatrics clinics and hospital wards. I was impressed by the preservation of ancient principles in the evaluation of children, such as examining the vein on the index finger to assess severity of illness. I learned about newer treatment modalities for children, and was especially delighted at the integration of Chinese and Western pediatrics. Some hospitalized children were receiving Western treatments, such as intravenous antibiotics, along with acupuncture and herbs. Preventive pediatrics is practiced following the ancient wisdom of "winter disease, summer cure," so that seasonal conditions—such as asthma—are treated during the summer before symptoms occur in later months. In China and many other Asian countries, acupuncture is being used to treat an entire spectrum of childhood illnesses, ranging from mild respiratory ailments to neurological disorders such as cerebral palsy and autism. However, pediatric acupuncture is only slowly being introduced to Europe and the United States.

Western pediatrics, on the other hand, is prevalent throughout the world, even though it has a very short history compared to its Chinese counterpart. While Chinese medicine began to recognize children as distinct from adults in 200 AD, Western medicine considered the child as an homunculus, a miniature adult, until the 1920s. In 1934, pediatrics became a subspecialty and has been growing at a phenomenal pace. Over a dozen subspecialties have been added over the past three decades, including pediatric nephrology (1974), neonatal medicine (1975), pediatric hematology and ontology (1974) and pediatric gastroenterology (1990).[2] Preventive medicine remains the mainstay of general pediatrics, with regularly scheduled well child visits, especially in the first two years of life. The pediatrician monitors nutrition, growth parameters and developmental milestones; performs routine physical examinations and laboratory studies, and administers immunizations as the essential components during well baby check-ups and physical examinations. Technological and medical advances enable the early diagnosis of congenital and hereditary abnormalities prenatally and shortly after birth, such as Down syndrome and hypothyroidism; the resuscitation of tiny premature babies of only a few hundred grams; and the prolongation of conditions that range from cystic fibrosis to childhood cancers. The majority of "bread-and-butter" pediatrics consist of treatment of viral illnesses, bacterial infections, and various skin rashes. Although there are pediatric medications that are specific for children, with incremental dosages calculated according to age or body weight, the majority of medications have very little data for young children under age 12. Dosages are frequently given as 1/2 or 1/3 of adult dosages.

The increasingly stressful lifestyle during the past decades has resulted in an increased incidence of "adult" conditions, such as hypertension and depression, in children. Complex neurodevelopmental conditions such as attention deficit disorder often necessitate a multidisciplinary approach by the pediatrician, psychologist, behavioral and educational therapist. In spite of modern technological advances and voluminous information about the physical aspect of disease entities, many pediatric conditions continue to be puzzling to Western medicine. Recent surveys indicate that alternative and complementary medicine, including acupuncture, are gaining increasing acceptance in the treatment of children.[3] This book hopes to introduce an integrative approach to children, to combine bioanatomic and biochemical information with the ancient wisdom of bioenergetics, for a more comprehensive understanding of all aspects of children: the energetic, physical, emotional, and spiritual aspects.

REFERENCES

1. *Nei Jing* (*The Yellow Emperor's Classic of Internal Medicine*), translated by Ilza Veith (1949). University of California Press, Berkeley, CA.
2. The American Board of Medical Specialties (2000) *The Official ABMC Directory of Board Certification 2000.*
3. Spiegelblatt L.S. (1994) The use of alternative medicine by children. *Pediatrics* 94, 811.

3 | The Beginning of Life

When life begins has been a controversial topic throughout the world. It is a complex issue with medical, philosophical, social, ethical, religious and even political ramifications. While sharing a few fundamental notions, Western and Chinese medicine offer vastly different perspectives for conception, pregnancy, birth, and the beginning of life. The differences are rooted in the anatomic and biochemical view of life versus the bioenergetic paradigm of individual and Universal Qi.

CONCEPTION

According to Western medicine, conception occurs when the father's sperm fertilizes an egg from the mother, forming a zygote. This fertilized egg implants in the uterus, and inherits two sets of chromosomes carrying genetic information from each parent. The transmission of genetic information based on the Mendelian model of dominant and recessive traits and the Watson–Crick model of DNA structures are well known to high school biology classes. The X and Y chromosomes determine the sex of the offspring: XX for girls, XY for boys; and the precise sequence and arrangement of nucleotides on the 22 pairs of autosomal chromosomes determine the child's physical characteristics, intelligence, temperament, and predisposition to some physical and emotional illnesses. While the specific genetic malformations have been deciphered in many conditions, such as trisomy 21 in Down syndrome, the majority of conditions with familial tendencies—such as migraines and depression—still do not have specific genetic mapping. A few conditions are associated with maternal age, such as increasing incidence of Down syndrome in children born to older women. On the whole, the genetic information is independent of the physical and emotional states of the parents at the time of conception.

The Chinese medicine perspective of conception reflects both individual and universal issues. The bioenergetic correlate to genetic inheritance is the transmittance of Essence or Jing from both the mother and father that form the basis of pre-Heaven Jing for the child. The qualitative potency of this Jing—the densest form of Qi—depends not only on the ancestral Essence that is transmitted through generations, but also on the parental physical and emotional health, as well as climatic and universal influences at the time of conception. Whereas Western medicine places importance on the physical health of the mother during conception and pregnancy, Chinese medicine emphasizes the physical and the emotional health of *both* the mother and the father.

Since Essence naturally decreases with age, older parents have less or weaker Jing to pass onto the fetus. Western medicine recommends amniocentesis for women over age 35 to rule out the possibility of a Down syndrome baby and does not take into account the age of the father. Chinese medicine posits that

Jing is affected by the age of both parents. In addition, physical factors—such as chronic illness, fatigue, drug or alcohol abuse—as well as emotional states—such as stress, depression, excess anger—of *both* parents are also important in determining the quality of fetal Essence.

Individually, the father's Jing is further affected by his history of sexual activity, while the mother's Jing is affected by her history of menstruation, number of pregnancies and miscarriages. In the man, Jing is lost through ejaculation. A promiscuous father has quantitatively less Jing for his child. In the woman, Jing is affected by blood loss during menstruation, pregnancy and miscarriage. A woman with heavier menstrual flow tends to lose more Jing each month. Childbirths, especially those that are close together, would seriously weaken the Liver, Kidney, and Conception Vessels, which would in turn affect the Jing.

Miscarriage in Chinese medicine is often considered to be more Jing depleting than childbirth because there is usually more blood loss and more abrupt alteration of hormone levels in a miscarriage than in childbirth. In addition, a miscarriage (especially a late one), is emotionally very distressing to the mother, who often has deep feelings of loss, and even failure. Numerous childhood conditions may be attributed to weak pre-Heaven Jing associated with parental health at conception. For example, children with elderly parents may develop Kidney deficiency headaches, enuresis, or a tendency to be fearful. Parents with fatigue from overwork may contribute to Spleen weakness that is transmitted to the fetus and manifests as digestive problems in the child.

In addition to familial and parental factors, the Chinese also take into consideration global conditions such as climate and the political atmosphere during time of conception. For example, it is considered inauspicious to conceive during a thunderstorm, and favorable to conceive on a day when a peace accord is reached between countries. This concept is based on the principle that man is a being between Heaven and Earth, is intimately related to one another and to all living beings, and is greatly affected by the Universal Qi. What happens in any part of the world affects everyone. Western culture is becoming more aware of man's relation to nature, such as the effect of rain forest destruction on global warming and massive changes in ecology. This awareness, however, does not carry over to individual human conception and birth.

PREGNANCY

In Western medicine, maternal physical health and well-being during pregnancy is the only crucial factor for development of the fetus. Any emotional stress is not considered detrimental if there are no physical changes, such as a rise in blood pressure.

The zygote undergoes rapid cell division. The first trimester—the first 13 weeks of gestation—is the critical period of organogenesis. This is the vulnerable period when any insult to the mother—such as illness, drugs (both prescription and abusive substances), alcohol ingestion, X-ray exposure—can result in fetal malformation. The brain and peripheral nervous system, heart and gastrointestinal system, as well as eyes and ears begin to develop within the first month of life. By the second month, all the other internal organs, arms and legs, and the musculoskeletal system begin to form.

By the third and fourth months of gestation, external genitalia and facial features begin to take shape. The fetus then continues to grow in size with gradual maturation of the organs, totally dependent upon the mother via the placenta for respiration, nutrition as well as excretion of carbon dioxide and waste material.

Chinese medicine emphasizes both the physical and emotional health of the mother during pregnancy. Contrary to Western medicine, Chinese medicine posits that emotional stress can directly affect the fetus energetically even without concrete physical changes in the mother. This bestows greater responsibility upon the father during pregnancy, as marital relationships could profoundly influence the mother's psyche during a time of emotional vulnerability. Fear and anxiety, for example, cause Qi to rise up. When this occurs in the mother during pregnancy, less Qi is available for the fetus. Excess emotions of any type can affect the Heart, which may result in a child afflicted with Heart deficiency.

BEGINNING OF LIFE

The Western model of conception and embryology has generated heated debate as to when life actually begins, particularly with regards to abortion. When is it medically safe and morally justifiable to perform abortions? At this time, drug-induced abortion can be performed as early as the first 72 hours of life with the "morning after pill," and up to 7 weeks of pregnancy with drug combinations. Mechanical and surgical procedures such as dilatation and curettage (D&C) are easily performed within the first trimester. Abortions in the second and especially the third trimester involve riskier surgical procedures that require hospitalization. Since the early 1970s, the US Supreme Court upheld a woman's right to have an abortion for any reason up to 24 weeks of fetal gestation. At this time, there are approximately 1.3 million abortions in the US and approximately 46 million women worldwide each year have an abortion.[1] Safety and medical indications aside, the question of when a fetus is a viable human life encompasses moral, ethical, religious and political implications. The Chinese medicine perspective merely presents another point of view and does not presume to offer easy answers for abortion.

Chinese medicine posits that the three treasures of life—Qi, Mind, and Essence—are present at conception. The pre-Heaven Essence from both parents is in fact the origin and biological basis of the Mind: "*Life comes about through the Essence; when the two Essences [of mother and father] unite, they form the Mind*"—Spiritual Axis.[2] Since Mind and Essence are both forms of Qi—Mind being the most subtle and nonmaterial Qi and Essence being the densest form of Qi—the integrated being of Energy, Mind, and Essence is therefore present from the moment of conception. As organs develop, so do the associated treasures: Qi with Lung, Stomach, Spleen; Mind with Heart; and Essence with Kidney.

We can further integrate Western embryology with Chinese energetics and extrapolate the development of meridians and human emotions. As early as the four-cell stage of the zygote, the Curious Meridians Chong Mai and Dai Mai that define the vertical and horizontal planes of the body are already coming into existence.[3] As the zygote continues to grow through cell division, it would be reasonable to assume that Qi channels form along with the organs within the first 2 months of gestation.

Besides the energetic and physical development, the question of when human emotions come into existence is also of paramount importance. It is emotions that determine our behavior, that are central to our interpersonal relationships, that motivate us to achieve our goals. Since emotions are part of the Mind and are associated with the organs, we can extrapolate that human emotions must also be present at conception and develop with the organs. The emotions have specific organ correspondences as follows: Heart, House of the Mind and all emotions, specifically is associated with joy and passion; Spleen/Pancreas (digestive system) with sympathy/worry; Lung with sadness; Kidney with fear; Liver with anger/frustration/irritability. This organ-related emotional development refers to the formation of normal range of human emotions that can be experienced by everyone, independent of heredity. Hereditary organ weakness can predispose a child to predilection of an emotion, such as a familial tendency toward depression with Lung deficiency or fearfulness with Kidney deficiency. This also means that the emotional states of parents during conception and mother's psychological state during pregnancy can give rise to *innate* emotional tendencies in the fetus that can manifest in behavioral patterns in infancy and childhood.

All of this is in sharp contrast to Western medicine, which has focused on the intellectual capabilities of children, and minimized their innate, emotional development. Developmentalists have long debated the issue of nature versus nurture, heredity versus environmental influences in shaping children's emotions. The nineteenth-century view of children as *tabula rasa*, blank slates upon which environment can etch its influences, has been held by psychologists until as late as 1950. Research into the emotional and psychological make-up of infants began in 1956, when a 30-year longitudinal study examined nine infant temperament characteristics. Drs. Chess and Thomas concluded that these are primarily genetic and innate attributes that can be categorized as: activity, biological rhythmicity, initial approach/withdrawal, adaptability, intensity, mood, persistence/attention span, distractibility, and sensory threshold.[4] These temperament characteristics can be assessed as early as 4 months of age. Some recent studies have extended these temperament characteristics to the fetus; e.g., a very active baby in the womb may become an active infant and child.[5]

BIRTH

Birth marks the indisputable emergence of a human life. Western medicine assesses the health of the baby immediately after delivery by using the Apgar score, a 10-point system that gives maximum of 2 points each for respiration, color, muscle tone, heart rate, and reflexes. At the present time, premature babies can be resuscitated as early as 22 weeks of gestation, although neonatal complications that include respiratory distress, cerebral bleed, and infections often necessitate an extended stay in the neonatal intensive care unit and require artificial support such as respirator ventilation, intravenous feedings, and administration of various medications.

Chinese medicine also celebrates birth as the emergence of the being of Qi, Mind, and Essence into the external world. After birth, Kidney stores the prenatal Essence which continues to provide nourishment for the Mind. This can correlate to the Western concept of innate intelligence or emotions that continues to manifest throughout a person's life. The Mind is also nourished by postnatal Essence produced by the Lungs, Stomach and Spleen so that our diet and lifestyle influence how we feel and our ability to think.

Just as universal influences are important in conception, the Chinese also take into account the auspiciousness for time of birth. Whereas conception marks the coming into existence of the three treasures of Qi, Mind and Essence, birth connotes the entry of Souls, the significant event that completes man as an energetic, physical, emotional, *and* spiritual being.

According to Chinese medicine, each person has two Souls: the Corporeal Soul, Po, and the Ethereal Soul, Hun. The Corporeal Soul enters the body at birth and returns to Earth upon the person's death. It resides in the Lung, pertains to the body, to the human physical form, and to all physiologic processes. It is the Po that enables us to breathe, to feel physical sensations, to have movement. It is interesting that the Western Apgar score is in a sense a measurement of how well the Corporeal Soul has entered the body. Po is Yin and quiescent. It is connected to Qi and to Yang. Disharmony of Po causes problems in vitality and symptoms during the daytime.

The Corporeal Soul brings with it the Ethereal Soul, Hun. Unlike the Po that is each person's individual Soul, the Hun comes from the Soul World, and returns to that Soul World upon the person's death. It resides in the Liver Blood and Yin, but is Yang and is the Qi of the Mind. It is closely linked with the Universal Mind. It is the Hun that brings images from the Eternal World. The Chinese concept of Hun is comparable to the Jungian idea of the "individual and collective unconscious." The Eternal Soul World is like the Collective Unconscious, made up of Individual Unconscious.[2]

Although this concept of Soul is foreign to Western pediatrics, it is incorporated into common expressions such as "the eyes are windows to the soul" and "soul-mates." Hun is part of everyday Chinese. A mother may call out to her impulsive son: "What's the matter with you? Did you misplace your Hun?" or "I was so frightened, my Hun left me." The eyes do in fact reflect the state of a person's Hun. In addition, by looking into each other's eyes, the Ethereal Soul enables us to become connected with one another. In this context, some pediatric entities can be categorized as Soul problems. Autism, which has the cardinal signs of poor eye contact and lack of social interaction, can be viewed as a problem of the Ethereal Soul; while babies born with low Apgar scores at birth can be viewed as inadequate entry of Corporeal Soul.

When we integrate knowledge from Western and Chinese pediatrics, we can have better understanding not only of conception, fetal development, birth, but also of physical, emotional vulnerabilities and behavioral tendencies in infants and children.

REFERENCES

1. US Census Bureau (1999), *Statistical Abstract of the United States*, 119th edition. Washington, DC.
2. Maciocia G. (1989) *The Foundations of Chinese Medicine, A Comprehensive Text for Acupuncturists and Herbalists*. London, Churchill Livingstone.
3. Helms J. (1995) *Acupuncture Energetics, A Clinical Approach for Physicians*. Berkeley, Medical Acupuncture Publishers.

4. Carey W.B. (1990) Temperament risk factors in children: a Conference Report. *Developmental and Behavioral Pediatrics*, 11 (1).

5. Cameron J. (2000) US Temperament researcher. Personal communication.

4 Understanding the Physiology and Pathophysiology of Childhood Illnesses

In both Western pediatrics and Chinese medicine, infants and children have unique physiological functions and pathophysiology of illnesses. This chapter discusses general pediatric physiology and pathophysiology, followed by detailed descriptions of each organ physiology and pathophysiology. The characteristics of each organ as coupled Yin–Yang organs of the same Element, and each organ relation to phases of childhood development are emphasized. Wherever possible, Western pediatric knowledge is integrated with Chinese theories of childhood health and diseases.

General Physiology and Pathophysiology

The general physiology and pathophysiology of children and childhood illnesses can be classified as follows.

- General physiology of children
    "Pure Yang"/maximum Yang
    "Young Yang and young Yin"
    "Clear Visceral Qi"

- General pathophysiology of childhood illnesses
    Easy onset—fragile and immature organs, pathogenic evils enter easily
    Rapid transformation—disease progression and changes occur quickly
    Rapid recovery

- Modified physiology and pathophysiology in the modern child
    Stressful lifestyle
    Bioenergetic lingering effect of illness, toxins, and medications
    Environmental toxins
    Exposure to electromagnetic fields
    Technology and imagination
    Diet.

Specific Organ Physiology and Pathophysiology

Table 4.1 shows the Yin organs and their links with the childhood constitution.

TABLE 4.1	The Yin organs and their links with the childhood constitution	
	Childhood constitution	**Yin organs**
	Lung deficiency	Lung
	Spleen deficiency	Spleen
	Blood and Fluid insufficiency	Heart
	Young Yin and young Yang	Kidney
	Liver vulnerability	Liver

Before discussing the physiology and pathophysiology of children, it is important to briefly review the basic health and healing concepts in Traditional Chinese Medicine (TCM). (The reader without a Chinese medicine background is encouraged to study basic textbooks on Chinese medicine for more detailed discussions.) The basic principles in TCM consist of Qi, Yin–Yang opposites and the Five-Element relationship of organ systems.

Qi is the fundamental concept in Chinese medicine. Qi has no equivalent in the English language. It can be roughly translated as "vital energy" or "vital force." Qi circulates unidirectionally in meridians and is also part of blood and moves within blood vessels. It permeates organs and tissues and is behind all physiologic processes. Health is the harmonious, uninterrupted flow of Qi, and disease ensues when there is disruption of Qi flow.

The homeostasis of Qi flow also balances the dynamic opposites of the human body: the Yin and the Yang. Chinese medicine views man as a small replica of nature, a microcosm to nature, the macrocosm. Everything in nature and within man is in a state of interdependence of Yin and Yang. The many correspondences of Yin include woman, femininity, Earth, the moon, darkness, emotions, rest; while Yang represents man, masculinity, Heaven, the sun, light, intellect, activity. The Yin–Yang opposites are not exclusive of each other, but each is moving along a continuum to be in balance with the opposite so that there is no absolute Yin or Yang, but within Yin there is Yang, and within Yang, there is Yin. Women can be feminine and intellectual, and men can be emotional and masculine. During the darkest of night is the beginning of dawn, and at the height of daylight is the beginning of evening. The dynamic balance between the opposites keeps all of Nature in equilibrium instead of chaos. The most common manifestations of Yin and Yang in diseases are excess and deficiency states. Health is defined as the balance of Yin and Yang.

The "building blocks" or vital substances of life are designated as Yang for Qi, Kidney Yang and Yin for Essence, Blood, Fluid.

- Yang
    Qi
    Kidney Yang
- Yin
    Essence
    Blood
    Fluid.

TABLE 4.2	The Five Elements		
Element		**Yin organ**	**Yang organ**
Water		Kidney	Bladder
Wood		Liver	Gallbladder
Fire		Heart	Small Intestine
		Pericardium (Master of the Heart)	Triple Energizer
Earth		Spleen	Stomach
Metal		Lung	Large Intestine

Kidney Yang is the basis of all Yang or physiologic fire in the body. Maciocia illustrates Kidney Yang as the firewood that burns and heats up the pot, which contains Kidney Yin—in the water. The steam from the boiling water represents Qi.[1] The Yin constituents in the "pot" are Kidney Essence, Blood and body Fluid.

The organs in the body are grouped as six Yin–Yang couplets. The Yin organs carry out the physiologic process of production and transformation of Qi and the hollow Yang organs carry out the lesser functions of storage and of transport of Qi. The couplet organs are further classified according to the Five Elements: Water, Wood, Fire, Earth, and Metal as shown in Table 4.2.

The meridians of the Yin–Yang organs connect with each other, so that the first point on the Large Intestine channel follows the last point on the Lung channel, and the last point on the Stomach channel connects to the first point on the Spleen channel. Each Element has numerous physical and metaphoric correspondences, such as emotions, voice, taste, color preferences; and universal correspondences that connect man with the natural world, such as seasons, directions, and climate. Table 4.2 lists the major correspondences of the Five Elements.

The Elements interact according to the natural laws governing nurturance and destruction. Each Element is the primary nurturer of another Element and at the same time is the primary controller or destroyer of another Element. Figure 4.1 illustrates the Five-Element Cycle.

The nurturing cycle operates with each Element nurturing the succeeding Element. The nurturer is the Mother Element to the nurtured, Son Element:

- Fire creates the ashes that become Earth
- Earth stores Metal
- Metal can be transformed into Water (this is true for metals physically being melted down to liquid, and for biological metabolism that yields water as the end product in the Kreb cycle)
- Water feeds Wood, as all trees need water to grow
- Wood provides the substance for Fire.

The destructive cycle operates with each Element controlling another Element. The controlling Element is the "grandmother," and the controlled Element, the "grandson":

FIGURE 4.1 *The Five-Element Cycle. (A) The nurturing cycle. (B) The destructive/controlling cycle. (C) The nurturing and destructive cycles combined.*

A

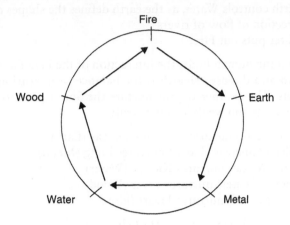

B

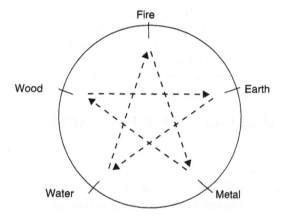

C

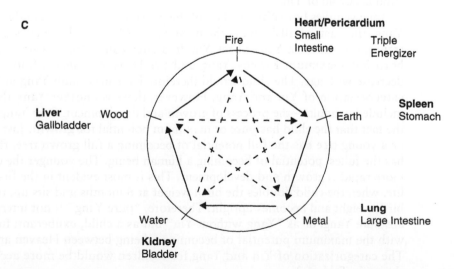

- Fire melts Metal
- Metal destroys Wood, as when an ax cuts down a tree
- Wood breaks up Earth, as when a root tears into earth
- Earth controls Water, as the earth defines the shapes of oceans, lakes, and the direction of flow of rivers
- Water puts out Fire.

Within the human body, the interaction of the Five Elements forms the basis for health and disease. Health is the balance of nurturing and controlling of the organs. The Mother organs nurture the Son organs to make sure that they do not become too weak, too deficient:

- Heart (Fire) nurtures Spleen/Pancreas (Earth)
- Spleen/Pancreas (Earth) nurtures Lung (Metal)
- Lung (Metal) nurtures Kidney (Water)
- Kidney (Water) nurtures Liver (Wood)
- Liver (Wood) nurtures Heart (Fire).

The controlling cycle is a sort of check-and-balance system to make sure that no one Element becomes too excessive or too strong:

- Heart (Fire) controls Lung (Metal)
- Lung (Metal) controls Liver (Wood)
- Liver (Wood) controls Spleen/Pancreas (Earth)
- Spleen/Pancreas (Earth) controls Kidney (Water)
- Kidney (Water) controls Heart (Fire).

GENERAL PHYSIOLOGY OF CHILDREN

"Pure Yang"

All Chinese pediatric textbooks list "pure Yang" as the foremost characteristic of children. The term is misleading, as the word "pure" does not imply that the child is devoid of Yin.

Yang signifies both Yang or Fire of the physiologic processes, and Qi. Kidney Yang, the basis of all Yang, is the most Yang. Although Essence is a Yin substance, it is the most Yang of the Yin. It is often called "fiery water." The newborn has maximum Kidney Yang and pre-Heaven Essence, both of which decrease with age. The child would therefore have maximum Yang in the usual categorization of Yin and Yang. However, there is another Yang that is not included in adults—the process of growth and development. Pure Yang refers to the fact that the child has pure or maximum potential for growth. Just as a seed or a young tree has the full potential of becoming a full grown tree, the zygote has the fullest potential of becoming a human being. The younger the child, the more rapid is growth and development. This is most evident in the first year of life, when the child doubles the birth weight at 6 months and sits up, triples the birth weight and becomes upright. Therefore, "pure Yang" is not interpreted as absolute Yang, or as "Yang without Yin" but as a child, exuberant, full of life, with the maximum potential of becoming a being between Heaven and Earth. The categorization of Yin and Yang for children would be more accurate, as shown in Table 4.3.

TABLE 4.3	Yin and Yang in children		
		Yang	**Yin**
	Maximum Yang	Kidney Yang	Essence = most Yang of the Yin
	Pure Yang	Growth and development	
	Young Yang	Yang functions	Blood
	and young Yin	Qi	Fluid

"Young Yang and Young Yin"

The Yang here refers to Qi and Yang functions, and the Yin refers to Blood and Fluid. The child's skin is tender and Wei Qi, the protective Defensive Qi that circulates under the skin, is weak. The internal organs are delicate and immature and Qi within them is insufficient. The physiological functions—both Yin and Yang processes of the internal organ—are not well developed. The corresponding Western medical principle is that the child has an immature physiology and a weaker immune system.

The child is Yin deficient, which means that Blood and Fluid are insufficient and are in delicate balance. Western medicine supports this concept. Pediatric textbooks tell us that young children are especially susceptible to the consequences of illness that affect fluid balance. Water constitutes 78% of body weight at birth but declines to approximately 60% (the adult value) by 1 year of age. However, the usual daily turnover of water in the infant is equal to almost 25% of total body water compared to approximately 6% in the adult. Thus, the effects of diseases that reduce fluid intake, such as vomiting, or increase losses, such as diarrhea, appear much more rapidly in infants than in adults. Hemoglobin (Hgb) level is lower in children: mean Hgb 3 months–6 years = 12, 7–12 years = 13, whereas adult female mean Hgb = 14, adult male mean Hgb = 16. Children are more susceptible to developing anemia. Growth process of the child is—as the famous Qing Dynasty physician Wu Jutong pointed out in *Solution of Child's Disease—Treatises on Differentiation and Treatment of Epidemic Febrile Diseases*—in "the development of Yang and Yin."

"Clear Visceral Qi"

Chinese pediatric classics tell us that children have "clear visceral Qi," which in ancient times means pure and strong Qi that is uncontaminated by improper diet and emotions. Unfortunately, this is less true for the modern child. With administration of medications—even *in utero*, in the newborn period, and in infancy; with additives in foods and improper diet; with environmental toxins; with increased emotional stress—the "visceral Qi" is becoming less "clear" as evidenced by increased incidence in children of adult illnesses, such as cardiovascular disease and adult diabetes. Nonetheless, compared to the modern adult with so much toxic and emotional "baggage," the "clear visceral Qi" in children can be modified as "relatively clear visceral Qi."

GENERAL PATHOPHYSIOLOGY OF CHILDHOOD ILLNESSES

The interplay of all the physiologic factors predispose the child to unique pathophysiologic characteristics of childhood illnesses.

Easy Onset

The child's skin is tender and delicate, and the pores are more readily open, Wei Qi is low, so pathogens can easily enter the child via the skin, further obstructing the flow of Wei Qi. Pathogens can also directly enter the respiratory and digestive systems via the nose or the mouth, and readily invade the fragile and immature organs.

Rapid Transformation

Childhood illnesses are characterized by rapid onset and change. Once the pathogen enters, because of the delicate Qi and fluid balance, "young Yang and young Yin", disease processes undergo easy and rapid transformation from cold to hot, hot to cold, excess to deficiency, deficiency to excess, or even the simultaneous exhaustion of both Yin and Yang. Take the case of the Western diagnosis of upper respiratory infection (URI) and the Chinese diagnosis of invasion of Wind-Cold. Initially the child develops simple common cold symptoms. However, because the body has so much Yang, so much "fire," the body responds to the cold by raising the body temperature which in turn consumes Yin so that the body in turn has less fluid, and high fever ensues. As the child's Qi is low, there is insufficient Qi to fight off the pathogenic influence which can quickly obliterate normal Qi and makes the child rapidly Qi deficient. The child becomes simultaneously exhausted of both Yin and Yang. Western pediatricians are trained to be apprehensive of a 2-week-old with URI symptoms, because that child can look robust one minute, and can quickly become septic with fever and lethargy—a Yang collapse picture that is compatible with meningitis—and may even develop seizures with high fever. As children become older, there is a gradual increase of Yin and of Qi, and fevers do not run as high, and URI does not quickly turn into meningitis.

Lingering Pathogenic Qi

In Chinese medicine, even after symptoms of an illness resolve, pathogenic energy may still linger in the body causing further injury to and transformation in the child. The acute illness weakens the child's body, diminishes Qi, and injures Yin, further predisposing the child to acute illness. Lingering symptoms such as persistent dry cough, or recurrent sore throat in spite of negative streptococcal cultures, point to the energetic residuals of pathogens.

Rapid Recovery

In spite of the above three pathophysiologic characteristics, children tend to recover rapidly from illnesses. The majority of pediatric conditions are acute illnesses caused by an attack of exogenous pathogens or an improper diet, involving more superficial responses without complex organ or emotional involvement. The relatively clear Qi in the Yin and Yang organs further enable children to recuperate quickly.

MODIFIED PHYSIOLOGY AND PATHOPHYSIOLOGY IN THE MODERN CHILD

The general physiological and pathophysiological characteristics are rooted in ancient times and have been used to describe children since the Ming Dynasty. Several aspects of the life of the twenty-first-century child modify traditional concepts of health and disease in pediatrics.

Stressful Lifestyle

Children today are living in a fast-paced lifestyle with enormous stresses both at home and at school. The divorce rate is approaching 50%, and the numbers of single-parent households are rising. Children are being placed in daycare centers at an early age and often for long hours. Pressure to enter college is the fiercest of all times. In some instances, parents begin to prepare children from preschool. Academic excellence no longer ensures acceptance by college of student choice. Children need to excel in sports, in extracurricular activities, and need to become involved in community affairs. The increasing number of divorces generates feelings of anger, sadness, abandonment, compounded by feelings of insecurity and uprootedness, all of which affect children's schoolwork and personal relationships. The increasing emotional difficulties in the pediatric population are reflected by the rise in behavioral and affective disorders, such as attention deficit disorder and childhood depression. Detrimental emotions are further injurious to the physiological functions of the organs.

Technology and fad obsessions erode the sense of value and tradition and further "uproot" children, so that a new watch full of gadgetry is preferred over the grandfather's heirloom watch. Stress is most injurious to the Liver, which is already vulnerable in children.

Prevalence of Medications and Their Adverse Qi Effects

Synthetic medications are being given to pediatric patients of all ages, including premature infants and young children. While some are no doubt lifesaving, many are often being given indiscriminately, injuring the child energetically and physically. Increasingly, very potent medications such as antidepressants are being administered to very young children. Chinese medicine posits that these powerful chemicals deplete Kidney Yang. Broad-spectrum antibiotics are energetically "Cold" to the human system, tend to disrupt the normal flora, and are injurious to Stomach and Spleen. Antipyretics are intended for the treatment of fever, which is often a necessary expression of Heat generated by the disease process. Medication may produce a paradoxical "trapping" of Heat within the body and further injures Yin. While some medications are carefully monitored with blood levels, topical creams, such as hydrocortisone cream, are given liberally to infants and young children without being monitored. According to Chinese medicine, children have very tender skin with wide open pores. It is therefore not known how much of topical medications are absorbed through the skin to the internal organs.

Bioenergetic Lingering Effect of Illness, Toxins, and Medications

Even after laboratory results return to normal or medications are no longer detectable in the blood, there is still energetic lingering of toxins and medications for weeks or months which may affect or potentiate the next dose of medication or illness.

Environmental Toxins

In ancient times children lived in environments free of industrial toxins. Children today are exposed to toxins from day 1 of life, from impurities in water to exposure to car exhaust, industrial fumes, and smog on the first car ride home. While some toxins, such as mercury and lead, are often tested in children, the majority of toxins are not detected.

Exposure to Electromagnetic Fields

Research has demonstrated that Qi has electromagnetic properties, similar to the electromagnetic force (EMF) of technological gadgetry such as TV, computers, and video games. Since energy is neither created nor destroyed, the EMF energy can enter a child's body and become transformed into Heat. This further depletes Yin in children who are already Yin deficient. When children exercise, this Heat can be converted into kinetic energy, which tonifies Lung and Spleen. The modern child, however, tends to spend hours in front of the TV or playing video games, gathering more Heat without a means to expend or convert it, causing further build-up of Heat and injury to the Yin.

The EMF also has a very important effect on the autonomic nervous system. Placing electronic gadgetry such as computers or video games directly in front of the face enables the EMF to directly penetrate the Yintang point, the important "third eye" acupuncture point which correlates to the autonomic nervous system. Electromagnetic waves yield "Yang" or "sympathetic" stimuli, which can cause potent disruption of autonomic balance.

Technology and Imagination

Cognitive development in children proceeds from preconcrete to concrete thinking; the preconcrete years are characterized by vivid imagination when children play with imaginary friends, and by non-temporal thinking that interprets the world according to the child's experiences. This precedes the concrete years when rational thinking begins to develop around age 7. Imagination is crucial and often considered superior to intellect for higher levels of awareness, such as in meditation, and for self-understanding. Even modern psychology places a great deal of emphasis on being in touch with the "inner child," when the adult imagines being at the age in childhood when physical or emotional trauma occurred.

Children today begin at a very young age—3–4 years or even younger—at playing computer games that have two characteristics: (1) children do not need imagination to play games that have built in sequences of actions; (2) children become accustomed to rapid firing of stimuli that require immediate response: e.g., an object bounces up and down on the screen ten times a second, and the child needs to respond each time by pushing a button. This is accompanied by sound effects each time the object is hit. The adverse sequelae from this are (1) stunting of crucial development of imagination, and (2) training children to be bombarded by visual and auditory stimuli that occur at an unrealistic pace so that when children are placed in a realistic environment such as the classroom they become easily bored.

Diet

Both diet and the manner of eating today are harmful to children's energetic system: prevalence of sweet and Phlegm-producing foods—such as milk products and peanuts—are injurious to Spleen; fried foods are harmful to the Liver; lack of fresh foods coupled with prepared foods containing food coloring, additives, and preservatives are deleterious to overall formation of Nutritive Qi. Chapter 8 discusses the importance of diet in health and diseases in children.

SPECIFIC ORGAN PHYSIOLOGY AND PATHOPHYSIOLOGY

Although most of the internal organs have the same names in both Western and Chinese medicine, there are major differences in physical characteristics, in physiologic functions, and in emotional and spiritual attributes (Table 4.4). The fundamental structures of Western organs are defined anatomically and biochemically as molecules, cells, tissues, organs, and organ/systems, with extensive blood and nerve supplies. The basic constituents of Chinese organs are Qi, Blood and Fluid. The specific organs are not recognized as concrete structures with distinct physical boundaries and attributes, but are energetic organs that have Qi channels extending beyond physical entities that are intimately interconnected with each other through Yin–Yang and Five-Element relationships.

The Chinese and Western organ models are complementary, and knowledge of both provides a more comprehensive understanding of human physiology and pathophysiology. The following discussion of individual organs gives both

TABLE 4.4	Chinese and Western organs	
	Chinese organs	**Western organs**
	Physical and energetic components	Primarily physical entities
	Have emotional attributes	No direct emotional correlation
	Have spiritual attributes	No spiritual correlation
	Some anatomic characteristics	Detailed anatomic characteristics
	No biochemical characteristics	Detailed biochemical characteristics
	Close connection to nature	Independent of nature
	Operate on laws of nature	Operate on laws of biochemistry
	Yin–Yang coupling, Five-Element interrelationship	Anatomic and physiologic interrelationship
	Organs cannot function independently	Mostly independent, segmentalized
	General ancestral weakness	Specific congenital anomalies
	No nervous system: brain as curious organ; part of marrow	Nervous system: sophisticated brain is important organ
	No nerve component	Nerve supplies to all organs

perspectives, and emphasizes their significance in pediatrics health and diseases. The organs are grouped as Yin–Yang couplets, presented in the order of principal meridians but starting with the more important Yin organs. Yin and Yang organs are shown in Table 4.5.

Lung

Western Lungs

In Western medicine, the lungs are part of the respiratory system, which extends from nostrils to the trachea, bronchi, and bronchioles to the lungs. The lung tissue consists of alveoli, thin-walled air sacs where exchange of oxygen and carbon dioxide occur.

By the sixth week of fetal life, the trachea, bronchi, and lung buds can be clearly differentiated. By the end of the third month, the lung is already formed. *In utero*, the fetal lung is filled with fluid and respiration is carried out by the placenta. At birth, clamping of the umbilical cord produces anoxia, which in turn leads to acidosis and the drop in pH provides the stimulus for the medullary respiratory center. Initiation of respiration and the associated changes are among the most important events occurring at birth. The weight of the lung is doubled by 6 months of age, tripled by age 1, and increased 20 times by adult life.

Respiration in infants is largely diaphragmatic (i.e., abdominal) and remains so until the fifth to seventh month of life. Respiration is initially irregular, and

TABLE 4.5	Yin and Yang organs	
	Yin organs	**Yang organs**
	Lung	Large Intestine
	Spleen	Stomach
	Heart	Small Intestine
	Kidney	Bladder
	Pericardium	Triple Energizer
	Liver	Gallbladder

respiratory rate drops from 30–80 in the newborn to 20–40 by age 1, 20–25 by age 5, 15–20 by age 15. Normal ventilation provides for maintenance of arterial oxygen, carbon dioxide, and pH for optimal physiologic function. The lungs have a heterogeneous cell population, with over 40 separate cell types that perform various functions, including synthesizing lipid and proteins, and protecting the lungs against external pathogenic agents.

Since the nose is the most important orifice opening to the outside, the respiratory tract becomes the most vulnerable system to become exposed to infectious and toxic substances in the environment. The respiratory system has elaborate defense mechanisms in order to protect the lungs and to ensure that the respiratory tract distal to the larynx remains sterile. There are four general defense mechanisms:

- Mucociliary clearance
- Warming and moisturizing of the respiratory tract
- Phagocytosis
- Cellular killing.

Mucociliary Clearance

The nose has a relatively large surface area lined with a richly vascular, ciliated epithelium. Gross filtering of particles greater than 10–15 μm is achieved by the coarse hairs at the nasal orifices, and most inhaled particles greater than 5 μm are impacted on the nasal surface.[2] Trachea and bronchi contain glands that secrete mucus and ciliated cells that move mucus toward the pharynx. Mucociliary clearance may be aided by cough, which provides an effective means by propelling excess mucus up the airways at pressures of up to 300 mmHg and at flows of up to 5–6 l/s. Mucus raised by the cough mechanism is usually swallowed by young children, but may be expectorated. The respiratory mucus contains about 95% water, 2% glycoproteins (mucins), 1% carbohydrate, and less than 1% lipid, DNA, and other substances.

Mucociliary clearance can be reduced by changes in body temperature: both hypothermia and hyperthermia. Cold air may irritate the tracheobronchial tree. Environmental irritants and inflammation from infections may damage the epithelial cells that line the respiratory tract.

Warming and Moisturizing of the Respiratory Tract

By the time the air column reaches the bifurcation of the trachea, up to 70% of the warming and humidification of the inspired air has occurred. The trachea and bronchi provide the final 25% of warming of the inspired air. During exhalation, heat and moisture are removed from the air stream.

Phagocytosis

Mucociliary clearance and the absorption of noxious fumes and gases by the vascular upper airway keep the respiratory tract distal to the larynx sterile. Reflexive laryngospasm and bronchospasm limit the depth and amount of penetration of infectious agents and foreign matter. When these protective mechanisms fail, the foreign particles may reach the alveoli of the lung tissue. The alveolar macrophages carry out phagocytosis of the particles, and the lymphocytes then clear them into regional lymph nodes or into the blood.

Cellular Killing

Phagocytosis and mucociliary clearance may not be sufficient protection from living microbial agents, such as bacteria and viruses. Additional factors include cellular killing of organisms and immune responses to assist in getting rid of the pathogens. Specialized cells rich in hydrolases such as lysozyme, acid phosphatase, and cathepsin are capable of digesting bacteria. The immune response consists of production of respiratory secretory antibodies, immunoglobulin A (IgA), which can neutralize certain viruses and toxins and help in the lysis of bacteria. Although serum IgA remains low during early infancy, it reaches adult levels within first month of life. IgA may also prevent antigenic substances from penetrating the epithelial surfaces. IgG and IgM are also found in secretions when lung inflammation occurs.

Western Lung Pathophysiology

Children are prone to infections of the respiratory tract: URI, the common cold, is the most common acute illness of childhood in the US and throughout the industrialized world. A preschool child has an average of 4–10 colds per year. The most frequent complication is otitis media. The larynx in young children is relatively narrow and is therefore susceptible to obstruction, particularly by inflammation and the resultant swelling of tissues. The obstruction produces the characteristic inspiratory stridor of croup, laryngotracheobronchitis. Recurrent pharyngitis and adenoid hypertrophy are also common.

Asthma is the most common lower respiratory tract condition in children, which may be due to either infection or allergens. The majority of the infections are caused by viruses and bacteria. The respiratory system is vulnerable to allergens, resulting in symptoms such as congestion and sneezing in the upper tract and asthmatic wheezing in the lower tract.

Foreign body aspiration is relatively common, especially in young children. The most common respiratory anomaly of serious clinical significance is a tracheoesophageal fistula. Other uncommon congenital malformations of respiratory tract include agenesis or hypogenesis of one lung, and congenital lung cysts.

Treatment is usually symptomatic: taking decongestants and cough medication, drinking extra fluids, using a humidifier. Antibiotics are given for bacterial infections, but are often overprescribed in viral infections.

Chinese Lung

The Chinese Lung complements the important physiologic functions of the Western lung by adding not only energetic components to the Lung system, but also emotional and spiritual components. The Lung governs Qi and respiration, controls the dispersal of Qi, defends the body, regulates water through sweat, and controls skin and hair.

Respiration is the process of taking in pure Qi from the air, from Heaven; and getting rid of impure Qi from our body, similar to inhaling oxygen and exhaling carbon dioxide. The pure Qi from the air combines with Food Qi to form the nourishing Qi that circulates in the meridians and organs. This close Qi relationship between the Lung and the digestive system supports the various respiratory and digestive system connections in the Western system. IgA and other antibodies are protein molecules, and mucus in the respiratory tract is primarily a proteinaceous substance. Even in Western pediatrics, parents are advised to eliminate mucus-producing foods such as milk products when the child has URI symptoms or cough.

It is important here to clarify the terminologies "phlegm" and "mucus" which have caused some confusion. Western medicine uses these two terms interchangeably to describe the concrete substance that can be coughed up. The Chinese term "phlegm" has a broader meaning that encompasses both energetic and physical forms, called non-substantial and substantial Phlegm. The Lung Phlegm is a substantial Phlegm, whereas non-substantial Phlegm encompasses non-visible disruption of energetic flow and functions. The Spleen is always the primary organ that is responsible for the formation of Phlegm. The Lung becomes involved in dispersing fluid and the Kidney in transformation and excretion of fluid. This concept is important in children, since Spleen dysfunction on an energetic Qi level can precede and predispose to respiratory symptom of mucus/phlegm production.

The Chinese Lung oversees the dispersion of Defensive Qi, Wei Qi, throughout the superficial layer of the body between skin and muscles. Wei Qi warms the respiratory tract, the skin and muscles, and protects the body from external pathogens—similar to the warming function of the Western respiratory system. At the same time, the Lung also spreads body fluids to the skin in the form of a fine "mist," which moistens the skin and regulates the opening and closing of pores and sweating.[1] While recognizing that the skin also "breathes," Western medicine considers the skin as a separate organ from the lungs. Chinese medicine considers the skin as the external aspect of the Lung. Their close relationship is evidenced by the frequent occurrence of both respiratory and skin symptoms even in the same Western diagnosis, such as eczema that often occurs simultaneously with asthma. There are further similarities in the functional approach in both Western and Chinese medicine. In Western medicine, the skin functions as a protective organ and a temperature regulator. The skin acts as a protective barrier against the physical environment, against chemicals and infections. The sweat glands within the skin regulate body temperature. When the internal temperature is high, the skin pores open to allow sweat to come to the surface. The evaporation of sweat cools down the body.

The Lung, as the uppermost organ in the body, is often referred to as the "lid" and governs the descending movement of Qi and body fluids to the Heart and blood vessels, the Kidneys, Bladder, and Large Intestine, which in turn respectively influence circulation, urination, fluid accumulation, and bowel movement. The external orifice for the Lung is the nose and Lung Qi also influences smell.

In Western medicine, the lungs and kidneys have a close relationship in maintaining acid–base balance for physiologic activities in the cells and tissues. The lungs contribute to this balance through exhaling carbon dioxide.

Hypoventilation can result in respiratory acidosis, whereas hyperventilation can result in alkalosis. The kidneys excrete hydrogen ions, H^+. An imbalance here can result in metabolic acidosis or alkalosis.

An intimate relationship between the Lung and Kidney also exists in Chinese medicine in the proper movement and flow of Qi. The Lung moves Qi downward and the Kidney "grasps it" to keep Qi from moving upward abnormally. Wheezing and vomiting occurs when Qi strays upward. In biochemical terms, wheezing can result in respiratory acid–base imbalance through inadequate air exchange, while vomiting can result in metabolic acid–base imbalance.

Lung corresponds to the Metal Element. Metal symbolically represents organization, and manifests as the rhythmic regularity of breathing, or as the specific molecular structure of metals. The corresponding taste is pungent or spicy, like the taste of fumes given off by burning metal. The corresponding emotions are sadness and grief. Through Lung Qi, Chinese medicine can correlate the increased incidence of respiratory illnesses such as asthma with increased incidence of depression.

The Chinese Lung has another important role which has no parallel in Western medicine. It houses the Corporeal Soul, Po, the Yin or counterpart of the Ethereal Soul, Hun. The Corporeal Soul enters our body at birth with the first breath and "dies" with us. Po affects breathing, and is the somatic manifestation of sensations and feelings. It is the Po that enables us to feel itchiness of eczema or the "heart pain" from immense sadness. Po is closely linked to Essence, which resides in the Kidneys and among its many functions is the transmission of ancestral information. The counterpart to Po is Hun, the Ethereal Soul that resides in the Liver Yin, also enters the body at birth, but is an Eternal Soul that connects with all the other Souls and returns to the Soul World upon the death of the physical body. When the Corporeal Soul is disturbed, there may be a vague, general feeling of physical uneasiness, a sense of "crawling under the skin."

Pathophysiology

The Chinese Lung in children is considered "immature," and vulnerable to Cold and Dryness, thereby predisposing children to frequent respiratory problems. Pediatric Lung Qi is "young," meaning weak and insufficient and often unable to carry out the Lung function of moving Qi downward. Reversal of Qi flow manifests as cough and wheezing. This Qi deficiency would translate into the Western biochemical concepts of decreased enzyme and IgA levels, decreased lung defense, since deficient Qi would impair all physiologic functions. When the Qi is insufficient to move Blood, respiratory distress maybe accompanied by cyanosis, agitation, cold limbs—the clinical picture of status asthmaticus.

In conventional pediatrics, diagnoses of Lung infections and disorders are substantiated by positive laboratory findings and/or positive chest X-ray. Usually, the disease is considered to be resolved when all the laboratory data return to normal. In Chinese medicine, however, pathogenic Qi can linger energetically in the body for an extended period of time, and manifest as persistent dry cough with minimal sputum; continual injury of Yin may manifest as dry mouth and tongue, scanty saliva, sweating, red cheeks; persistent Qi depletion can manifest as fatigue.

The digestive system is closely linked to the respiratory system—children with Spleen deficiency (see below) are ensnarled in a Spleen–Lung deficiency cycle, especially with unhealthy modern day lifestyle and diets.

Large Intestine

Western Large Intestine

The large intestine begins embryologically as early as the 4th week of gestation. The major function of the colon is to receive wastes from the small intestine, extract more water from the contents in the intestinal lumen in order to partially or completely solidify the stools. The rhythmic contraction of the intestinal muscles propels wastes down the large intestine.

Pathophysiology

The most common pediatric symptoms are abdominal pain and diarrhea, which are most often attributed to infections such as virus, bacteria, or parasites. Constipation occurs frequently and is often diet related. Ulcerative colitis is a chronic condition in which the colon wall becomes inflamed and forms ulcers. Symptoms include diarrhea, bleeding, stools with mucus, and pain. The most common congenital anomaly is Hirschsprung's disease, a condition of absence of nerve cells that result in megacolon and accounts for about 1/3 of obstruction in newborns. Other anomalies include stenosis, agenesis, and fistulae.

Chinese Large Intestine

The Chinese Large Intestine performs the same task of excretion as its Western counterpart.

Pathophysiology

Large Intestine symptoms are generally attributed to other system imbalance or causes. The Spleen/Pancreas controls the transformation and transportation of food and fluid throughout the entire digestive system, including the Large Intestine. Many of the symptoms attributed to the Western large intestine, such as diarrhea, abdominal pain are usually due to Spleen/Pancreas deficiency. Other symptoms, such as constipation, are secondary symptoms to Qi deficiency or Cold stagnation.

The Large Intestine is the Yang coupled organ to Lung. When Lung Qi is deficient, there is less Qi being sent to the Large Intestine, and a person may become constipated. On the other hand, if Large Intestine does not function well, food stagnates. Lung Qi cannot descend and the symptoms of cough or shortness of breath ensue. This may explain why children often develop flu symptoms that include both upper respiratory symptoms and gastrointestinal symptoms. The Large Intestine has no mental–emotional role.

Spleen: Spleen/Pancreas

Western Spleen

The spleen in Western medicine is primarily a hematologic and immunologic organ. *In utero*, the spleen is responsible for hematopoiesis, or active blood formation in the fetus. Postnatally, bone marrow forms red blood cells and the spleen is the principle organ for destruction of old red cells. The spleen is also a major immunologic organ, both in its lymphoid components, as well as in its synthesis of humoral antibodies.

Pathophysiology

The most common disorders of the spleen in children are splenomegaly due to viral infections, traumatic rupture, and hemolytic diseases. Less common disorders include storage diseases, congenital anomalies, and rarely, neoplasms. Splenectomy or removal of spleen is sometimes indicated in traumatic rupture and as treatment for certain hemolytic diseases, such as spherocytosis.

Western Pancreas

The spleen is in close anatomic proximity to the pancreas, which has both exocrine and endocrine functions involved in digestion. The exocrine cells secrete digestive enzymes, fluid and electrolytes. The endocrine cells secrete insulin that regulates glucose metabolism.

Pathophysiology

Appetite fluctuates enormously in children. In periods of rapid growth during infancy and adolescence, appetite is usually voracious. During the intervening years some children appear to eat almost nothing while growing and gaining weight normally. The most common digestive disorders are constipation, abdominal pain, vomiting, and diarrhea. The most frequent causes are viral infections, the "stomach flus." Less common causes are congenital anomalies, inflammatory bowel disease, and rarely tumors. Regurgitation of gastric content is very common in infants before 9–12 months (which Western medicine attributes to positioning and TCM explains as Spleen deficiency). Gastrointestinal symptoms can also be secondary to problems in other systems, such as vomiting associated with urinary tract infection.

In children, the Western spleen is frequently involved in all sorts of infections: viral, bacterial, parasitic, etc. It is easily traumatized in sports and in accidents, and is sometimes surgically removed because of excess hemorrhage.

Chinese Spleen

The Spleen in Chinese medicine is really the incorporation of both Spleen and Pancreas as one entity, and would be more appropriately termed Spleen/

Pancreas. It carries out hematologic and digestive functions attributed to the two separate Western organs. The Spleen/Pancreas is the Yin organ with Stomach as the Yang organ of the digestive couplet. Food "rots and ripens" in the Stomach, which correlates to the Western concept of breaking down of food by stomach acid and enzymes. The Spleen/Pancreas has six major physiologic functions.

Transformation and Transportation of Qi

The Spleen has the important function of transforming food into Gu Qi, which combines with Lung Qi to form Rong Qi, the Nutritive Qi that is the basis for Qi and Blood. Spleen directs Gu Qi to the Heart to form Blood. Spleen then transports Gu Qi and other refined food parts, the "food essences," to organs and all parts of the body, to muscles and limbs. Because the Food Qi extracted by the Spleen is the material basis for the production of Qi and Blood, the Spleen together with the Stomach are often called the Root of post-Heaven Qi.

Spleen also separates "clear" from "dirty" fluid, moves the former to the skin via the Lung and the latter downward to the intestine. Since Spleen usually sends Qi upwards, it has an "uplifting" effect to hold organs in their place and prevents prolapse.

Spleen/Pancreas corresponds to the Earth Element, as Mother Earth is the provider of nourishment to all living beings. It corresponds with late summer—the harvest season.

Production and Regulation of Blood

The Spleen controls Blood both in production and in prevention of hemorrhage. Food Qi, assisted by Original Qi from the Kidneys, forms Blood in the Heart. Blood circulates in blood vessels, and it is the Spleen that "holds" the Blood in the blood vessels and prevents hemorrhage.

Taste

The Spleen opens into the mouth and manifests in the lips, and is responsible for taste, for chewing and preparing food for further digestion, and for moistness of lips. The flavor associated with Earth organs, Spleen and Stomach, is sweetness. Children naturally develop a preference for sweet taste as early as 1 month of age. Sweet is the predominant flavor in fruits and vegetables. Modern medicine advises the feeding of solids after age 6 months, with preference for introducing fruits and vegetables first. Early introduction of solids has been associated with abdominal discomfort and allergic gastrointestinal symptoms. Eating normal amounts of naturally sweetened food is healthy, while consuming excess sweet foods—especially artificially sweetened foods, which are the major constituents of a modern child's diet—can induce digestive imbalance.

Spleen is the "Residence" of Thought

The Spleen influences our capacity for introspection, for thinking, studying, focusing, and memorizing data. Overwork can be injurious to Spleen Qi. When

Spleen Qi is deficient, children do not feel centered, cannot think clearly, and have difficulty with concentration and school work.

Emotions

The emotions associated with Earth are sympathy and worry, and are the characteristics of the mother. When Spleen Qi is in balance, the child is capable of giving and of being sympathetic. When Spleen Qi is out of balance, the child may worry excessively, and even become obsessive in extreme circumstances.

Phlegm

The Spleen is the major organ for production of substantial and non-substantial Phlegm, the physical and energetic Phlegm. Spleen likes "dryness" and is injured by "dampness" and "coldness."

Pathophysiology

The Spleen/Pancreas in children is "immature" and constitutionally weak. There is impairment of all of the above six functions, but especially in the transforming and transporting of food and fluids. Insufficient Nutritive Qi and Blood are formed, along with a tendency toward accumulation of Phlegm. These account for the predominance of digestive symptoms in children. The diet of the modern-day child further contributes to Spleen deficiency: a diet rich in Phlegm-producing foods, such as milk products; ice-cold drinks and foods, such as ices and ice cream; and excess artificially sweetened foods, such as candies, cookies, and cakes. The stressful lifestyle of children and excess school pressure can cause further deterioration of Spleen function. The vicious cycle of Spleen Qi deficiency and digestive symptoms begins with colic in infancy, and includes a wide range of symptoms: poor appetite, indigestion, abdominal pain and distension and loose stools; fatigue, paleness and blood deficiencies, such as anemia. While Western medicine considers poor appetite in toddlers as a normal phase, Chinese medicine attributes it to insufficient and immature Spleen Qi.

Spleen versus Lung

The most common disorders in children are respiratory and digestive illnesses. Both of these systems have orifices that are in direct contact with the external environment. Pathogens can easily and directly enter the respiratory and digestive systems via the nose or the mouth, and invade the fragile organs internally. Fluid in the Lung accumulates and transforms into Phlegm, which in turn blocks airways—bronchi and bronchioles. The child has more difficulty getting air in and out, resulting in signs of respiratory distress, such as nasal flaring, tachypnea (rapid breathing), intercostal retractions (pulling in of muscles in the rib cage). Children's "young Yin" further predisposes them to easily becoming fluid depleted, the phlegm becomes thicker, the fever tends to rise higher, which in turn causes more Yin deficiency. Since the Lung breathes in Heavenly Qi to form Nutritive Qi, when the Lung function is compromised, all the other organs—especially the Spleen—are also affected.

Liver and Spleen have a controlling or destructive relationship in the Five-Element Cycle. Spleen deficiency can in turn result in Liver excess. The subsequent sections will discuss the significance of "liver vulnerability" and Wood phase of development in relation to Spleen deficiency.

Stomach

Western Stomach

The stomach begins to form in a 4-week-old fetus. The stomach functions as a reservoir with cells that secrete mucus, acid, and digestive enzymes. It delivers liquefied, blended, but minimally digested portions of the diet to the intestine.

Pathophysiology

The most common gastrointestinal disorder, the "stomach flu," clinically presents with abdominal pain, vomiting and diarrhea, and is an anatomic and biochemical condition affecting the intestines.

The majority of disorders of the stomach in children are due to congenital anomalies that include atresia, hypoplasia, and gastric duplications. The most common congenital condition is infantile hypertrophic pyloric stenosis, a thickening of the pylorus that results in obstruction of the gastric outlet. It must be surgically corrected before age 6 months. Peptic ulcers occur primarily in the duodenum, and less frequently in the stomach in children. They can present in early infancy from congenital excess gastric acid secretion. Acute stress ulcers may develop in older children in trauma, sepsis, shock, or critical illness.

Chinese Stomach

The Chinese Stomach is the most important Yang organ, an Earth organ that couples with Spleen. It "rots and ripens" food, which is comparable to the Western concept of acidic and enzymatic breakdown of food. To do so, the Stomach needs sufficient fluids, which are derived from food and drink. Stomach incorporates some fluid into food essences, and others are condensed to form body fluids. Stomach is therefore vulnerable to dryness. This is compatible with the biochemical explanation of the digestive process, when breakdown of macromolecules or polymers into monomers is a hydrolysis reaction that requires water.

The Spleen–Stomach couplet is often called the "Root of post-Heaven Qi," since together they are responsible for all the Qi produced after birth. This is also the closest of all the Yin–Yang couplets, working closely together to digest food, to extract Qi from food, and to transport Nutritive Qi throughout the body, including the muscles of arms and legs.

Pathophysiology

Like the Western model, the Stomach sends food and fluid to the Small Intestine, therefore, Stomach Qi must move downward. When the Stomach is healthy, food and Qi move downward from the Stomach to the Small Intestine to the Large Intestine. When the Stomach is unbalanced, the downward Qi movement is poorly directed and Qi starts to come upward. This may result in symptoms such as burping, regurgitation, nausea, vomiting, and a sense of full-ness. Regurgitation is a common symptom in infants. In Western medicine, this is treated by positioning the infant in a more vertical/sitting up position to allow gravity to "pull" food downward. In Chinese medicine, regurgitation is due to immature and insufficient Stomach and Spleen Qi, and upright position-ing in effect engenders gravitational downward pull of Qi flow. Chinese medi-cine can treat regurgitation with tonification of Stomach and Spleen.

The Stomach plays a minor role in the mental–emotional realm, compared to the pervasive influence of the Spleen/Pancreas. Stomach imbalance may induce confusion. This is in sharp contrast to the Western stomach as being the most common target organ for "psychosomatic" symptoms, because stomach dis-comfort that occurs frequently—especially in children—usually has no physical or biochemical findings and is diagnosed as "functional abdominal pain." Chinese medicine can contribute to the understanding of functional disorders as having energetic disturbances. In children, inappropriate diet and manner of eating can also induce a variety of Stomach symptoms that are difficult to explain in Western medicine.

Heart

Western Heart and Pathophysiology

The heart in Western medicine is a mechanical pump that is responsible for cir-culation of oxygenated blood throughout the body. In pediatrics, cardiac prob-lems consist mostly of congenital anomalies, occurring in approximately 8/1000 live births[2] such as ventriculoseptal defect (VSD); atrioseptal defect (ASD), and pulmonary stenosis. Arrhythmias are infrequent in children. Cardiovascular disease is becoming more prevalent in children.

Chinese Heart

Chinese medicine regards the Heart as the most important of all the internal organs. It is the "Emperor" that rules over all aspects of physical, emotional, and spiritual being. On a physical level, the Chinese Heart is comparable to its Western counterpart in governing the movement of blood in the blood vessels, and the Heart is closely related to the Lung in that Qi and blood nourish each other. However, Chinese medicine also posits that the transformation of Food Qi into Blood takes place in the Heart, and it is the vitality of Qi within the blood vessels rather than the Heart as a mechanical pump that moves blood. Facial complexion reflects the condition of the Heart: rosy cheeks indicate good blood flow, healthy Heart, while a pale complexion indicates anemia, poor blood flow, and an unhealthy Heart. Through the interaction of fluids and Blood, the Heart also influences sweat and other body fluids.

The Heart opens onto the tongue and therefore influences speech. A child with a calm Heart is articulate. Children with disturbed Hearts can have a hard time finding the right words, stutter, or forget what they want to say.

The most important function of the Heart is being the House for Shen, which embodies both the Mind and the Spirit. This reflects the closeness of Ethereal Soul (discussed under Liver) and the Mind. Through the Soul, the Chinese Mind extends to more than just the individual mind, but to thoughts and ideas of eternity from the Soul World. In this way all the Minds and thoughts are connected with each other. When the Heart is in a state of balance, the Shen is said to be properly housed. The Emperor rules wisely. The child can think clearly and creatively, can have articulate speech, can experience joy and passion, and is at peace with himself. He can also connect with others. When the Heart is in a state of imbalance, the Shen is not properly housed, and the child becomes restless, easily distracted, inarticulate, irrational, has poor memory, and becomes disconnected with others. In severe cases, the child can become hysterical and delirious or even completely lose consciousness as in a coma. The emotional Chinese Heart is very vulnerable, and can easily become imbalanced by all emotions.

The Heart corresponds to the Fire Element. The primary emotion that corresponds to Heart is no surprise: joy or passion. The Fire phase of development comprises the teenage years; therefore, Heart conditions in Chinese pediatrics correlate mostly to teenage behavioral issues (pointed out in Chapter 5). The emotions are volatile, like a spark that becomes explosive, or fiery passion. Since all other emotions—sadness, anger, fear, worry—will eventually also affect the Heart, Heart Fire can become out of control because of chronic emotional problems, giving rise to excess symptoms of agitation, restlessness, and physical symptoms of excess Heat. Therefore the Heart is at the center of our emotional being. The teenager who cannot become motivated in something because his or her "heart is just not in it," or can become bitter and rebellious, which is metaphorically represented by the bitter taste. When the heart is hurt, the fiery passion can turn into bitterness. The color corresponding to the Heart is red—the color of blood, passion, and fire.

Small Intestine

Western Small Intestine

The human small intestine begins to form at 4 weeks of gestational age. Intraluminal ingestion depends largely on the exocrine pancreas. Digestive enzymes are secreted by the small intestine in response to food and fluid in the lumen. Digestion is facilitated by bile salts, and is usually completed in the upper small intestinal segment, where sugars, proteins, and carbohydrates, and fats are broken down into smaller components for absorption. Electrolytes, minerals, and fluids are selectively absorbed and wastes are then sent down to the large intestine.

Pathophysiology

Small intestine disorders in children include various infections, such as viral, bacterial, *Giardia* and other parasitic infections; malabsorption syndromes; Crohn's disease, inflammatory bowel disease of the small intestine; stress ulcers, and motility disorders.

Congenital anomalies include atresia, duplication, and various anatomic defects. Symptoms often appear during early infancy, but sometimes a congenital small intestine defect may not be discovered until adulthood. Symptoms include diarrhea, abdominal pain, weight loss, and fever.

Chinese Small Intestine

On a physical level, the Chinese Small Intestine also performs digestive functions, and separates "clean" from the "dirty." It receives food and fluids after digestion by the Stomach and Spleen, and separates clear food which is transported by the Spleen to nourish all the body tissues. The separation of fluids is controlled by Kidney Yang, which provides Qi and Heat for this process.

Unlike other Yang organs, the Small Intestine plays an important emotional and psychological role. As the Yang couple organ of the Heart, which stores the Mind and governs mental capacities, the Small Intestine metaphorically separates the "clear" from the "dirty" as the ability to distinguish right from wrong, what is needed from what is not needed: to "sort things out," in order to think clearly to make life's decisions.

Pathophysiology

Physical symptoms in children associated with Small Intestine tend to be secondary to Spleen deficiency, such as diarrhea; or to Kidney dysfunction, such as disorders in fluid separation manifesting as excessive or scanty urination; or when Heart Fire is transmitted to the Small Intestine, resulting in tongue ulcers, bitter taste, thirst, or blood in the urine. Since Small Intestine is a Fire organ and therefore corresponds to teenage development, its balance would influence teenagers' ability in sorting out right from wrong, which may have significant consequences in their behavior, especially when the Heart Fire is out of balance.

Kidney

Western Kidney

In Western medicine the kidneys have many responsibilities. They form and excrete urine. They secrete the hormone renin that regulates blood pressure and erythropoietin that stimulates the production of red blood cells. The kidneys and lungs share the important responsibility of maintaining acid–base balance. The kidneys maintain proper pH balance by controlling the excretion of salt and hydrogen ions. Insufficient kidney function may result in metabolic acidosis or alkalosis, whereas lung dysfunction may cause respiratory acidosis or alkalosis.

Pathophysiology

Kidney disorders in children include infections such as glomerulonephritis or pylonephritis, disorders of kidney functions in filtration and in concentration of urine, congenital anomalies such as polycystic disease, and secondary involvement of the kidneys in systemic illnesses, such as lupus or diabetes, and trauma.

Renal symptoms are due to inadequate formation or excretion of urine, and to the toxicity from accumulation of waste products. Bilateral kidney failure necessitates dialysis to remove toxic waste products. Kidney transplants, which can come from both live donors and cadavers, are rare in children.

Chinese Kidney

The Chinese Kidney shares some of the physical attributes of Western kidney. Anatomically, the kidneys are located at the first to fourth lumbar vertebrae. The acupuncture back Shu points for the Kidneys, BL-23, and Mingmen, the Gate of Life and Vitality, GV-4 situated between BL-23, are at lumbar 2 level. The Kidneys are Water organs, and therefore are the major physiologic organs for fluid regulation. However, Chinese medicine ascribes characteristics and importance to the Kidneys that have no parallel in Western medicine.

The Kidney is the foundation of life. Kidney is the origin of both Water and Fire, of Primary Yin and Yang, of all the organs. Kidney Yin is the foundation of all Yin energies of the body, especially that of the Liver, Heart, and Lung; and Kidney Yang as the foundation of all the Yang energies or the Fire of the body, especially that of the Spleen, Heart, and Lung.

FIGURE 4.2   *Relationship among Kidney Yin, Kidney Essence, Kidney Yang and Kidney Qi. (Adapted with permission.[1])*

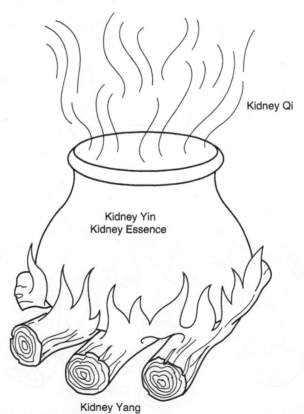

Kidney Qi

Kidney Yin
Kidney Essence

Kidney Yang

Maciocia illustrates Kidney Yang as the firewood that burns and heats up the pot, which contains Kidney Yin and Kidney Essence in the water (Figure 4.2).[1] The steam from the boiling water represents Qi. Figure 4.3 carries this imagery one step further to illustrate the relationship between Kidney Yang and Kidney Yin with the Yang and Yin of all the other organs. Kidney Yang is the main stack of firewood with a very big Kidney Yin pot in the middle. The other organs have their own smaller stacks of firewood sitting on top of extensions of the Kidney firewood so that the Kidney Yang is underlying all the Yang. When Kidney Yang is deficient, it does not matter how much wood each organ has, it would be deficient since the base stack that provides the fire is deficient. On the other hand, when Kidney Yang is tonified—which means making the center fire bigger by burning more of the existing wood, since Kidney Yang cannot be increased (that is, there cannot be more firewood added)—the other organs would be tonified by receiving more fire from the Kidney. Each organ can have its own deficiency—a smaller, individual stack of firewood. Each organ also has a "pot" that is connected to the central Kidney Yin pot. If the Kidney pot is full,

FIGURE 4.3   *Kidney relationship to other organs. When Kidney Yang and Yin are tonified, all the other organs are tonified. Each organ's Qi is related to Kidney Yang and Yin, as well as directly to its own.*

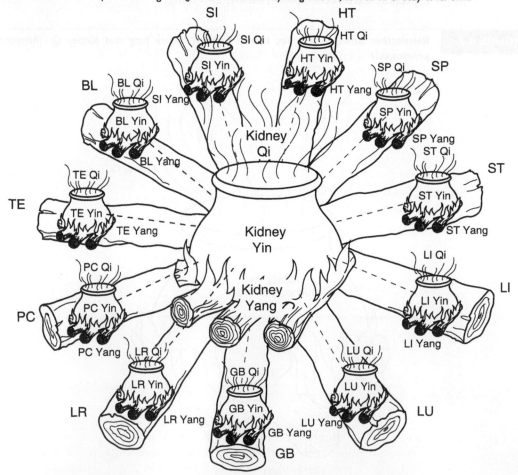

it can fill the smaller "pots." When the central pot is deficient, all the other pots would have less "soup."

Kidney stores Essence, Jing, a substance without equivalence in Western medicine. Jing is called both the "fiery Water" and "densest form of Qi." This translates into Western terminology as the impossibility of Jing being both particle (liquid water molecules) and energy (Qi) at the same time. The illustration in Figure 4.4 can help clarify this confusing concept for the scientific mind. Basic high school physics indicates that there are three physical states: solid, liquid, gas. The molecules in a solid are in a compact state; they are further apart in the liquid state, and have the most kinetic energy in the gaseous state, moving farther apart from each other. The heat from the fire is transferred to the water molecules and becomes kinetic energy that increases movement of the molecules. The hottest part of the water or "soup in the pot" is the layer right at the bottom of the pot. As these molecules gain kinetic energy and move around, the heat or energy is transferred from the molecules at the bottom of the pot upward to heat up the rest of the soup molecules, eventually causing the top layer of molecules to gain sufficient kinetic energy to become "steam or vapor," the gaseous form of water—the Qi. Essence can be thought of as the molecules at the bottom of the pot: they are the "hottest" with the most heat

| FIGURE 4.4 | Jing is the densest form of Qi. The molecules of soup at the bottom of the pot have the most amount of kinetic energy, which is comparable to the kinetic energy of Qi, but, because they are at the bottom of the pot, they cannot evaporate. The kinetic energy is transmitted upwards so that the molecules at the top gain sufficient energy to move away from the pot as steam, comparable to the action of Qi. |

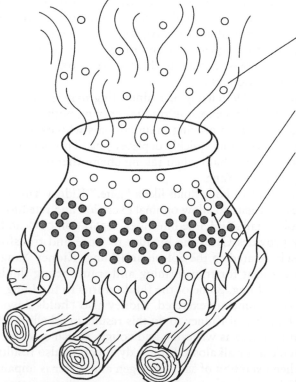

"Steam molecule" with kinetic energy to move away from pot

Transfer of kinetic energy to other molecules

Molecules at bottom of pot (the Ying molecules) closest to fire are hottest, i.e. have the same amount of kinetic energy as the "steam molecules" (the Qi molecules), but cannot escape because of the molecules above them. The "steam molecules" have the most amount of kinetic energy for moving away from the pot

that can become kinetic energy but they are still in the liquid state, prevented from vaporizing by the molecules further up in the pot. Essence is therefore both the "fiery Water" and the "densest Qi."

This imagery can also illustrate the powerfulness of Essence or Jing. Just as all the molecules in the pot depend on the heat or energy in the bottommost molecules, Jing exerts global influence of Yin (Blood and Fluid), the "soup" and of Qi (the vapor), which are the Yin–Yang building blocks of life. Therefore, Jing is said to exert global effects on life: conception, pregnancy, childbirth, growth, development, maturation, sexual function, fertility, and aging. Pre-Heaven Jing carries ancestral genetic information, comparable to the chromosomes. Jing is at the maximum at birth and naturally declines with age. Jing is quickly expended with stress, with aging, and with ejaculation in the male and menstruation in the female. Jing can be preserved by Qi exercises, such as Qigong or Tai Chi; better diet and lifestyle.

Kidney produces marrow, which encompasses both bone marrow, and the "Sea of Marrow" that correlates to the brain and spinal cord. The Western marrow is responsible for the production of antibodies, red and white blood cells and platelets—blood components that are influenced in Chinese medicine by Spleen and Heart, but are dependent on Kidney Yang. Whereas the brain in Western medicine is the most important organ that distinguishes man as a superior, intellectual being, it is just a "curious organ" in Chinese medicine that depends on Kidney Qi and Essence. Since Kidney nourishes the brain, it therefore influences memory, concentration, and thinking.

Kidney also nourishes the ears, enabling normal hearing. Western medicine regards the ear and kidneys as separate organs, and cannot provide an explanation for the many associations between the two. For example, children born with low-set ears often have congenital kidney anomalies; some familiar syndromes have nephritis and deafness (e.g. Alport syndrome); some antibiotics, such as gentamicin that are frequently given intravenously to premature babies and young infants for sepsis, can be both ototoxic (toxic to the ears) and nephrotoxic (toxic to the kidneys).

Kidney nourishes hair. Deficiency of Kidney Jing may manifest as brittle, dull, and graying of hair. This explains gradual graying with aging as Essence depletes over time, and sudden graying in individuals who experiences severe physical or emotional shock that quickly depletes Jing. This is most striking in cancer children who become bald when taking chemotherapy—potent drugs that deplete Kidney Jing and Yang.

Kidneys govern the flow of body fluids like a "gate." Kidney Yin "opens" and Kidney Yang "closes" the gate to allow optimal excretion and retention of fluids. Kidney Yang controls Small and Large Intestines' separation of clean from dirty fluids, and Kidney provides Qi to the Bladder to store and transform urine. Kidney is also closely related to the Spleen and Lung: Kidney Yang provides Spleen with necessary heat for transforming and transporting fluids; Kidney receives fluids from the Lung. Some of the fluid returns to the Lung as mist to keep them moist, while some are excreted. Kidney also "holds down" Qi that Lung sends down. Inability of Kidney to do this results in rebellious flow of Qi upward, which can manifest as wheezing and cough, which can biochemically cause respiratory acidosis or alkalosis. Kidney dysfunction also results in metabolic imbalance; when excretion of salt, hydrogen and water is impaired, metabolic acidosis or alkalosis may ensue, which in turn can influence respiration.

The Kidney is associated with the Water Element. The taste corresponding with Water/Kidney Qi is salt, which has a profound effect on fluid volume in the body. Taste for salt develops in children as early as 1 month of age, during the Water phase of development.

The emotions associated with Kidney are willpower and fear. When Kidney is weak, children do not feel motivated, are fearful and lack willpower. A healthy dose of fear can keep them from taking foolish risks. Excessive fear can prevent them from making decisions. Unlike the indecisiveness due to lack of direction associated with Gallbladder deficiency, there is an ebb-and-flow, push–pull Water quality to this indecisiveness from fear, best exemplified by a young child in the Water phase of development. For example, it is natural for toddlers to want to become more independent and yet still needing attachment to their mother, so that they rebel by not wanting to hold their mother's hand, yet become afraid and cry for their mother when she is out of sight. Fear from Kidney deficiency in older children may become so excessive as to prevent normal emotional growth or to be overly concerned about insignificant things.

Pathophysiology

Disorders of the Chinese Kidney encompass energetic, physical, and emotional attributes of the Kidney.

The Water phase of development extends from prenatal period to early childhood. The Kidney vulnerability of this age group is reflected in the ease of injury to the brain, so that infections may easily lead to meningitis and encephalitis; metabolic disturbances may frequently result in seizures and even mental retardation.

Congenital and hereditary disorders are attributed to deficiency of Kidney Jing. Potent medications, especially when given to very young children, induce a strong "jolt" to the system that is similar to "shocking the system." Kidney Yang is released in response, and therefore becomes prematurely depleted. Because of the abundance of Kidney Yang in children, the effect may not be seen until years or even decades later. The majority of metabolites of medications are excreted in the kidneys—resulting in increased renal load that translates into weakening the Kidney.

Enuresis may be primary due to Kidney Yang deficiency or secondary to Spleen and Lung deficiency and the resultant fluid imbalance, or overall Yin deficiency with resultant heat in Bladder. In Western medicine, nocturnal enuresis is considered to have strong correlation with emotions, especially fear. Since fear is associated with Kidneys, it can cause an abnormal flow of Qi, called "sinking of Qi" in the Bladder which manifests as bedwetting. Just as the Kidney is the root of all organs, it can in turn become affected by all chronic conditions in the other organs.

Bladder

Both Western and Chinese medicine consider Bladder as the organ for storage and excretion of urine formed by the Kidney. The symptoms, and even causes, have strong correlation.

The most common pediatric disorder is bladder infection, or urinary tract infection, most frequently caused by bacteria, sometimes by viruses. Congenital malformations include duplication of the urinary collecting system. As the Yang couplet organ of the Kidney, Bladder disorders are usually secondary to Kidney imbalance, resulting in alteration of urine output. Bladder infections are usually attributed to excess Damp Heat in the Bladder.

Pericardium

Western Pericardium Physiology and Pathophysiology

The pericardium in Western pediatrics is the covering of the heart and may infrequently develop an infection, usually viral or bacterial pericarditis; or may be secondarily involved in chronic conditions such as rheumatoid arthritis, lupus, or other generalized illnesses.

Chinese Pericardium

In Chinese medicine the Pericardium is also called Master of the Heart and assumes the important role of protecting the Heart. As protector of the Emperor, it wards off external evils and pathogens. The Pericardium is analogous to the sympathetic nervous system of the autonomic nervous system, which controls involuntary functions such as heart rate and sweating. The sympathetics stimulate the heart, whereas the parasympathetics have the reverse effect.

Pathophysiology

There is a great deal of overlap between the Heart and the Pericardium, as both are associated with the Fire Element. The Pericardium channel runs next to the Heart along the inside of the arm. The Pericardium is considered to be the "centre of the thorax"[1] and therefore has a great deal of influence on the chest. While the Heart is influenced by all emotions, the Pericardium is more affected by difficulties in relationships. This channel is therefore important in the teenager, who is in the Fire phase of development and is beginning to explore the ups and downs of sexual relationships.

The sympathetic association of Pericardium is useful for treating arrhythmia in children, either associated with congenital heart disease or iatrogenically induced by medication.

Triple Energizer

The Triple Energizer, formerly known as the Triple Heater or Triple Burner, is a difficult concept for Western medicine. It is not really an organ but a designation of three divisions of the body. As such, it has no corollary in Western medicine.

The Triple Energizer is considered a Yang organ, although it has no specific form. It is the Yang couplet organ of the Yin organ—Pericardium/Master of the

Heart. Its overall function is regulation of body fluids and it controls fluid circulation. With the fluid, it nourishes, moistens, warms and cools tissues. It acts as a sum total of all the Yang organs and gives unity to the different organs. The fluid has a different form in each division, reflecting physiology of the organs.

Just as the Pericardium is the sympathetic nervous system with overall stimulatory effect on physiology, the Triple Energizer is the parasympathetic nervous system, with a calming physiologic effect.

The three divisions of the Triple Energizer are:

- Upper Energizer
  - location: thorax or chest area, above the diaphragm
  - organs: Heart, Lung, Pericardium
  - fluid form: mist or vapor—the Lung distributes fluid as a fine mist or vapor to skin, muscles, and fluid circulation
- Middle Energizer
  - location: abdominal cavity above the umbilicus
  - organs: Spleen/Pancreas, Stomach, Gallbladder
  - fluid form: foam, turbid pool—food and drink from digestion
- Lower Energizer
  - location: lower abdominal cavity below the umbilicus
  - organs: Small and Large Intestine, Liver, Kidney, Bladder
  - fluid form: "swamp" or "drainage ditch"—separates clean from the dirty.

Pathophysiology

There are no specific disease entities of the Triple Energizer. The Triple Energizer points are used to maintain balance in the three energizers, the three divisions of the body, and to treat a variety of disorders for fluid balance. In children, routine stimulation of the master points of the three energizers has been found to be useful in general health maintenance.

Liver

Western Liver

The liver is an important metabolic organ that is one of the most commonly involved/frequently affected organs in childhood. The liver and biliary system begin to form as early as 18 days of fetal life. It becomes the largest internal organ in the body, and its long list of metabolic and secretory functions make it the main organ for maintaining a stable internal environment. It gets oxygenated blood from the heart, and nutrients from the digestive system. The liver absorbs raw materials which it transforms into metabolically useful compounds or unusable end products; it selectively secretes the former into blood or bile and the latter exclusively into bile. The liver stores carbohydrate as glycogen, a polymer readily degraded to monomeric glucose. The newborn depends entirely on hepatic glycogen to maintain the supply of glucose suddenly interrupted at delivery.

The liver is the main source of proteins in the circulation, including plasma proteins, enzymes, and clotting factors. During postnatal development certain proteins reach adult values within days while others take 1–2 years. The liver also stores vitamins, iron, and minerals.

The liver is involved with the biotransformation and elimination of metabolites: the oxidative, reductive, hydrolytic, and conjugative reactions, which include the breakdown of bilirubin, secretion of bile, metabolism of carbohydrate, fat, drugs and hormones. The liver is also involved in the immune function and detoxification of the body. The liver synthesizes cholesterol. Many of these processes generate heat for maintaining body temperature.

Liver contains about 10% of the blood in the body, and carries blood from the pancreas and spleen.

Pathophysiology

Disorders of the liver that can affect the child from birth and early infancy include congenital malformations, atresia/hypoplasia, cystic malformations of bile duct, and metabolic disorders, such as galactosemia. Hepatitis (inflammation of the liver) is the major disorder in children that can occur at any age. It is usually caused by viral infection, but may also be due to bacteria, parasites, chemical agents, or drugs. While most cases of hepatitis are self-limiting, a small percentage may lead to chronic hepatitis and cirrhosis.

Liver is often the secondary organ involvement, as in cystic fibrosis, or chronic inflammatory bowel disease. As the main organ responsible for drug metabolism, liver is particularly susceptible to injury from drugs and environmental toxins. The possibility of liver damage increases when two agents are administered together, since one drug may inhibit or induce hepatic microsomal enzymes necessary for the metabolism of the other. In addition, predictable dose-dependent or unexpected dose-independent (idiosyncratic) drug reactions may affect the liver.

When the liver is diseased, bilirubin cannot be broken down, and jaundice ensues. Newborn jaundice may be physiologic, secondary to liver immaturity, caused by breast feeding, or blood type incompatibility. Liver transplant has been successful in children in the past two decades.

Chinese Liver

Chinese medicine concurs about liver's importance and calls Liver the "General" of the Qi system. It is Liver that directs smooth and proper Qi movement in all directions, and profoundly influences digestion, secretion of bile, and emotions. When Liver Qi flow is smooth, Stomach and Spleen can carry out digestive functions harmoniously, with Stomach Qi flowing downward and Spleen Qi flowing upward. Liver Qi also affects the flow of bile. Chinese medicine associates Liver Qi stagnation with frustration, irritability, and anxiety—the emotions of an impatient child. When the Liver Qi is out of balance, the emotions become exaggerated. Smoldering anger is most characteristic of Liver, and can be accompanied by resentment and even withdrawal. Accompanying physical symptoms may include heavy sensation in the chest, a "lump" in the throat, abdominal distention.

The Chinese Liver stores blood, regulates the quantity of blood and fluid according to activity, and also regulates menstruation.

The biochemical description of the liver is complemented by the Chinese metaphoric and symbolic description of Liver. Liver is a Wood organ, represents youth and springtime, and is also the organ that occupies the longest period of childhood development. All the metabolic processes are essential for pediatric growth and maturation, just like a seedling blossoming into a tree.

The Chinese Liver has another very important role in that the Liver Yin or Liver Blood houses the Ethereal Soul, Hun. It enters the body with the Corporeal Soul, Po, at birth. Unlike the Corporeal Soul which "dies" with the physical body, Hun returns to the Eternal Soul World and enters another physical being. Dreaming is interpreted as Hun visiting the Soul World and bringing back images from the Soul World. Whereas the Corporeal Soul is concerned with the physical being, Hun is the Spirit that is associated with the Mind. It is, therefore, closely related to the Heart, which houses Shen that is both Spirit and Mind. Hun influences thinking and emotions of the Mind. Through the Ethereal Soul, individual Minds become connected with each other, and can access thoughts and ideas from eternity. In this way, it is closely related to the Jungian concept of the collective unconscious made up of individual unconscious.[1]

The external orifices associated with Liver are the eyes. The taste associated with Wood/Liver is sour—the taste of bile. The external susceptibility is Wind, just as a small tree would sway back and forth in strong wind.

Pathophysiology

All Chinese pediatric textbooks point out that the Liver in children is vulnerable, which means that the Liver is prone to develop disorders. Liver is the Wood organ, and the majority of childhood is in the Wood phase of development, lending support to the theory that the Liver is vulnerable during childhood.

Liver vulnerability generally indicates Liver Yin deficiency and Liver Qi stagnation or Yang excess. Since children are constitutionally Yin deficient, a growing "Wood" child is more prone to have Liver Yin deficiency. Liver Blood and Fluid deficiency can manifest as dizziness, muscle spasm and weakness. Since Liver Yin nourishes and lubricates tendons and ligaments, deficiency can manifest as both gross and fine motor incoordination, which can affect children's athletic abilities. The Chinese Liver is susceptible to Wind. When Wind combines with Liver Fluid deficiency, young children are prone to develop febrile seizures, when Heat from febrile illnesses dries up the Liver Yin and stirs up Liver Wind, resulting in contraction and tremor of the sinews.[1] The more serious Liver Yin deficiency would manifest as disturbance of Hun. When the Ethereal Soul is not properly housed, the Shen is affected, the child may appear confused, impulsive, and unable to focus. In China, whenever a child does something without thinking, such as abruptly running into the street, one would often hear a familiar yell from the mother: "What is the matter with you? Have you lost your Hun?" Behavioral problems, then, are often due to Hun not being at peace.

On the other hand, Liver Qi and Yang usually become stagnant, but not deficient. In these circumstances, children would manifest physical symptoms such as headaches (Yang rising to the top) and behavioral symptoms such as low frustration tolerance, ease to anger, and aggressiveness. Excess medications, which are metabolized in the Liver, can result in various Liver imbalances. Liver opens into the eyes, which explains why the appearance of jaundice in liver disease first manifests as yellowness in the eyes.

Gallbladder

Western Gallbladder and Pathophysiology

The gallbladder is a muscular sac that stores bile secreted by the liver. When the bile is needed for digestion, the gallbladder empties into the duodenum. While the gallbladder is frequently the cause of discomfort in adults, such as formation of gallstones, it seldom causes diseases in children.

Chinese Gallbladder

The Chinese Gallbladder also functions as storage for bile and secretes bile but has other important physiologic and mental/emotional functions. Together with its Yin couple organ Liver, the Gallbladder also controls movement of tendons and sinews. Liver nourishes tendons with blood, while Gallbladder nourishes them with Qi. As the Wood organ, Gallbladder is also predominant in children's Wood phase of development. In the mental–emotional realm, the Liver as General gives directions and the ability for planning, the Gallbladder enables children to make decisions, to have courage to make changes in their lives. When the Liver and Gallbladder are in harmony, children make decisions and carry them out, to have the courage in facing life's vicissitudes.

Pathophysiology

The Gallbladder can be affected in children, especially in Liver imbalance. Together with Liver, Gallbladder provides agility and coordination for gross motor and fine motor development in children, which can influence athletic abilities that are an important component of the school age child. The "clumsy" child is often relentlessly teased in school, develops low self-esteem, becomes easily discouraged and becomes timid to participate in sports, has difficulty making decisions; this in turn injures Gallbladder.

REFERENCES

1. Maciocia G. (1989) *The Foundations of Chinese Medicine: A Comprehensive Treatise for Acupuncturists and Herbalists*. Edinburgh, Churchill Livingstone.

2. Nelson W.E. *et al*. (eds) (1996) *Nelson's Textbook of Pediatrics*, 15th edition. Philadelphia, W.B. Saunders, Co.

Childhood Development According to the Five Elements

INTRODUCTION

This chapter is subtitled "An Original Theory Proposal: Yellow Emperor Meets Piaget and Freud."

Childhood is a wondrous progression of acquiring new skills, and especially of achieving new understanding of oneself, of one's relationship with the world, with nature and the universe. Children develop by assimilating the world into their own mental and physical frame of reference, which in turn changes over time as they progress through different stages of development. An understanding of children necessitates a thorough comprehension of childhood development. In the past century, conventional theories abounded in describing all developmental aspects of children: cognitive, psychological/emotional, social, physical/motor. Of these, Piaget's cognitive and Freud's psychoanalytic theories continue to be the most influential in Western thinking.

An exhaustive search in both Chinese and Western literature revealed that to date there has not been any formal discussions of childhood development in Chinese medicine. Dr. Maurice Mussat briefly touched upon this topic in one of his lectures, but did not correlate development to conventional stages. This chapter presents an original theory of integrating conventional developmental theories with the Five Elements, a meeting of East and West, Yellow Emperor with Piaget and Freud. This theory helps to identify vulnerable organs in different age groups, and the organ of origin of chronic illnesses.

CHILDHOOD DEVELOPMENT

Childhood can be divided approximately into four developmental stages that correlate with the Five Elements. It is important to note that the transition from one stage to another is not abrupt or sharply demarcated. One Element is predominant in each phase, and gradually transitions into another Element but never completely disappears, resulting in each phase containing characteristics of at least two Elements simultaneously:

1. Infancy to early childhood: birth to 2–3 years
   Metal (mother of Water) transition to Water phase

2. Early childhood: 2–3 to 6–7 years
    Water transition to Wood phase
3. Early child to pre-teen: 6–7 years to 12 years
    Wood phase, transition to Fire phase
4. Teenage and early adulthood
    Fire phase, transition to Earth phase
5. Adulthood
    Earth phase, transition to Metal phase (middle age), Water phase
    (old age).

Infancy to Early Childhood (Birth to 2–3 Years)—Metal Transition to Water Phase

Cognitive and Psychoemotional Characteristics

Piaget describes birth to 2 years of age as the *sensorimotor* phase of development.[1,2] Children at this age perceive reality by what they can see, grab, touch, or put in their mouths. Objects are initially perceived as an extension of themselves, that is, objects are spatially related to the body. Mother, the warmest and most perceived "object," is a part of the self. In a positive emotional climate, the child progresses to the concept of object permanence: when they learn that objects—beginning with mother—continue to exist even when they can no longer see them.

Freud defines this stage as a closed monadic, psychological system, a symbiosis.[3] The child's identity is firmly attached to the mother, and mother and child are perceived as one entity. With the acquisition of motor skills, the child begins physical separation from the mother, but still "checks back" to the mother as a point of orientation and reference.[3]

Freud designates this as the oral phase of development. From the psychoanalytic standpoint, the infant and young child needs psychological oral gratification as "sexual drive first manifests itself through the mouth."[4] The baby at this stage is primarily the "Id," the embodiment of instinctual and impulsive drives.[3]

Emotionally, the baby's first expression is crying at the moment of birth. Crying becomes the all-encompassing emotional outburst for all the baby's instinctual needs: hunger, warmth, comfort, fear, as well as physical discomfort, such as a wet diaper. Social smile occurs at approximately 2 months, laughter at 3 months, and true expression of fear can manifest as early as 4 months of age. For example, when an infant is frightened by a loud noise, he wrinkles his face into a fearful expression before bursting out in tears.

Five-Element Development: Metal Transition to Water Phase

In Chinese medicine, this stage can be characterized metaphorically as the Metal transition to Water phase of development. Metal is the "Mother Element" to Water. Birth marks the entry of the Corporeal Soul, the Soul of the physical being. The Apgar score is in fact a good indication of the "health or strength" of the Corporeal Soul: a high Apgar score indicates a healthy, strong baby, and a low Apgar score indicates a physically compromised baby (see

Chapter 3). The Corporeal Soul resides in the Lung, the Metal organ. Skin corresponds with the Lung, and majority of the baby's sensations are from the skin, such as touch, wetness, coldness or warmth. The concept of the Corporeal Soul correlates well with both sensorimotor and Freudian interpretations. When babies express their needs by crying, they can cry with and without tears. Crying with tears corresponds to the Lung, while crying without tears is associated with the Water organ, Kidney.

Water is the beginning of life. The infant and young child is like a seed, the beginning of a tree. It is submerged under water, buried within Earth. It does not yet have its own identity; it is at one with Mother Earth. The infant and young child has the Water body habitus: puffy hands, short arms and legs. The predominant Water emotion is fear, which encompasses all facets of fear: the instinctual fear of hunger and the psychological fear of abandonment.

The vulnerable organs during this phase are Lung and Kidney, as respiratory illnesses are prevalent in the infant and young child, and the marrow, the brain, is sensitive to nourishment and any form of insult. Since the mother is in symbiotic relationship with the child, the digestive system, the Spleen, is also susceptible to insult and injury.

Early Childhood (2–3 to 6–7 Years Pre-operational)—Water Transition to Wood Phase

Cognitive and Psychoemotional Characteristics

Piaget's pre-operational or preconcrete stage describes the child from approximately 2 to 6–7 years of age. During this period, the child manifests specific cognitive characteristics: egocentrism, illogical transformations, vivid imagination, and animism.[1,2,5]

The pre-operational child is egocentric and is at the center of the universe. Everything happens because of them and for them. For example, when a 4-year-old boy is asked, "Why is it snowing?" He may answer, "It snows because *I* want to build a snowman." "Why is it sunny outside?" "It is sunny because *I* want to play outside." While the egotistical child takes credit for everything good that has happened, he also takes the "responsibility" and blames himself for everything bad that is happening: "Mommy and Daddy are fighting because I'm bad."

Accompanying this sense of being at the center of the universe is also a feeling of magical power: "When I walk, the sun follows me." The child feels as if everything notices him: the wind, the stars, the clouds.[2] He then interprets the world around him from an illogical, distorted viewpoint based on his own time, space, and experience.[5] When father does not feel well and comes home from work at 2:00 p.m., 5-year-old Jonathan says: "Daddy's home, it's dinnertime," because Jonathan usually associates eating dinner shortly after Daddy walks in the door. When father lies down to take a nap, Jonathan pulls him out of bed to "have dinner," unable to understand that "Daddy's not feeling well and it is not yet time for dinner."

This illogical thinking also makes it difficult for the young child to separate reality from fantasy,[5] so that TV shows, movies, and commercials can make a very powerful impact on the young mind. Jessica insists that mother buy her a

Susie Talking Doll, because the TV said ". . . every little girl wants a Susie Talking Doll." Anna was frightened by the wicked witch in the Wizard of Oz, and wanted to know when the witch might come to take her away.

This distorted reality is further accentuated by vivid imagination and animism. The preschool-aged child plays with imaginary friends and invisible toys. When mother tells 4-year-old Amanda to get in the car, she runs into the house to get her friend "Dino," "I wouldn'da left ya, Dino," she tells Dino, who is invisible to adults. The imaginary friends may also be inanimate objects infused with human qualities. Children endow stuffed toys or inanimate objects with the abilities to talk, laugh, play. The "Calvin and Hobbes" cartoon illustrates this point well. When there is an adult in the cartoon frame, Hobbes is a stuffed tiger sitting on the couch; when Calvin is alone with Hobbes, it is the perfect playmate who sings, runs, plays.

This magical, egotistical, illogical thinking is one-dimensional: everything revolves around the child, the self. Reality is distorted when there is only one point of view and all other perspectives are not being taken into account.

The Freudian anal stage of development begins around 2–3 years of age, when basic psychological energy, libido, begins to be invested in the anus.[5,6] Toilet training, therefore, becomes the most important developmental milestone for the young child. Traumatic toilet training experiences may have psychological ramifications that can persist into adulthood.[3] The neo-Freudian, Dr. Margaret Mahler, characterizes the toddler as struggling with separation–individuation issues:[3] the toddler wants independence from the mother, begins to have an increasing sense of self as a separate individual, yet is still very attached to the mother and has difficulty separating from her. For example, a 3-year-old may defiantly say "no" when mother wants to hold his hand, and throw a temper tantrum, yet cries unconsolably when she leaves the room. By 3–4 years of age, the child has achieved intrapsychic perception of mother, of object constancy, so that there is an internal image of her even when she is not physically present.[3] Amanda starts crying all of a sudden in preschool and calls for "mama," because she is now capable of thinking of mother and misses her.

Id still predominates in pre-operational children to drive them toward instant gratification and pleasure. The majority of behavior can be explained by instinctual fear: fear of separation, fear of abandonment, fear of losing mother's love. Fear is the underlying emotion of enuresis—persistent bedwetting when toilet training fails.

Both toilet training and separation–individuation have the characteristic of a push–pull, to-and-fro struggle. The child has to learn when to hold on, when to let go. (These are the actual words used by Milton Ericksonian hypnotists for treating enuresis.) The same "hold on, let go" paradigm operates with separation–individuation: wanting to leave and walk away from mother, yet returning to check back with mother, afraid of losing her love.

Five-Element Development: Water Phase, and Water Transition to Wood

The pre-operational child, like a seed and young sprout, metaphorically corresponds to many characteristics of both the Water and Wood Elements. The identity of the Water child is still very much defined by mother, as all bodies of water are defined by Mother Earth: the lake, the ocean, the river. The junction between Water and Earth illustrates well the push–pull, separation–individuation relationship the young child has with mother. At any junction between Water and Earth, there is the ebb and flow, to-and-fro movement of water. Waves crash onto shore, recede into the ocean; tide rushes in, tide rushes out. Even on river beds, there is that constant to-and-fro movement of water onto and receding from land. Toilet training is both a "water" milestone as well as the holding on/letting go of nourishment, which is provided by mother, by Earth.

Piaget's pre-operational cognitive characteristics are well illustrated by Water children. Egocentricity is manifested by reflection of the self in the water: When young children look in the water, they see first and foremost a reflection of themselves. Everything else around them is defined in relation to them: how far it is from them, to the left of them, to the right of them. While their reflection is clear, everything else is distorted—the far-away mountain appears to be right behind them, the nearby trees have hazy outlines. The world is equally distorted if the child, like a seed, is submerged in the water—the view of the outside world through the water surface is blurred and indistinct. It also changes depending on where they are or how deep they are in the water. Thus Water children see the world as they interpret it: from their point of view, distorted, unrealistic.

Within the water, the children are all powerful. By moving their arms, they can cause swirls in the water, making the fish swim in the direction of the swirl, and making the underwater plants sway as if they have become "animated."

But the omnipotence is tempered by fear, as Water children need to feel the firm support of Mother Earth under their feet. They can float for only a short period of time, before becoming very anxious and fearful and need to feel the touch of earth under their feet. They are exhibiting the Freudian fear of losing mother's love, of abandonment, of letting go.

The corresponding Water organ is Kidney, the foundation of all the Yin and Yang of the body; of the marrow, the brain; of Essence—the ultimate life defining force that determines development, sexual function, and aging. Life begins with the Water, with Kidney. Fear is the corresponding emotion of Kidney. When the child is not overcome by fear, willpower—the healthy Kidney emotion—helps in the decision of when to let go, when to hold on.

The vulnerable organs in this Water to Wood phase are the Kidney and the Liver. The most important person in the Water child's life is the mother. According to Mussat, if the mother is overbearing, the child feels confined and may be delayed in the natural progression toward individualization,[7] just as Earth "locks in" a body of water, giving rise to the images of stagnant water, of swamps where seedling cannot grow. If the child is overly attached to mother; the all-consuming relationship with mother induces further "distortion" of reality, just as the view from deep within a stagnant body of water.

Mussat calls this type of mother one that has "breasts that are too big."[7] This conjures up the image that the child feels suffocated when breastfeeding. The child ends up eating too much, and is unable to perceive what is around as the breast fills the entire sensorimotor world. Mussat further points out that this predisposes the child to obesity, to gastrointestinal disorders such as colitis, and to obsessional neurosis.[7]

The undernourishing mother, on the other hand, cannot give shape to Water, and the seed washes away. According to Mussat, the child constantly, obsessively looks for mother, for the breast, for Earth. This is like Water flowing everywhere, without a definite shape, "looking" for Earth boundaries, for identity.

Childhood disorders may reflect the importance of Earth. Respiratory symptoms of cough with phlegm often begin with Spleen Qi deficiency. Gastrointestinal symptoms can be colic, vomiting, or diarrhea. Feeding disorders range from failure to thrive (which sometimes reflects poor mother–child bonding) to obesity (constant need for the nipple) to eating disorders (push–pull characteristics in eating/purging). Congenital and developmental anomalies are often genetic, which is transmitted through Kidney Jing. Brain is marrow controlled by Kidney, so that central nervous system development is most vulnerable during this stage, when any severe illness can result in mental retardation.

Early Childhood to Preteen (6–7 Years to 12 Years)—Wood Phase, Transition to Fire

Cognitive and Psychoemotional Characteristics

According to Piaget, the child progresses from the pre-operational to concrete/operational stage at 6–11/12 years of age. During this developmental stage, the child learns to operate mentally on a rational basis. The child is capable of learning right from wrong, and of relating to the world on a more realistic level defined by time and space.[1,2,5] Nine-year-old Jason now knows it is wrong to hit his friend Tommy as he did when he was 4 just because he wanted Tommy's toy robot. He also knows to go to daycare on Tuesdays and Thursdays because mother works late on those days and cannot pick him up until 6:00 p.m. However, the thinking must be on a concrete level that readily relates to their everyday experiences. Math problems involve adding or multiplying numbers of pencils or notebooks, not the abstract algebraic unknown, x. The thinking is now linear, two-dimensional, cause and effect, right and wrong. Thus, the one-dimensional imaginary thinking of the pre-operational child is the precursor of the two-dimensional rational thinking of the operational child.

With these new cognitive skills, the operational child needs direction and information as he learns to negotiate in the real world. Parental nurture, guidance and discipline steer the child toward the right moral and ethical path. Schooling provides the child with factual information to prepare for the future. Children are confronted more and more by decision-making, ranging from what they would like to pack for school lunch, to which of their parental rules they would obey and which they would rebel against. Maturation of motor skills enables the child to not only physically leave the mother with ease, but also participate in more sophisticated activities, such as bicycle riding and sports.

Psychologically, the child also becomes more independent due to the maturation of the Ego, the Freudian reality-oriented facet of the personality.[1,3,4] The Ego provides the child with a sense of self-awareness, an identity that is separate from the mother and others so that they are now capable of describing themselves or comparing themselves to others. The focus of the identity, however, is primarily on concrete, physical characteristics. Jason describes himself as being tall and having brown eyes, and says that Tyler is taller but he is a faster runner. In order to be an entity and get along with others, the Ego needs to control the Id impulses that were driving the younger child toward immediate pleasure and gratification. The behavior of the school-aged child now follows the reality instead of the pleasure principle. Jason does not hit his friend not only because he cognitively knows right from wrong, but also because psychologically his maturing Ego can now control his Id. Whereas instinctual fear was the underlying emotion of Id, anxiety underlies the formation of Ego—which institutes various defense mechanisms in response to perceived danger or threat to existence.[1,3,4]

Five-Element Development: Wood Phase, and Wood Transition to Fire

From the Five-Element perspective, the operational child is a young tree, growing above ground. Most of it is still underground, strongly attached to and therefore identified with Mother Earth. The part above ground is gradually developing a distinct identity, like an Ego, with definitive physical characteristics that can be compared to others: a taller tree, brighter colored flowers.

The tree is the Taoist symbol for man, rooted in Earth, reaching upward toward sky, coming into being between Heaven and Earth. Heaven is symbolic for father, who provides guidance and direction for the child, the tree, to grow straight and upward. Thus, nourished by Mother Earth and guided by Father Heaven, the child learns Yang and Yin, right from wrong, which correlates to the rationalization process of concrete thinking.

The corresponding Wood organ is the Liver. The emotions associated with Liver are frustration, irritability, smoldering anger, and anxiety—the emotions of an impatient, operational child, of Ego. Healthy Liver Qi enables the child to understand and take proper directions for growth, so that the tree grows straight and upward. The increasing motor activities are also associated with the Liver, which rules the tendons and sinews and controls movement.

The Liver Yin houses Hun, the Ethereal Soul. Hun is the the Soul from the Eternal Soul World that enters our body along with the Corporeal Soul at birth. Whereas the Corporeal Soul resides in the Lung and is the soul of our physical being, the Ethereal Soul resides in the Liver Yin and is the soul of our Mind, of Shen. It therefore influences our thinking, our reasoning, our mental abilities, our emotions. When we dream, it is our Hun that brings back images from the Soul World. Through the Ethereal Soul, our Minds become connected with each other, and all of us can access thoughts and ideas from eternity. In this sense, the Hun is psychologically comparable to the Jungian concept of our Collective Unconscious, which is made of Individual Unconscious from each and every one of us. Whereas the Corporeal Soul dies when the body dies, the Ethereal Soul returns to the Soul World and becomes the Hun of another physical being.[8]

The vulnerable organ is Liver, which is especially susceptible to Wind, just as a small tree would sway back and forth in the wind, and may even be uprooted by strong wind. Chinese pediatrics posits that children have "vulnerable Liver,"[9] which primarily means that children's Liver Yin is immature and vulnerable, as Liver Yang even in adults usually becomes stagnant and never becomes deficient. Young children prior to age 6 are susceptible to seizures which are "internal wind" disorders. When the Liver Yin is deficient, Liver Yang may become excessive, resulting in excess physical symptoms such as hyperactivity; or excess emotional symptoms such as increasing irritability, frustration, anger. When the Ethereal Soul is not properly housed, the Mind does not function well, so that the child can manifest cognitive difficulties and appears to be impulsive and "out of it." An old traditional Chinese expression describes this state as acting as if

"Hun is not there." The child is inattentive, cannot focus, cannot follow direction, cannot think clearly. A well-balanced Liver enables the child to make decisions, to take more charge of his life, to becomes his own "General."

Mussat calls this the crucial moment of establishing equilibrium between Yin and Yang.[7] The father is an important balance for mother. From both parents the child gets masculine and feminine perspectives and incorporates the Yin and the Yang. The Wood child still has a very close relationship with mother, needing nurture and foundation for "growing roots," and looks to the father, to Heaven, for direction and guidance. From a monadic, symbiotic entity, the mother/child and father become a dyad: one begets two.

During this phase of development, if the mother is weak, the child is unable to root properly, lacks centeredness, becomes easily influenced by external influences, like a tree bending or even toppling by strong wind and rain. The child has difficulty distinguishing right from wrong, becomes anxious in not knowing which direction to take. Mussat calls this "anxiety with disorientation."[7] The Wood qualities of making decisions and taking directions do not become fully developed. In mild cases, the child manifests behavioral problems, as negative behavior is essentially the child crying out for help, for nurturing, for guidance. In more severe cases, the unrooted child may manifest more severe behavioral problems of a juvenile delinquent. As Spleen/Earth is the seat of learning information, versus Kidney/Water as the seat for learning life's experiences, a child with weak Spleen/Earth/Mother may have difficulty grasping concepts, as in a child with learning disability.

A weak father or absent father leaves the child without Yang guidance. This is like a tree without sunshine; it grows crookedly looking for the sun. This child may be easily swayed by opinions, constantly looking for guidance. According to Mussat, a child without orientation will begin to follow any whim and is at risk of developing borderline personalities.[7] On the other hand, an overpowering mother is dictatorial and does not allow the child to make any choices. The child is afraid to ask, becomes nervous, anxious, and easily frustrated.

A domineering father is a dogmatic General that allows little or no flexibility. The child follows strict guidelines, cannot ask questions, and does not have the opportunity to become his own General. According to Mussat, this kind of a child is anxious due to "non-liberation of self-expression."[7] The child is stifled, but still does not know right or wrong as he is not allowed to experience for himself.

Adolescence and Early Adulthood—Fire Phase, Transition to Earth Phase

Cognitive and Psychoemotional Characteristics

This is Piaget's stage for Formal operation, when children progress from linear to abstract thinking.[1,2,5] They can now ponder over hypothetical problems that are beyond their concrete realm of experience, such as ideas, philosophies, and abstract events. They become increasingly more aware of their possible role in society and make plans for college, career, the future, and possibly for marriage and family.

Psychologically, the child enters Freud's Genital phase of development.[4] Teenagers experience dramatic hormonal and bodily changes and gradually discover their sexual identity. Accompanying the physical changes are drastic behavioral manifestations: They distance themselves from their parents and prefer peer interactions and approval. They are fearless and drive recklessly. They feel invincible and freely experiment with sex, drugs, and alcohol. There can be moments of tremendous emotional upheaval which may precipitate identity crisis and self-destruction.

On the other hand, emotionally balanced teenagers contribute to society and plan for the future. They are involved in community, and begin to piece together their adult identity and make college and career choices.

Five-Element Development: Fire Phase and Fire Transition to Earth

The teenager and young adults in their early 20s correspond metaphorically to the Fire Element. The Fire organ is the Heart, the House of Shen, which is both the Spirit and the Mind. Through the Ethereal Soul, the Mind can perceive far beyond the concrete boundaries of human experiences into the abstract: the infinite, the eternal, the universal. The predominant emotion that corresponds to the Heart is passion. As teenagers develop sexual identity, they enter into intimate relationships that are in reality infatuations consumed by "fiery" passion. This is the archetype of romantic love, exemplified by Tristan und Isolde, Romeo and Juliet—young, passionate love with life-and-death intensity.

Teenage Fire children establish themselves as the Emperor of being, no longer dependent on Heaven or Earth, Father or Mother. They are rebellious, scorching Mother Earth and following their own directions, rejecting direction toward Heaven.

When Fire children are out of control, they behave recklessly, sending sparks flying everywhere, igniting whatever they touch. They feel fearless, indestructible, the exact opposite of the fearful Water child. When they are in a state of balance, they can provide warmth to others. They contribute to the future by providing nurturing ashes for the Earth.

Whereas the Water child is in symbiotic oneness with mother, Wood child reflects the dyad of mother/child and father, the Fire child is in a triad: mother, father, child. Thus, one begets two, two begets three, three begets everything.

The vulnerable organ during this phase is primarily the Heart. However, if the previous developmental phases were well balanced, there is the appropriate amount of wood for a warm fire, appropriate rational preparation for formal operation so that the teenager, though driven by passion, is still able to distinguish right from wrong. When the previous phases were not well balanced, the Fire child goes out of control, sexual exploitations and reckless behavior may lead into compromising situations with serious sequelae.

Adulthood—Earth Phase, Transition to Metal Phase (Middle Age), Water Phase (Old Age)

From the Fire phase, teenagers progress to the Earth phase of adulthood, when they can become the nurturer. The middle years corresponds to Metal phase, while old age declines into Water phase, and life cycle begins again. The Five-Element Developmental Theory is summarized in Figure 5.1.

FIGURE 5.1   *The Five-Element developmental correspondences to cognitive and psychoemotional phases: summary of the Five-Element Developmental Theory.*

Age	Cognitive	Psychoemotional	Five Element Developmental Phase	Vulnerable organs	Taoist correlation
Birth–2 years	Sensorimotor Object permanence	Oral stage symbiotic relation with mother	Metal—Corporeal Soul: senses, limbs, movement, "Mother" of Water Water—beginning of life (seed) Strong attachment to Mother (Earth) = identity of one mother/child	**LU** **KI** SP	One
Age 2–6 years	Pre-operational—one dimensional thinking Egocentric Illogical transformations Vivid imagination Animism	Anal stage Separation/individuation Id—instinctual, pleasure principle Fear: letting go, holding on	Water Child: distorted perception of reality; fear Water–Earth junction: to-and-fro, push–pull, letting go–holding on Identity of one (seedling still under water) = mother/child Water transition into Wood	**KI** **LR** LU SP	One begets
Age 6—preteen	Concrete operational rationalization two-dimensional, linear cause–effect thinking	Ego formation Reality principle Gradually more independent, needs guidance Still strong identification with mother, looks to father for advice/guidance	Wood Child—Taoist tree symbolic of man: rooted in earth, reach upward toward sky Heaven & Earth = father/mother, right/wrong, Yin/Yang decision making Identity of two = mother/child, father Hun—Ethereal Soul, resides in Liver Yin Wood transition into Fire	**LR** HT SP	Two begets
Teenage–young adult	Formal operational abstract thinking	Genital phase, sexual identity Drastic changes: hormonal, physical, emotional Preference for peer Fearless, reckless, rebellious behavior Sexual identity; passion	Fire Child—coming into own identity Identity of three: father, mother, self Shen—Mind, through Ethereal Soul—perceives infinity Fiery passion Reckless sparks Rebellious—scorches earth, follows own direction Fire transition into Earth	**HT** SP LR	Three begets
Adult			Earth = center; mother = own nurturer and nurturer of others Identity = everything Transition into Metal = declining years, Water = old age	**SP** **HT** LR KI, LU	Everything

DEVELOPMENTAL CONSEQUENCES THAT PERSIST INTO ADULTHOOD

Modern psychology tells us that adults are essentially grown-ups still "stuck" at various ages in childhood during times of physical or emotional trauma. Freudian psychology considers the first 5 years as being crucial for adult behavior and personality formation.[1,3,6,10]

The Five-Element Developmental Theory provides another perspective of the possible origins of physical and emotional disorders. It has been the author's experience that adults who manifest certain Elemental characteristics would often relate a traumatic experience during that phase of development. For example, a 30-year-old man who has difficulty making commitment—wanting intimacy yet being afraid of it, one day proposes marriage and the next day backs down; he behaves with the push–pull quality of Water and Earth interaction. He later reveals that his parents were divorced when he was 3 years old. Some adults traumatized in the Wood phase of development may have difficulty determining right from wrong; they may be more prone to develop anxiety disorders.

APPLICATION OF THE FIVE-ELEMENT DEVELOPMENTAL APPROACH

The importance of the Five-Element developmental phase in chronic disorders are twofold: first, it identifies the vulnerable Element according to the age and development of the child; second, it provides a means to trace the Element of the *origin* of chronic illness. This is especially helpful in sorting out which Element to treat in complex disorders with multiple symptoms, such as attention deficit hyperactivity disorder (ADHD).[11–14]

The protocol for using the Five-Element phases is as follows:

1. Identify and treat the vulnerable Element that corresponds to the phase of development, e.g., Wood in the school-aged child.
2. Identify and treat the *origin* of the disorder according to the developmental age of onset. For example, a child who develops asthma as an infant needs to have Water points treated along with Lung points, whereas a school-aged child needs to have Liver points treated along with Lung points (Liver–Lung in the controlling cycle relationship). Since one Element is the precursor of the succeeding Element, it is necessary to treat all Elements in the nurturing cycle from the origin to the manifestation of symptoms. For example, the older asthmatic child who had bronchiolitis at age 3 months needs to have Lung, Kidney, and Liver points balanced. This explains the progressive difficulty in treating older children with more Elemental imbalance so that the older the child, the more complex is the disorder and management.
3. Identify the corresponding Element during time of trauma. For example, a recalcitrant teenage boy was abused in the second grade. His Fire symptoms are rooted in the Wood phase of development, in the injury to the Liver Yin.

4. Treating children entails well child care, prophylactic preventive care. Balancing the corresponding vulnerable Element helps to maintain well-being and prevent development of disorders.
5. Childhood disorders often reflect family dynamics. For example, in treating a child who has recurrent digestive symptoms and goes home to a caregiver that fits Mussat's "big-breasted mother," it would be beneficial to look at the family interaction and treat the parents as well.

TREATMENT OF THE MODERN CHILD

One final word of caution regarding difficulties facing treatment of the modern child and family. An inadequate diet and use of medications can prematurely weaken the Spleen and Liver so that, regardless of age, medical management needs to include proper dietary counseling and overcoming side-effects of medications, tonification of Spleen and Liver Yin. Family structure has become more varied and complex, as single parents and divorced households are often the norm rather than the deviation. The single-parent assumes both the guidance and nurturing roles of father and mother, while a child shifting between two sets of parents may encounter conflicting rules and regulations. The prevalence of computer games that promote eye–hand coordination stunt imagination, the cognitive characteristic of the Water child, the precursor to rational thinking.

CONCLUSION

The conventional cognitive and psychoemotional theories of Piaget and Freud correlate well to the Chinese medical model of the Five Elements. Childhood development can be divided into Elemental phases, which can identify the vulnerable Element/organ of a particular age and the Element/organ of origin of a chronic condition.

REFERENCES

1. Lecture Notes, Postdoctoral Fellowship in Behavioral and Developmental Pediatrics. UCSF, 1989.
2. Piaget J. (1930) *The Child's Conception of Physical Causality*. New York, Harcourt.
3. Mahler M.S. (1970) *On Human Symbiosis and the Vicissitudes of Individuation*. New York, International Universities Press, Inc.
4. Kline P. (1972) *Facts and Fantasy in Freudian Theory*. London, Methuen & Co. Ltd.
5. Flavel J.H. (1963) *The Developmental Psychology of Jean Piaget*. Princeton, D. Van Nostrand Company, Inc.
6. Freud S. (1908) *Character and Anal Eroticism*, Vol. 9.
7. Mussat M. Acupuncture Energetics Lecture—part of video film library for UCLA Acupuncture course (no date).
8. Maciocia G. (1994) *The Practice of Chinese Medicine, The Treatment of Diseases with Acupuncture and Chinese Herbs*. London, Churchill Livingstone.
9. Cao J. *et al.*, (1990) *Essentials of Traditional Chinese Pediatrics*. Beijing, Foreign Language Press.
10. MacIntyre A.C. (1958) *The Unconscious, A Conceptual Analysis*. New York, Humanities Press.
11. American Psychiatric Association (1994) *Diagnostic and Statistical Manual of Mental Disorders*, 4th edition, DSM-IV. Washington DC, American Psychiatric Association.

12. Shaywitz B., Fletcher J.M. & Shaywitz S.E. (1997) Attention deficit hyperactivity disorder. *Advances in Pediatrics* 44, 331.

13. Levine M.D. *et al.* (eds) (1999) *Developmental and Behavioral Pediatrics*, 3rd edition. Philadelphia, W.B. Saunders, Co.

14. Meninger W.C. (1943) Characterologic and symptomatic expressions related to the anal phase of psychosexual development. *Psychoanalytical Quarterly* 12, 161–93.

6 Evaluation of Children

Western pediatrics follows a systemic assessment of children based on both subjective information obtained from history and objective information based on a general physical examination and more definitive laboratory reports. Chinese pediatrics is particularly sensitive to specific physical findings that reflect the child's physiology and pathophysiology, substantiated by some history but without any technical information.

Comprehensive evaluation of children can incorporate both systems of healing to encompass detailed history taking, physical examination that focuses on significant features unique to children, and formulation of impressions that can follow specific pediatric guidelines for acute and chronic disorders.

HISTORY

Conventional medicine posits that 80–90% of diagnoses can come from proper history taking. Western medicine focuses on specific segmental, organ/system involvement; while Chinese medicine emphasizes the overall imbalances in the child. Although many categories are the same in both disciplines—such as dietary history, perinatal history, family history—the contents are vastly different.

The following list integrates the salient features of both forms of history for a comprehensive evaluation of the child:

- Chief complaint
- History of present illness
- Detailed dietary history
- Sleep
- Activities
- Prenatal and perinatal history
- Past medical history
- Review of systems
- Family history
- Social history.

Chief Complaint

The chief complaint is the *major* symptom or reason that the child is being seen, e.g., cough, stomachache, and its duration. It should be limited to just one or at most a few words, and the duration as specific as possible, e.g., cough for 3 days. This immediately alerts the physician to the specific problem and organ/system involvement.

History of Present Illness

More detailed information is given that centers around the chief complaint.

- *Symptoms*: more detailed information about the symptoms, such as dry cough versus cough with phlegm.
- *Course*: nature of the course of the illness: waxing and waning, progressively worsening, complications, etc.
- *Precipitating events*: what brought on the symptoms, e.g., knee pain noted after exposure to cold; earache started 3 days after URI symptoms; headache started when taking an examination at school (knee pain, earache, and headache are the chief complaints that brought the child in). Also important is what types of food the child was eating around the time of onset of illness.
- *Treatment received so far*: medications, herbs, acupuncture, etc. Any relief with the treatments.
- *History of similar symptoms or illnesses*: the number of similar episodes and age(s) of occurrence; severity of previous illness: home treatment, outpatient clinic visit, emergency room visit, hospitalization; complications and residual effects from illness, such as seizures, or persistent abdominal pain.
- *Current medications or herbs*: any remedies taken on a regular basis.

Detailed Dietary History

Chapter 8 discusses in detail various aspects and effects of foods on health. In taking a dietary history in children, focus on the following items:

- *Types of food*:
  - Ask if the child's diet routinely consists of fresh foods or of frozen, packaged foods.
  - Ask which of the common unhealthy foods the child consumes regularly: energetically "Cold" foods, greasy, fried foods; Phlegm-producing foods; artificially sweetened foods; excess salty foods.
- *Flavors of food*: ask if there is one or two predominant flavors that would point toward specific organ disharmony.
- *Seasonal variation of food*: ask if the child routinely eats foods that are in season.
- *Thermoregulatory properties of food*: prepare a list of foods with various thermoregulatory properties. The child or parent can check off foods on the list to indicate if the child's diet has a preponderance of energetically Hot, Warm, Neutral, Cool, or Cold foods.
- *Manner of eating*: ask about any manners of eating that predispose to Qi imbalance:
  - Eating too fast, not chewing properly, eating while studying or watching TV
  - Times for meals
  - Poor eating habits: nibbling, sudden change in eating habits, signs of possible eating disorders
  - Appetite variations: poor appetite, picky eater, irregular appetite, good appetite but irregular bowel movement

- Emotional state while eating
- Any disturbance after eating: vomiting, dry heaves, abdominal distension and pain.

Sleep

Ask about the child's sleep in terms of postures during sleep, amount of sleep, insomnia, and dreams, and if there is snoring. Sleep disturbances in Western pediatrics consists of sleep apnea primarily in infants and young children and night terror and insomnia in older children. Chinese pediatrics places import-ance on the following aspects of sleep for determining possible imbalances.

- *Position of sleep*:
  - *Curled up, fetal position* indicates coldness.
  - *Lying on abdomen* can cause food stagnation.
    It is interesting to note that Chinese babies normally sleep on their backs while American babies are routinely placed on their abdomens in the nursery. In 1992 the American Academy of Pediatrics (AAP) recom-mended that infants be placed on their backs to sleep. Since this recom-mendation was issued, the incidence of sudden infant death syndrome (SIDS), has reduced by 15 to 20% in the United States. The Chinese theo-ry of food stagnation is a possible explanation: when infants are placed on their abdomen, food stagnation may result in regurgitation of stomach contents, which in turn may choke the baby.
    Preference for sleeping on the abdomen may indicate Stomach deficiency.
  - *Inability to sleep supine* (on the back) is suggestive of Lung excess condi-tion.
  - *Sleep with arms and legs thrown outward*, covers and bedclothes thrown off suggests Heat.
  - *Preference for sleeping on the side* is suggestive of Qi Blood deficiency on that side with an excess on the opposite side. For example, a child may prefer to sleep on the right side when there is right Lung deficiency and left Lung excess.
- *Amount of sleep*—the number of hours varies from child to child. A child has had sufficient sleep when he wakes up feeling refreshed and does not need to take extra naps during the day.
  - *Not enough sleep* may temporarily lead to Qi deficiency and chronically to Kidney deficiency.
  - *Too much sleep* may lead to Spleen Yang deficiency and accumulation of Damp.
- *Insomnia*—insomnia in children can be either an excess or a deficient state.
  - *Excess insomnia* is usually characterized by restless sleep and sometimes by an inability to sleep on the back, waking up during the night with men-tal and/or physical restlessness, sometimes accompanied by a stuffy sensa-tion in the chest. This often occurs after a Wind-Heat illness, with residual Wind-Heat settling in the diaphragm.
    A modern diet with drinking caffeinated soft drinks or eating chocolate before bedtime can also cause an excessive type of insomnia.

- *Deficient insomnia* is usually characterized by problematic sleep rhythms. Children may experience the night terror type of insomnia due to Liver Yin deficiency with several of the following characteristics: wakes up during the night, talks in sleep, walks in sleep, appears irritable, appears frightened and confused, breathes fast, has fast heart rates and excessive dreams.
- *Excessive dreaming*—usually indicates Yin deficiency.
  - *Kidney deficiency*: the dreams tend to be disturbing.
  - *Liver Yin deficiency*: the dreams are filled with anger, frustration, agitation.

    The dreams may be quite vivid, as the Ethereal Soul, Hun, which resides in Liver Yin is not properly housed, therefore does not feel peaceful, leaves the body when the child is asleep and brings back vivid images from the Soul World that manifest as dreams.[1]

    The child may report feeling a light, floating sensation as he or she is falling asleep, which correlates to the Hun leaving the body.

    The child may take a long time to wake up, which indicates that the Hun does not want to come back to a deficient home.
  - *Spleen Cold deficiency*: dreams of fighting things. This can sometimes be brought on by watching too many violent shows on TV.
- *Snoring*—indicates Spleen deficiency resulting in Phlegm in the Stomach channel.

Activities

Ask about the general amount of activity during the day: such as always on the go or usually prefers to do very little. Ask about the types of activities that the child regularly engages in: such as video games, sports, reading, and if the child is physically aggressive.

The opposite of sleep is activity, which should occur appropriately during the day: the Yang phase of the biologic cycle that balances the Yin sleep cycle. Yang cannot function well when Yin is out of balance, and vice versa.

The degree or appropriate amount of activity is difficult to assess, because of the wide range of normal behavior, the multitude of variables as well as subjectivity of the person evaluating the child. A child may be appropriately active when surrounded by 30 other children, but appears exasperatingly hyperactive to an exhausted, burnt-out teacher. Therefore, the hyperactive or "excess" state and lethargic or "deficient" state are relative and vary with circumstances.

Some types of activity are indicators of specific imbalances:

- *Playing video games*—an activity primarily involving eye–hand coordination without much thinking or large motor activity; an excess may lead to Liver Qi stagnation.
- *Playing sports*—is an appropriate outlet for the child's usual excess Yang state during the day, the Yang part of the biologic cycle. It is also good for large motor movement which helps to balance Liver Qi. This is especially important for children in the Wood phase of development.
- *Excess reading or thinking* may lead to Spleen Qi deficiency and Damp and Phlegm accumulation. Each child should have a balance of reading/thinking

with rest and playing. Therefore, Chinese theories of medicine are supportive of the old saying "all work and no play makes Johnny a dull boy."

- *Inappropriate aggressive behavior*, such as hitting, fighting, indicates Liver Fire or Heart Fire rising.

Prenatal and Perinatal History

Chapter 3 discusses the significance of prenatal and perinatal events. Taking a thorough history on conception, pregnancy, and birth provides important information about the child's pre-Heaven Essence that can have significant influence on his health.

- *Conception*
  - Ask about both parents: age, general physical and emotional health, stress, consumption of alcohol or drugs during conception.
  - Questions about the father: possible history of promiscuity.
  - Questions about the mother: menstrual history; previous miscarriages or abortions.
  - Also ask about the general climate and the state of the country and the world (e.g. war or peace) during the time of conception.
- *Pregnancy*
  - Ask about the mother's physical and emotional states during pregnancy; alcohol, cigarettes or drug consumption; ascertain degree of emotional stress: e.g. mild depression to needing antidepressants or psychotherapy.
  - Ask about parents' relationship during the pregnancy as an indication of degree of support or stress on mother.
- *Birth circumstances*
  - Ask about the type of delivery: vaginal delivery versus Caesarean section; any complications, birth weight, Apgar scores, climate and general state of the country at the time of birth.

Past Medical History

The past medical history of previous illnesses is important for information of the child's general state of health and of vulnerability of organ/system.

- *Previous hospitalizations*—an indication of the child's vulnerability to and potential severity of subsequent illnesses.
- *Previous operations*—Chinese medicine posits that surgery is traumatic and stressful to the system, and surgical scars continue to interrupt meridian flow to the area so that the location of scars may be associated with the disorder.
- *Any serious accidents*—significant physical trauma can also cause disruption of energetic flow.
- *Previous fevers*—the degree of fever the child usually has with illnesses provides information about tendency toward Heat accumulation and Yin depletion.
- *Vulnerable organ(s)*—which organ/system has had the most recurrent illnesses.

- *Duration of previous illnesses*—especially those similar to the present illness; longer illnesses usually indicate Qi deficiency; complications that point to other organ involvement, e.g. febrile convulsion indicates Liver Yin deficiency.
- *History of medications taken*—names, types, side-effects or reactions; duration of medications. Both the effects and side-effects may indicate injury to organs.
- *History of immunizations*—ask about the type(s) of vaccinations, single or combined; dates given; age of immunization, any reactions (see Chapter 9).

Review of Systems

Ask about symptoms in other organ/systems that were not expressed in the chief complaint. Focus on the Five-Element relationships that connect symptoms in different organ/systems, e.g. a child with productive cough has mild Spleen deficiency symptoms such as slight abdominal distension and loose stools.

Family History

- Age of grandparents at time of parents' birth provides information of ancestral Jing that parents inherited.
- Significant familial illnesses—detailed history of significant illnesses in the family, specifically look for familial tendencies of the child's illness.

Social History

The child's social situation provides information on the level of stress and support the child experiences: a single-parent household, parents' marital status, number of siblings, parents' occupation(s) and levels of education, drug and alcohol abuse, cigarette smokers in the family.

PHYSICAL EXAMINATION

A thorough pediatric examination consists of four parts:

- General appearance
- Observation/inspection
- Palpation
- Examination.

General Appearance

In both Western and Chinese pediatric examination, the first step is "eye-balling" the child, i.e. assessing the general appearance. Western pediatricians would specifically note if the child is lethargic or vigorous; is in any acute distress; has cyanosis; has any obvious signs of dehydration; has any obvious abnormal physical features, especially dysmorphic features that would suggest a genetic or chromosomal syndrome, such as the readily recognizable facial features of Down syndrome. An experienced pediatrician would be able to glance at a child and tell a sick, possibly septic child from a well child.

In 1575 a well known Chinese pediatrician Zhou You-fan compiled a list of 15 steps for diagnosing children. Eleven of those 15 steps are looking or inspection.[2]

The most important feature of the general appearance for the Chinese pediatrician is the child's Spirit reflected in the eyes. Whereas the Western physician includes the eye examination as part of the physical findings of structures of the head, looking for pupillary light reaction, for any abnormalities such as nystagmus, or for eye infections, the Chinese pediatrician looks in the eyes for the child's Shen and Hun, the Spirit and Soul. Even Western literature calls eyes the "windows to the soul." When the eyes are clear and shining, the baby is aware and intelligent, and the disease is not all that serious. A child who looks frightened and is crying in pain is not as worrisome as a child with a dull, distant, empty look in the eyes that gives one the impression that the Shen and Hun are no longer with the child. A classic pediatric condition reflected in the eyes is autism, when one of the cardinal signs is poor or fleeting eye contact. Even when the autistic child is looking at someone, he gives the eerie feeling that "nobody's home," that he is looking through another person without being connected on a human level. When a child has a "distant look" with an infection, it indicates that the infection has progressed to a serious level.

After the eyes, the child's overall coloring suggests general conditions:

- Redness is indicative of Heat
- Paleness of Cold, of Blood deficiency
- Whiteness of Qi deficiency
- Yellowness of Spleen deficiency
- Greenish hue of Liver Qi stagnation.

After the general appearance, the two examinations begin to diversify with the Western physician using instrumentation to help with physical findings, such as the otoscope and stethoscope, and laboratory analyses to confirm diagnostic impressions; the Chinese physician continues to rely on what is seen and felt to gain an understanding of an overall imbalance in the child.

Observation/Inspection

Color

- *Normal*—a healthy child's face is pink, lustrous, and shiny.
- *Redness*
  - Redness indicates presence of abnormal Heat. When the child is ill, redness indicates the presence of pathogenic Heat. When the child is otherwise well appearing, redness may be due to transformation of food stagnation into Heat. This is an excess condition, so look for other signs and symptoms of Yang excess.
  - Deeper or darker red indicates more intense Heat which has resulted in Yin deficiency, therefore, this is false Heat, and the child may have other Yin deficiency symptoms, such as dryness; or Blood deficiency symptoms, such as paleness.

- Unilateral red cheek:
  - Right side indicates Lung Heat, left side indicates Liver Heat or stagnation.
  - In infants and young children indicates teething on the same side as the redness.
  - Localized: nonsystemic, localized inflammation due to insect bite, localized infection.
- *Paleness* indicates presence of Cold, or Blood deficiency such as anemia.
- *Whiteness*
  - White facial color indicates Lung deficiency
  - Qi deficiency: face is somber white
  - Yang deficient: bright white
  - More severe Yang deficiency: bright white with cold limbs
  - Yang or Qi deficiency with Dampness: white face with signs of edema, such as swollen eyelids.
- *Yellow facial complexion*
  - Yellow hue: Spleen Qi deficiency presenting as Dampness
  - Sallow yellow: Qi and Blood deficiency
  - Bright yellow: presence of Damp Heat
  - Dull, pale yellow: presence of Damp Cold.
- *Qing-greenish tinge*—this color is always dull. Liver stagnation—Qing is Chinese for pale green that is like the color of veins. The veins appear more prominent in Liver Qi stagnation because of Liver's function for storage of Blood. Veins are especially prominent around and between the eyes, the external orifice for Liver.
- *Dark bluish tinge*
  - Dark bluish tinge indicates Kidney involvement.
  - Qing-bluish, cyanotic, indicates Cold with contraction of Blood and Qi; this correlates with ischemia causing blood desaturation manifesting as cyanosis.
  - Purplish discoloration indicates Blood stasis, bruises.
  - Bluish around the lips indicates obstruction or stagnation of Lung Qi resulting in Blood stasis (in Western medicine, perioral cyanosis indicates hypoxia or right-to-left shunting of blood as in congenital cyanotic heart diseases so that blood bypasses lungs for oxygenation, resulting in circulation of desaturated blood).

Special Facial Areas

- *Shan Gen, root of mountain: between eyebrows.* Shan Gen, "root of mountain," is the area at the root of the bridge of the nose between two eyes, (the nose being the mountain of the face). This area is below the Yintang point. *Greenish veins* visible on the face indicate weak Spleen in infants and small children. The more prominent the vein, the weaker is the Spleen. This is a very reliable diagnostic sign that is easy to determine. *Veins with bluish tinge* indicate Kidney involvement, possibility of intrauterine insult or congenital Kidney anomaly.
- *Yintang area*: The Yintang correlates to the autonomic nervous system. Red and dry skin in children indicates localized internal Heat, with tendency toward febrile convulsions.

Hair

- *Normal* healthy hair in children is lustrous.
- *Withered, brittle* hair indicates Qi and Blood deficiency.
- *Sparse, bald spots* indicates Kidney Essence deficiency; may be congenital; secondary to medication, toxins; presence of infection, e.g. fungal.

Tongue

The tongue can be examined in the infant and young child by using a tongue blade. A *normal* tongue in children is pink, moist but not boggy, younger children usually do not have a coating. Redness of the tongue in children is a different shade from the red tongue seen in adults.

- *Red* tongue generally indicates Heat. However, children today tend to normally have internal Heat, so that the baseline tongue is several shades redder than usual.
- *Red tip* indicates Wind-Heat; in children with behavioral problems, it can also indicate mental irritation and agitation as the tongue reflects conditions of the Heart, of Shen.
- *Deep red* indicates Heat having entered the Blood.
- *Thorny red* like red bayberry indicates toxic Heat in the Blood, exhaustion of Yin fluids.
- *Purple* indicates Blood stagnation and stasis.
- *Pale* tongue indicates Qi, Blood deficiency.
- *Coating* is generally unreliable in children. A thick coating usually indicates food stagnation that has transformed into internal Heat.
- *Dry, scanty, peeled* tongue indicates Yin deficiency.
- *Geographic* tongue indicates Kidney deficiency. Western medicine considers geographic tongue as a normal variant without significance.
- *Patchy* tongue that comes and goes indicates Spleen or Stomach weakness.

Eyes

The eyes reflect the Spirit of the child.

- *Normal* eyes should be bright, giving the sense that the child is connected with the person he is looking at, with the world.
- *White of the eyes* showing while sleeping indicates Spleen Yang deficiency.
- *Eye discharge*
  - Watery indicates Wind, such as URI, allergies.
  - Thick eye discharge indicates presence of Phlegm, Dampness.
  - Dry eyes without tearing indicates Liver Yin deficiency.
  - Yellow discharge indicates Damp Heat.
- *Eyelid*
  - Pale inner eyelid indicates Blood deficiency, anemia.
  - Puffy under eyelids indicate Kidney and/or Spleen deficiency.
  - Dark circles around eyes indicates Kidney deficiency.
  - Brown color around eyes indicates steroid poisoning.
  - Sunken eyes indicates moderate dehydration (early, mild dehydration manifested by dry lips and mouth). Western medicine assesses sunken eyes as a sign of approximately 5–7% dehydration.

- *Pupil*
  - Normal pupils are round, equal, and reactive to light.
  - Abnormally dilated/constricted pupils indicates Kidney Qi deficiency, coma, drug toxicity—sympathetic stimulant drug overdose causes pupil dilation; parasympathetic stimulant drug overdose causes pupil constriction.

Nose

- *Normal nasal membrane* is moist, intranasal fluid is clear.
- *Nasal discharge*
  - Clear nasal discharge indicates possible Wind-Cold URI; allergies.
  - Thick white discharge indicates presence of Phlegm.
  - Yellow, thick discharge indicates presence of Damp Heat.
- *Nasal flaring* indicates respiratory distress from Lung deficiency or Lung Heat.
- *Nosebleed* indicates Lung Heat if accompanied by URI symptoms; Stomach Heat if it occurs after eating, especially after eating greasy, fatty, and/or spicy, hot foods.

Mouth

- *Normal mucous membrane* in children is pink to light red.
- *Red, swollen throat/tonsils* are due to Wind-Heat with Heat toxins, Yin deficiency, or Stomach Heat.
- *Red, swollen gums* with erosion indicate Stomach Heat.
- *Deep red lips* are from internal Heat.
- *Canker sores* indicate Spleen Damp Heat.
- *Sores on tongue* indicate Heart and Spleen Heat.
- *Patchy white covering with red satellite lesions* is oral thrush, due to Damp Heat, is usually associated with Spleen deficiency.
- *Dental caries* is the result of Stomach Fire and/or Spleen Damp Heat.
- *Delayed growth of teeth* is indicative of Kidney Qi deficiency.
- *Dribbling at the mouth* suggests internal Dampness.
- *Mouth hangs open* is indicative of extreme Qi deficiency, often associated with mental deficiency.
- *Pale lips* are signs of Cold from deficiency.

Ears

A very helpful pediatric instrument in Western medicine is the otoscope, which now can be purchased by anyone, including parents who wish to examine their children's ears. *Normal* tympanic membrane, the ear drum, is pearly grayish white with a light reflex.

Otitis externa is inflammation in the external ear canal distal to the ear drum. The otoscopic examination would show normal eardrum with redness in the canal, sometimes accompanied by white or purulent discharge. Western treatment is instillation of antibiotic ear drops. Chinese medicine distinguishes white discharge as due to Spleen deficiency, and purulent discharge as due to Wind-Heat invasions.

Otitis media is inflammation in the middle ear. There are two types in Western medicine: acute serous otitis media (ASOM) is fluid in the middle ear and acute otitis media (AOM) is infection in the middle ear. In serous otitis, the otoscopic examination would reveal a dull tympanic membrane with fluid behind the ear drum. In AOM, the ear drum is red, inflamed, and sometimes can be bulging. When the ear drum ruptures, there can be purulent discharge from the middle ear into the external canal. Recurrent AOMs with incomplete resolution can lead to chronic build-up of fluid in the middle ear as chronic serous otitis media. Chinese medicine would designate serous otitis as due to Spleen Qi deficiency, and purulent discharge is from Damp Heat specifically localized in the Gallbladder, Triple Energizer and Small Intestine channels. The three ear points in front of the tragus: GB-2, TE-21 and SI-19 are usually tender, and often would have a red discoloration.

Low-set, small ears are a sign for a poor constitution or Kidney Jing deficiency; this is compatible with Western pediatrics associating low-set ears with congenital anomalities, especially kidney abnormalities, and with mental retardation.

Posterior auricular adenitis (swollen glands) indicates Wind-Heat toxins invading the Shao Yang channel.

Two Yins

The two Yins refer in the male to the urethra and anus; in the female, to the vagina with the urethra and anus. The anterior Yin being the urethra, urethra with vagina; and the posterior Yin, the anus.

- In girls, red and moist external genitalia is a sign for Lower Energizer Damp Heat.
- In boys, a flaccid scrotum indicates Kidney Qi deficiency, and inguinal hernia is due to Spleen Qi deficiency, when Spleen cannot hold organs in place.
- *Yellow skin* in genital area indicates Dampness.
- *Anal itch* is indicative of pinworms.
- *Diaper rash* is due to *Monilia*, which is Damp Heat; recurrent diaper rash in spite of careful hygiene indicates Damp Heat in the Liver channel.
- *Anus sore and irritated* is due to Heat in Intestines.

Skin: Rashes and Eruptions

- *Erythematous, maculopapular rash* usually is viral exanthema, measles, rubella, or scarlet fever.
- *Vesicular rash* is varicella, i.e., chickenpox.
- *Hives* are due to Blood Heat.
- *Hemorrhagic rash* is indicative of severe Blood Heat that has turned to Fire; it is seen in terminal stages of Wind-Heat invasion.

Urine

- *Normal* urine in children is pale, clear, light yellow.
- *Cloudy, yellow* urine with clinical presentation of increased frequency and dysuria indicate cystitis or Damp Heat in the bladder.
- *Grossly bloody urine* can be associated with trauma to the urethra, and the possibility of foreign objects.

Stools

- *Newborn and breast-fed babies* normally have frequent, yellow, stools that are not too dry or too wet.
- *Constipation* is due to Heat in Yang Ming or Yin deficiency due to Heat depleting fluid.
- *Loose stools* is indicative of food stagnation, Spleen Qi deficiency.
- *Blood, mucus* in stools is Damp Heat and Fire in Intestines; the amount of blood is proportionate to the Heat, so that more profuse bleeding indicates an increasing amount of Heat.
- *Pus* indicates Damp Heat.
- *Dark stools*, melena, indicates bleeding from higher up in the Intestine, may be due to ulcers, gastritis, or Small Intestine obstruction; currant-jelly stool indicates intussusception.

Special Inspection: Vessel of Three Bars at the Tiger's Mouth

Since the Tang Dynasty, Chinese pediatricians have inspected the vein at the base of the side of the palmar surface of the index finger in children under age 3, mostly under age 2 years, to determine severity of illness. *Hu kou san guan zhi mai* means "vessel of the three bars at the tiger's mouth." It is located between the thumb and index finger when both are fully extended. The three bars are the three joints of the index finger. Look for any visible vein.

- *Wind bar* is at the metacarpophalangeal (MCP) joint.
- *Qi bar* is at the proximal interphalangeal (PIP) joint.
- *Life bar* is at the distal interphalangeal (DIP) joint.

Traditionally, examine the left hand on boys and right hand on girls. Currently in China, the right hand can be examined for both boys and girls, because left also means pre-Heaven, and right means post-Heaven.

Look at the depth, color, size, and location, for indications of Heat, Cold, deficiency, excess, progression, and seriousness. Moistening the palmar surface of the finger and hyperextending the finger would make the vein more visible.

- *Depth*
  - Normal depth is dimly visible.
  - Superficial is close to the surface of the skin, easily seen; indicates less serious, exterior condition.
  - Deep is deeper under the skin, less distinct; indicates more serious, interior condition.
- *Color*
  - Pale or pale red indicates Qi and Blood deficiency or internal Cold.
  - Red indicates Heat.
  - Dark red indicates Heat congestion.
  - Bluish-purple indicates spasm, pain, Blood stasis.
- *Size*
  - Broad suggests excess condition.
  - Narrow suggests deficient condition.
- *Location*
  - *Wind bar* is often seen in healthy children, or in children with a mild condition.

- Prominent indicates exterior invasion, but is not severe.
- Engorged indicates food stagnation.
- Red indicates Heat.
- *Qi bar* indicates more serious channel invasion. The child may present with high fever, no appetite, fatigue, somnolence, or diarrhea. Look for accompanying symptoms in specific channels.
- *Life bar* indicates more serious visceral involvement, it may be life threatening with very high fever, delirium, or convulsions. Look for other accompanying symptoms that would point to specific visceral involvement.
  - Redness indicates presence of pathologic Heat.
  - Purpleish red is presence of toxins, Blood stasis.
  - Wet, weepy lesions indicates Dampness.
  - Pus indicates presence of Damp Heat toxins.
  - Paleness indicates severe deficiency, Cold, even shock.

Listening

The child's strength of voice and characteristics of cough are often indicative of internal imbalances.

Voice

- *Strong voice* is suggestive of excess condition.
- *Weak voice* is suggestive of deficiency, especially of Lung Qi which controls the strength of the voice.
- *Low pitched voice* is indicative of Kidney deficiency, as Kidney Essence controls timbre.
- *Hoarse or raspy voice* indicates Wind-Heat invasion or dryness from Yin deficiency.
- *Loss of voice* may be due to invasion by external pathogens or due to dryness from Yin deficiency.

Speech

- *Normal* speech development depends on healthy Kidney and Spleen Qi.
- *Articulate* speech reflects strength of Heart Qi.
- *Delayed speech development* indicates Kidney or Spleen deficiency.
- *Incessant talking* that is intelligible indicates excess condition of the Heart, such as Heat affecting the Heart.
- *Incoherent speech* as in delirium indicates chaos and confusion of Shen.

Cough

- *Strong cough* is excess; *weak* is deficiency.
- *Wet, gurgling cough*, or *wheezy cough* indicate presence of Phlegm due to Spleen deficiency.
- *Dry cough* indicates Yin deficiency resulting in insufficient Lung fluid.

Smell

- *Food stagnation* in the Stomach from poor digestion can cause burping and breath that smells like rotten eggs.
- *Foul smelling stools and urine* are from Damp Heat, which correspond to the Western diagnosis of bacterial infection.
- *Odorless stools and urine* are due to Spleen deficiency.
- *Copious urine* without smell is due to Kidney Yang deficiency.

Palpation

Palpation is done at both the superficial and the deep level.

Superficial Palpation

Superficial palpation consists of simply feeling the skin of the child for subtle temperature differences.

Triple Energizers

Gently touch with the back of the hand on the master points of the Triple Energizer—CV-17, CV-12, and CV-6. The subtle temperature differences can reveal relative imbalances in the three areas of the body. For example, when CV-17 feels much warmer than the other two points, the Upper Energizer, and hence the corresponding organs of Heart and Lungs (usually Lungs in children), have either Heat or an excess condition.

Abdomen

The abdomen is a microsystem reflecting the Five Elements arranged in a clockwise direction (with the child as the clock). The Heart/Fire is placed at the 12 o'clock position (below the sternum), and the other four Yin organs arranged as in a Five-Element diagram around the umbilicus. Any area that feels cooler or warmer relative to the other areas may indicate Coldness/deficiency or Heat/excess in the corresponding organs. For example, if the child's left lower abdomen, about 4–5 o'clock position, which corresponds to Lung/Metal, feels cooler than other areas of the abdomen, this may suggest Lung deficiency.

Back

In older children, temperature variations may be felt in individual back *Shu* points that suggest pathology in corresponding organs. In younger children, general areas of palpation similar to the Triple Energizer palpation may suggest an imbalance in the corresponding Energizer. For example, a cool feeling of the middle back which has back *Shu* points to the Middle Energizer organs may suggest deficiency in the digestive organs.

Palms and Soles

- Colder than rest of body indicates deficiency, frequently Kidney Qi deficiency.
- Warmer than rest of body indicates excess Heat or Yin deficiency.

Skin Overall Feeling

- Cold with sweating indicates insufficient Qi or Yang.
- Hot without sweating indicates fever in superficial excessive patterns.
- Children's skin should feel smooth; areas of "lumps" indicate Qi stagnation or Phlegm accumulation.

Fontanelles

Babies' fontanelles should feel soft. The posterior fontanelle usually closes at 2–3 months of age, and the anterior fontanelle closes between 12 and 18 months of age. Delayed closure may reflect Kidney Essence deficiency, as Essence influences growth and development. In Western medicine, a bulging fontanelle may indicate increased intracranial pressure as in meningitis, which is Damp Heat of the brain. A sunken fontanelle may be associated with dehydration, which correlates to Yin (fluid) deficiency or Yang excess.

Firm, Deep Palpation

Ear Points for Otitis Media

Palpation of the three ear points in front of the tragus: GB-1, TE-21 and SI-19 for tenderness in older children can indicate presence of Wind-Heat or residual pathogenic influence.

Glands (Lymph Nodes)

Children usually have palpable glands in the cervical, postauricular areas because of frequent URI, sore throat, and ear infections.

Nontender nodes indicate lingering pathogens. The shoddy, "benign" nodes dismissed by Western pediatric examination is interpreted in Chinese medicine as sites where the energetic residual of previous infection/inflammation is still present so that the gland is more vulnerable to become infected again. Nontender nodes are also considered to be sites of Phlegm accumulation where Qi flow is sluggish, and are often found in chronic illnesses.

Red, swollen, tender glands indicates presence of Heat or toxin.

Abdomen

Abdominal pain or tenderness relieved with palpation indicates Cold or deficiency. Abdominal pain or tenderness aggravated with palpation indicates excess.

Muscle Tone

Normal tone is difficult to assess, especially in young children. Low muscle tone in the extremities may indicate overall Qi deficiency, more specifically Spleen Qi deficiency. This may manifest as inability to bear weight for an extended period of time. However, in children between 3 and 5 months of age, there is normal flexion of the knees without bearing as the child progresses from primitive reflexive leg straightening, which should disappear by 3 months of age, to the normal development of pulling to stand up.

Increased muscle tone, hypertonia, is indicative of Liver Yin deficiency. In children under age 1, this can be manifested subtly as curling of toes upon placing the child in the standing position.

Weak muscles in the lower back is suggestive of Kidney deficiency. This may be done by palpation, or by placing the child on the side, with the legs extended, pulling the legs toward the back (dorsiflexion). Usually this is difficult or even impossible. Excessive "folding" of the lower back indicates weak trunk muscles.

Pulse

Pulse-taking can be done in children over 3 years of age (the vein on the finger is examined prior to age 3). In young children or small children, the three positions of the pulse may be too close together to be palpated by individual fingers, so that the examiner can use the thumb to get an overall impression of all three positions. In older children, it is often possible for the examiner to place fingers close together for three-finger palpation.

Generally, a much more simplified pulse-taking is used in children: pulses are classified as strong or weak, fast or slow, superficial or deep, regular or irregular. Strong pulses are seen in excess conditions when Blood and Qi are strong; weak pulses in deficient conditions when Blood and Qi are weak; fast pulses in Heat, slow in Cold conditions; superficial pulse in exterior conditions whereas a deep pulse signifies penetration into the interior.

- Strong/weak: Blood and Qi states
- Fast/slow: Heat/Cold
- Superficial/deep: exterior/interior conditions.

The pulse rate in children is faster than adults and varies with age as follows:

- Newborn   120–140 beats/minute
- 1 year old   110–120
- 4 years old   110
- 8 years old   90
- 14 years old   75–80.[3]

Heart rate varies with respiration:

- Normal is 7 beats/respiration in 3–5 year old
- Presence of Heat is 8–9 beats/respiration
- Presence of Cold is 4–5 beats/respiration.

The rhythm varies physiologically with respiration: increases during inspiration and decreases with expiration. Irregularity in the rhythm, such as skipping beats, indicates a cardiac disorder. In Chinese medicine, since the Pericardium channel correlates to the sympathetic nervous system that regulates heart rate, the irregular rhythm may point to a disturbance of the Pericardium as well. In this situation, it would be best for the child to have an electrocardiogram with a rhythm strip to see what type of a heart rate irregularity it is. The physical findings in children are summarized in Tables 6.1 and 6.2.

DIAGNOSIS: FORMULATION OF IMPRESSION

Formulation of an impression or diagnosis combines information obtained from the history and evaluation—keeping in mind the basic physiology and pathophysiology of children, and the developmental phase of the patient. The diagnosis consists of two parts: assessing the general state of the child, and assessing specific organ imbalance. (Specific treatment guidelines are provided in Chapter 10.)

GENERAL IMPRESSION

General Yin/Yang State

First form an impression if the child is in an overall state of excess Yang/Yin deficiency or excess Yin/Yang deficiency (see Table 6.3).

Acute versus Chronic

Next, determine if the child has an acute or a chronic condition. Approximately 80–90% of afflictions in children—the bread and butter of pediatrics—consist of acute illnesses.

Acute Illnesses in Children

External Pathogens: Wind, Cold, Heat

The majority of acute illnesses in children consists of viral and bacterial infections. Western medicine assesses the extent of involvement based on history, physical findings and laboratory data. The Chinese call these "invasion by Wind-Cold and Wind-Heat pathogens."

Wind, Cold, and Heat are the three major external pathogens. Each has distinct individual characteristics; when combined as Wind-Cold and Wind-Heat, the pathogens have definitive patterns of invasion.

Wind

Wind is a Yang pathogen. It has a tendency to injure Blood and Yin. Children with Liver imbalance or in the Wood phase of development are especially sensitive to Wind. In general, Wind does not act alone in causing an acute illness. It is the vehicle that carries the Cold or Heat pathogen into the body, resulting in Wind-Cold and Wind-Heat illnesses.

TABLE 6.1 Physical findings in children

Physical findings	Cold	Heat	Damp	Phlegm
Facial complexion Normal = pink, lustrous, shiny; one cheek red = teething	Pale Qing (light, venous green) with parts of face white	Red Always red = food stagnation; undigested food → Heat Deep red with white forehead = LU deficiency → Heat Deep red with green/yellow around mouth = LR Yang rising	Yellow; white & puffy Red cheeks in p.m. = Damp Heat Bright yellow = Damp Heat Dull yellow = Damp Cold	
Eyes—spirit Normal = clear, shining		Red = Wind-Heat; internal Heat Photophobia + watery = womb-Heat	Watery discharge	Gluey discharge
Between eyes		Red = localized internal Heat +/- convulsions	Green, greenish/blue	
Sclera		Blue = Liver Heat	Yellow	
Mouth		Red = HT, SP Heat Red gum = ST Heat	Excess saliva	
Lips	Pale	Deep red = internal Heat		
Throat		Red = Wind-Heat		
Tongue—normal = light red, wet	Pale	WH slight red side +/- front, red points = greater int. Red dots = patho. Minister Fire, organ distribution	Swollen	
Coating—unreliable			"Thicker" coating	"Thick" greasy
Ears			Purulent discharge = Damp Heat	Thick discharge
Hearing			Decreased	Decreased
Nose			Nasal discharge	
Two Yins		Red anus = intestinal Heat	Yellow genital skin = Damp, Damp Heat Recurrent diaper rash = LR Damp Heat	Recurrent
Urethra, anus				Monilia

TABLE 6.1	Physical findings in children (contd.)				
Physical findings	**Cold**	**Heat**	**Damp**	**Phlegm**	
Finger veins < age 3 Superficial = acute, exterior Deep = chronic, interior	Pale red	Dark red, purple Black = Heat congestion		Black = food stagnation	
Pulse > age 3	Slow, superficial	Fast, superficial		Slippery	
Voice Strong = excess Weak = deficiency		Hoarse = Wind-Heat Loss of voice = external ST		Gurgling	
Speech		Incessant = HT Heat Incoherent babbling-Heat nutritive level	Poor grammar, forgets words, late speech development = Phlegm clouding Heart Excess saliva = Dampness		
Breathing			Gurgling = bronchial Phlegm Sniffling, snoring = nasal Phlegm		
Smell	Copious urine without smell = Cold SP/KI def.	Bad like eggs = ST Heat	Foul smelling stools = Damp Heat Foul urine = Damp Heat	Burping gas = food injury; stagnation Sour = food injury	
Rashes	Itching = Wind; Blood/Qi stagnation	Red; purple = Blood Heat	Raised; watery fluid		
Stool—normal babies = yellow/soft	Green = Wind-Cold	Dry = excess Heat Watery, foul smelling = Damp Heat (infectious)			
Urine		Dark, painful, bloody = Damp Heat Dark yellow = Damp Heat rising (jaundice)			

TABLE 6.2 *Acupuncture physical findings in children*

Physical findings	Yang excess	Qi deficiency	Yin deficiency	Accumulation/stagnation
Facial complexion	LR Yang excess = green/yellow around mouth	Pale Dull yellow = SP Qi deficiency Deep red with white forehead = LU Qi deficiency Qing—cyanotic lips with respiratory difficulty = LU Qi obstruction	Red cheeks in p.m.	
Eyes		Puffy below eyes = KI, SP deficiency Dark circles = KI deficiency	Dark circles + red cheeks Dry = LR Yin deficiency Pale eyelid = Blood deficiency	Brown around eyes = steroid toxicity
Sclera		Whites of eye visible during sleep = SP Qi deficiency		
Mouth		Mouth hangs open = extreme Qi deficiency often seen with MR	Red = floating Heat	
Lips				Lower lip protrudes
Throat			Red	
Tongue	"Yin deficient"	Cracks in corresponding areas	Red; antibiotics = ST Yin Xu = coating falls off, thinner, partially peeled Geographic = constitutional ST Yin Xu	
Ears			Low set, small = KI Jing deficiency	
Finger veins	Dark	Pale		
Pulse > age 3	Fast, strong	Slow, weak, deep (irregular = Qi stagnation) Low pitch = KI deficiency (Jing controls timbre) Weak voice = LU deficiency (LU controls strength)	Fast, weak, deep	
Voice			Loss of voice	
Stool	Mucoid = ST stagnation	Green = SP injury from overeating Thin, watery = SP deficiency Currant-jelly stool = SP deficiency, intussusception (prolapse)	Dry	Irregular, foul smelling
Urine		Turbid = SP deficiency		

TABLE 6.3	Yin/Yang states	
Excess Yang = Yin deficiency	**Excess Yin = Yang deficiency**
Dryness: dry skin, throat, mouth	Moist skin; edema
Thirsty	Not thirsty
Constipation	Loose stools
Decreased urine	Copious urine, enuresis
Dry cough or thick sputum	Moist cough, watery sputum
Hypermetabolic symptoms:	Hypometabolic symptoms:
– fast heart rate, nervousness;	– slowness, tendency toward weight gain
– tendency toward weight loss	
Red complexion, red tongue	Pale complexion
Red cheeks, red eyes, sores in mouth	
Nosebleeds	
Feels hot, dislikes heat, likes cold	Feels cold, likes warmth, dislikes cold
Warm hands and feet; often sweaty; more spontaneous sweating	Cold hands and feet
Backache	
Heaviness or pain in the head	Heaviness—lower part of body
Red rashes, hives	Pale rashes
Mentally more agitated, impatient	Mentally sluggish
Insomnia, irritable, excess thoughts	
Menstrual disorders in teenage girls	Overall: fatigue, slow growth
Overall Heat symptoms: easily excitable, loud	Slow movement; not excitable
Pulse is strong, superficial	Pulse is weak, deep
Underweight	Overweight

Wind characteristically causes illnesses to come on quickly and change rapidly. In Nature, Wind has the most effect on the top of the tree, is roughest on the younger trees with slender trunks, and can make the thin branches sway this way and that. In the child, Wind similarly tends to affect the top part of the body first by causing headaches and upper respiratory tract symptoms. It enters the body via the skin and therefore interferes with Wei Qi circulation. It is therefore more detrimental to the infant and younger child who have immature Wei Qi. Since one of the Wei Qi functions is warming the skin, Wind invasion results in aversion to cold, chills, and myalgia. In advanced stages, when the Wind becomes internal, it can cause stiffness or flailing of the extremities; the tonic–clonic movements of the arms and legs as in a convulsion.

Cold

Cold is a Yin pathogen and tends to injure Yang. Cold in Nature causes contractions. It has the same effect on children: causing Qi channels and Blood vessels to constrict, resulting in decreased Qi and Blood circulation. When confronted by Cold, the body physiologically contracts the more exposed, external Qi and Blood channels, in order to preserve these treasures for the more internal structures. Unfortunately, this means contraction of pores and circulation of Wei Qi. As Chapter 4 points out, the child's skin is tender and Wei Qi is weak, Cold invasion therefore immediately compromises the child's first immune defense against external pathogens and the child is unable to sweat. Usually accompanied by Wind, Cold quickly enters the internal channels and penetrates the muscle and organs, the most vulnerable ones being the Lungs, the Stomach and the Spleen. Cold can manifest as severe headache, aversion to cold, myalgia, upper respiratory tract infection with cough, watery nasal discharge; abdominal pain, vomiting, and diarrhea. Because of children's delicate balance between Yin and Yang, this Cold can quickly transform into Heat. Cold induces shivering, which Western medicine explains as the physiologic response that raises body metabolism and therefore raises the body temperature, the Yang. The increased Yang can in turn quickly dry up the Fluid, the Yin, resulting in further elevation of body temperature manifesting as fever.

Heat

Heat is Yang and injures Yin, which is already deficient in children. Heat is a more harmful pathogen than Cold because it can quickly dry up fluid and manifest as high fever. As optimal cellular metabolism operates within a narrow range of body temperature, higher temperature can rapidly damage tissues and organs versus the less detrimental decreased delivery of Qi and Blood in Cold invasion. Heat usually rises and therefore can prevent Qi descension, resulting in diminished Qi circulation to the important digestive and Kidney functions. Heat usually couples with Wind and can spread quickly through the body.

Wind-Cold and Wind-Heat Pathogens

Wind-Cold and Wind-Heat pathogens correlate well to the Western concepts of viral and bacterial infections. Chinese medicine delineates specific patterns of invasion of these pathogens into the channels and organs. A simple metaphor that compares the pathogenic attack to a burglary has become a favorite tale of many teachers of Chinese medicine. The image of a child struggling with a burglar helps students to understand and remember not only the signs and symptoms at each level of illness, but also treatment rationale and principles.

The characteristic Wind-Cold invasion occurs in Six Stages, while the Wind-Heat pattern follows a more aggressive Four Level progression.

Wind-Cold Invasion: the Six Stage System

This is based on the classical text, *Shang Han Lun* (*Treatise on Febrile Diseases Caused by Cold*), written in approximately 200 AD. Wind-Cold invasions correlate to Western diagnosis of viral infections, the most common infections in childhood. They are less virulent, and advance relatively slower than bacterial infections. The initial clinical picture is usually mild. However, if the infection is unresolved in early stages, it can become complicated with secondary bacterial infection in the later stages.

The Six Stage System describes the Wind-Cold pathogen as it progressively invades the body from the most superficial Yang channels and organs to the deepest Yin channels and organs. At each stage, the child's Qi struggles with the external pathogen, the burglar. The health of the child versus the virulence of the pathogen determines the channels and organs invaded and the degree of excess or deficiency symptoms.

The Six Stages are as follows:

1. Tai Yang: Bladder, Small Intestine (only exterior level)
2. Shao Yang: Triple Energizer, Gallbladder
3. Yang Ming: Large Intestine, Stomach

4.   Tai Yin: Lung, Spleen
5.   Shao Yin: Heart, Kidneys
6.   Jue Yin: Pericardium, Liver.

In the three Yang stages the burglar or Wind-Cold invasion affects the more superficial, less important Yang organs and channels. The body's Qi is still relatively strong in the presence of the pathogenic factor, i.e., the child still has a lot of options to ward off the burglar. The signs are excess—which correlates with the struggle at the various stages: turning on the radio loudly, slamming doors, etc. The ultimate goal is to eliminate the pathogen, to chase out the burglar.

In the three Yin stages, the body's Qi and defense have markedly weakened and the pathogenic factor has invaded further into the body, affecting the more important Yin organs and channels. The signs are now of interior deficiency and interior Cold. Deficiency is the result of the expenditure of a great deal of energy fighting in the first three Yang stages. Cold is the result of depletion of Qi, but can quickly transform into Heat.

The Tai Yin level is the last effort to eliminate the pathogen. At the Shao Yin level, the child is too weak and the pathogen is too far into the interior to be chased out. Rigorous treatment—integrating both Western and Chinese medical treatment—would be needed to "kill the burglar," to bring the child out of danger, repair damage, and restore health and balance.

Tai Yang Stage

This is the only superficial, exterior level of the body, and corresponds to the initial attack by external Cold—the burglar is still outside the house. The child's symptoms manifest aversion to the presence of the pathogen—such as the smell of the burglar, dislike of Wind and Cold, shivering, or headaches. The signs are excesses, as the child is still relatively healthy and struggles with the pathogen: running around, closing windows and doors, general myalgia, occipital neck pain, low back pain, shortness of breath, and may begin to show some heat signs such as sweating and low grade fever (Figure 6.1).

The Tai Yang channels are rich in defensive Wei Qi, which circulates between skin and muscles, controls the opening and closing of pores, and protects the body from invasion by external pathogens. The pathophysiology of Wind-Cold is the contraction of the pores of the skin and of the Tai Yang channels, thus decreasing the circulation of Wei Qi. Cold symptoms permeate the Bladder and Small Intestine channels, resulting in headache, neck and back pain. The child shivers, which is the body's response to Cold by increasing metabolic rate. This may slightly raise the body temperature, manifesting as a low grade fever with some sweating. The conflicting clinical picture of a child complaining of being cold, yet runs a fever and sweats is explained by Chinese medicine as the manifestation of weak Wei Qi in children: the skin is not warmed and the pores are not controlled, resulting in flaccid pores that allow sweat to come out (Figure 6.2).

This stage correlates to Western diagnoses of the common cold, mild viral infections, and localized bladder infection. Mild viral meningitis can present with stiff neck and low grade temperature, but the child does not appear very ill and the blood and spinal fluid cultures are negative. The Western treatment consists of symptomatic treatment, such as decongestants and antipyretics, and letting the illness "run its course." At this time, there are no specific treatments for viral infections. Bladder infection is usually treated with a course of antibi-

FIGURE 6.1   *Tai Yang stage of Wind-Cold invasion or Wei Qi level of Wind-Heat invasion. The burglar has one foot in the door, the window is open, and the child smells and sees the burglar.*

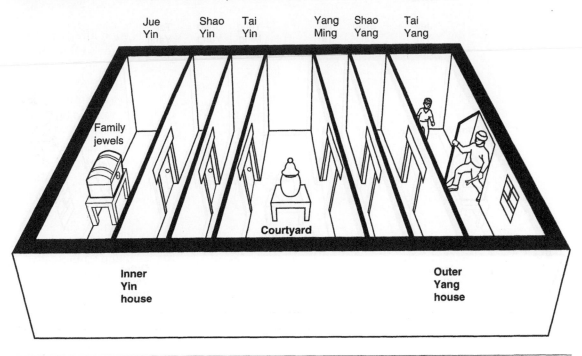

FIGURE 6.2   *Scenario 1: The child kills the burglar and now has to deal with the body and smell.*

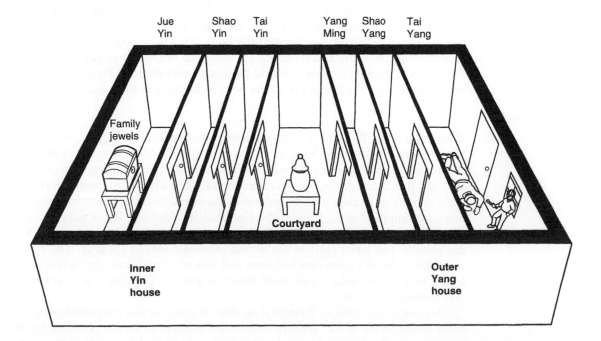

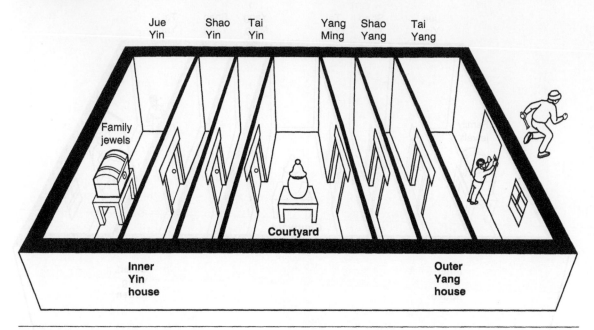

FIGURE 6.3   *Scenario 2: Strengthening Wei Qi. The child scares away the burglar and locks and bolts the windows and doors.*

otics, preferably with one that localizes in the bladder and has minimal systemic effect.

The Chinese treatment is to keep out the pathogen by tonifying Wei Qi, to scare away the burglar and lock the door (Figure 6.3). It would also be import-ant to tonify any other weaknesses, such as Lung or Spleen deficiency, that the child may have so that in the event the pathogen passes through the Wei Qi bar-rier, it cannot penetrate further into the body. This is comparable to taking an inventory of the house and repairing any doors to bedrooms or storing the fam-ily jewels in the safe so that it would be much more difficult for the burglar to enter further into the house even if he were to break into the house.

Shao Yang Stage

When the child's Wei Qi is not strong enough to expel the pathogen, Wind-Cold would enter into the next Yang level. Shao Yang is the beginning of the inside of the body—the hallway of the house. Cold symptoms persist along with progres-sion of Heat transformations, manifesting as chills alternating with fever. The child complains of pain and tenderness in the costal and hypochondriac regions due to disruption of Qi flow in the Gallbladder channel. There may be Shao Yang Heat symptoms appearing in the eyes and mouth as blurred vision and dry mouth. The bitter taste in the mouth induces a loss of appetite. The child's usual lively facial expression becomes dull due to diminished circulation of Qi to the facial Gallbladder and Small Intestine points. The child has less energy and becomes irritable.

This stage correlates to Western diagnoses of otitis media, mononucleosis, and more severe forms of flu. Western treatment continues to be symptomatic for flu symptoms and mononucleosis. Antibiotics are indicated for acute otitis media

(AOM). Chinese treatment consists of dispersing Cold and Heat, expelling the pathogen from Shao Yang through Tai Yang to the exterior, followed by tonification of Wei Qi. Contrary to tonification of Wei Qi as the initial treatment in the Tai Yang level, doing so in the Shao Yang level would be "trapping" the burglar. It is only after the pathogen is expelled—the burglar is chased out—should the immune system be strengthened—bolt the doors and close the windows.

The different philosophical approach to infection is illustrated by the contrasting approaches to the treatment of AOM. While some AOM are caused by bacteria, many are viral in origin. However, Western physical examination using the otoscope cannot distinguish between the two, as both manifest with red ear drums. Because of concern of possible complications with untreated bacterial AOM, such as the progression to mastoiditis and even meningitis, the current practice is to treat all AOM with antibiotics. From the Chinese medicine perspective, treatment with antibiotics is like killing the burglar inside the house: there will be lingering pathogenic, energetic effects from the dead bacteria (lingering smell of the dead body, or nightmares of killing the burglar). This may explain the development of chronic serous otitis media that persist for months or even years after recurrent AOMs.

Yang Ming Stage

The Wind-Cold has now penetrated into the Yang Ming level. Whereas the previous two stages were characterized by the pathogen affecting primarily the channels—the burglar is in the hallway—this stage signals the beginning of pathogenic invasion of the organs, the Stomach and Large Intestine—the house proper, the living room (Figure 6.4).

The Heat from the Shao Yang stage quickly dries up the Yin, which is already physiologically deficient in children. Fever becomes markedly elevated, accompanied by other pronounced Heat symptoms: very dry mouth, profuse sweating, thirst, a preference for cold drinks, red face, irritability, and restlessness. Temperature can now enter the 104–105°F (40–40.5°C) range, and the child may become delirious, which Western medicine explains as the inability of the cells of the central nervous system to function in the presence of high temperature. Chinese medicine explains this as the loss of Fluid affecting everything, including the marrow, i.e. the brain. The Yin deficiency fever is present throughout the day, but characteristically peaks at a higher temperature in the afternoon. Heat in the Stomach and Liver channels show up as red face and restlessness, and irritability. The interior Heat pushes body fluid outward as sweat. The biochemical explanation is that Heat imparts energy to the molecules of the Fluid, so that there is more Fluid movement through open pores. If sweating is profuse, temperature may temporarily decrease as sweating dissipates Heat, giving the false impression that the child is getting better. The pulse would reflect the continuing presence of Heat: strong and superficial, a Yang pulse.

These signs are often referred to as the "four bigs": big fever, big thirst, big sweating, big pulse. The priority here is to clear the Heat from the channels in order to prevent further weakening of the body.

When Heat enters the Yang Ming organs, the Stomach and Large Intestine will develop Fluid and Yin deficiency. Heat in the Stomach causes the child to have little or no appetite. The tongue and throat are red. Heat in the Large

FIGURE 6.4 *Yang Ming: the burglar is in the living room, the "outer" Yang part of the house.*

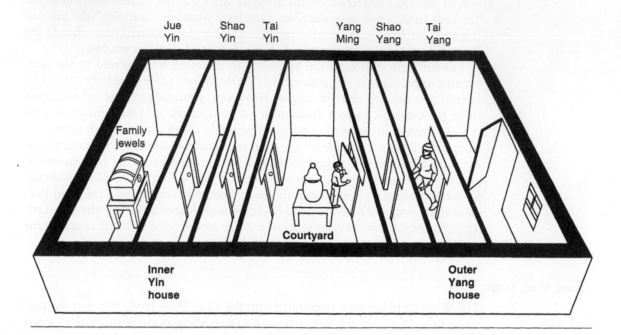

Intestine results in dry, constipated stools, which in turn obstruct Qi flow in the abdomen, causing abdominal pain that becomes worse with pressure (Yang pain).

The Western diagnoses that correlate to this stage are otitis media, pharyngitis, adenitis, and further progression of flu to involve the gastrointestinal tract. Western treatment focuses on symptomatic lowering of fever with antipyretics and on prevention of dehydration. The child would be on antibiotics, as high fever generally signals the presence of bacterial infection. The priority in Chinese treatment is to vigorously clear the Heat, replenish fluids, and continue to try to expel the pathogen.

The struggle in the three Yang stages markedly weakens the child's Qi and defense system. If unsuccessful, the pathogenic factor can advance further into the more important Yin organs and channels, the "inner house." The excess signs and symptoms give way to those of Qi depletion, of interior Cold and deficiency. The Cold is unstable and can transform quickly into Heat when the child engages in any further struggle. A last effort can still be made to eliminate the pathogen in the Tai Yin level—the living room of the inner house. At the Shao Yin level, the child is too weak and the burglar is too far into the house to be chased through the courtyard and various rooms and hallway to the outside. There is now no other choice but to kill the burglar and rescue the child. Rigorous treatment—integrating both Western and Chinese medicine—would be needed if the child is to survive the pathogenic invasion.

After the child recovers from the illness—the burglar is no longer in the house, the child can then be tonified—build stronger doors, put in bolt locks—in order to be in a stronger position against the next invasion.

Tai Yin Stage

This is the beginning of the Yin channels and organs, the inner sanctuary of the child's body. The traditional Chinese house has a courtyard that separates the "outer" house from the "inner" house. The "outer" house is for visitors, and the "inner" house is the private living quarters that only family members and intimate friends are allowed to enter. A burglar in this part of the house is indicative of a weakened host, as the child begins to manifest interior Cold and deficiency symptoms in the Spleen and Lung. These are dramatically different from the four big Yang Ming symptoms.

A Cold and deficient Spleen cannot carry out transformation and transportation of food into Qi. There is now vomiting and diarrhea. The excess abdominal tenderness becomes a deficient fullness that is relieved by pressure. Cold quickly enters the Intestines where it interferes with the sorting of clear from turbid, and with absorption of fluid. The stools are watery and often contain undigested particles. The child appears lethargic, has no appetite, and no desire for fluids. The tongue is pale and moist, and the pulse is now deep and slow. Lung deficiency coupled with Spleen deficiency results in deep cough with clear or white phlegm.

Western diagnoses that correlate to this stage are persistent viral infections with possible beginning of secondary bacterial complications, such as bacterial gastroenteritis, bronchitis, or pneumonia. The treatment is symptomatic with cough suppressant, dietary and fluid management, and sometimes antidiarrheal medications in more severe cases. Physicians often prescribe antibiotics to prevent bacterial complications.

In Chinese medicine, this is the last stage in which the pathogen can be expelled. Treatment consists of vigorously dispelling Cold and warming the Middle Energizer, while continuing in the attempt to force the pathogen to leave the body and go to the exterior. This is difficult as the weakened child must expel the pathogen through many stages—chase the burglar out from the "inner" house through the courtyard, the various rooms and hallway of the "outer" house to the outside. This is especially difficult in a child weakened by previous infections—in a house weakened by previous "invasions" with cracks in the walls and broken doors. A treatment would be considered partially successful if it can at least warm up the interior enough—strengthen the child enough—to "chase" the "burglar" back to the more superficial Yang levels. The child remanifesting Shao Yang or Yang Ming symptoms is therefore improving.

Shao Yin Stage

The Wind-Cold pathogen has passed the first line of Yin defense and entered the next critical level to injure the Heart and Kidneys. The burglar is now deep into the "inner" house. The child at this stage is very feeble, and the illness can alternate between Shao Yin Cold or Heat symptoms (Figure 6.5).

The Cold symptoms continue with added Shao Yin symptoms due to Kidney Yang deficiency: the child complains of being cold, has chills, wants warm fluids and sleeps in a curled up, fetal position; the arms and legs are cold, and the diarrhea contains a lot of undigested food. Previous lethargy progresses to persistent drowsiness, listlessness and sleepiness. The cough continues as a weak cough. The increasing abdominal coldness manifests as more severe abdominal

FIGURE 6.5 *Shao Yin: the child is very weakened and the burglar is close to the family jewels.*

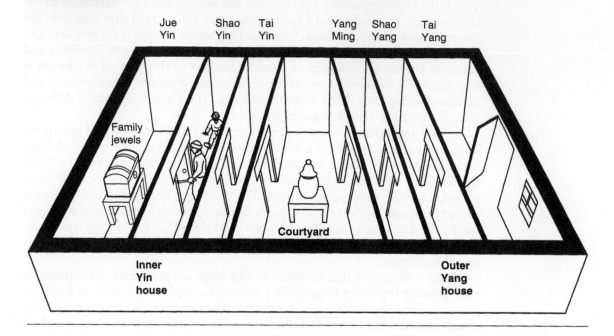

pain and discomfort. With Kidney Yang deficiency, the child urinates profuse, clear urine. The tongue is very pale, and the pulse is weak and deep.

As the child develops Yin deficiency in Shao Yin Kidney and Heart, Heat symptoms begin to manifest as high fever, dry mouth and throat; scanty, yellow urine. The disturbance of Shen is seen as irritability, and insomnia. The tongue is red to reflect both Heat and Yin deficiency; the pulse is weak but rapid.

This stage correlates to Western diagnoses of the presence of more serious infections. The viral illnesses have now developed secondary bacterial infections. The ear infection has developed complications, such as mastoiditis. An earlier bladder infection has now spread to the kidneys causing pyelonephritis. Stool cultures can be positive for *Salmonella* or *Shigella*. The blood culture is often positive for bacteria, indicating sepsis.

The best treatment at this stage would be integrating Western medicine with Chinese medicine. The child is now gravely ill, and the priority is to institute life-saving treatments. Potent intravenous antibiotics are indicated to quickly clear the bacterial infection—to "kill" the burglar and rescue the child. The child's vital signs of temperature, heart rate, respiratory rate, and blood pressure need to be closely monitored. An integrated approach, as that adopted by some hospitals in China, is to give antibiotics through one intravenous line and herbs through another line, and acupuncture treatment. The herbs and acupuncture clear Heat and Cold, tonify Yin, and sometimes also counteract the side-effects of antibiotics. Western technology would also be helpful for continual assessment of progress, such as monitoring white blood count, X-ray, blood culture, etc. After the child recovers, Chinese medicine would be best used to tonify the child, and to balance any side-effects induced by Western treatment, such as any lingering pathogenic effect from dead bacteria.

Jue Yin Stage

This is often called the Terminal Yin Stage, when the pathogen has clearly won the battle and the child is critically ill, fighting for his life. The burglar is within reach of the family jewels, and the child is too weak to protect them. The imbalance of Yin and Yang with involvement of Liver Heat and Yin results in greater swings between the extremes of Heat and Cold symptoms: Yang energy and Heat rise to the top leading to very high fever with very cold limbs (Yang energy is directed away from the limbs) and severe chills alternate with fever. The child clutches the chest because of an uncomfortable sensation of fullness and heat in the chest; or doubles over because of more severe abdominal pain. The diarrhea is very watery and may even be bloody. The child has persistent thirst and hunger with little or no desire to eat, and vomits frequently. The cough is weak with moderate to severe signs of respiratory distress, such as tachypnea, substernal and intercostal retractions. Liver Yin's vulnerability to Wind leads to the manifestation of internal wind as generalized, grand mal convulsions with tonic–clonic movements of all extremities. The pulse is thin and may be either fast or slow.

This stage correlates to the Western diagnoses of sepsis, meningitis, and encephalitis. Blood culture and cerebral spinal fluids are positive. This child should be in a pediatric intensive care unit on intravenous fluids, antibiotics, or seizure medications. The vital signs and blood oxygen levels are closely monitored. If the child cannot keep anything down orally, nutrition may need to be given through a hyperalimentation line. The child may need to be placed on a ventilator if there is progression of respiratory compromise. Chinese medicine can again assume a complementary role in using intravenous herbs and various other treatment modalities for dissipating Heat and Cold, and for counteracting the side-effects of medications. After the child recovers, Chinese medicine would be invaluable in restoring balance and tonifying the child to prevent similar episodes in the future.

Wind-Heat Invasion—the Four Level System

The Four Level System was developed in the seventeenth century for the evaluation of external Wind-Heat invasion, which correlates to the Western concept of a bacterial infection. The Four Level System follows the Wind-Heat pathogen as it progressively invades the body from the most superficial Wei Qi level to the deepest Blood level.

The Wind-Heat or bacterial pathogens are very contagious, and usually enter the body through the nose and mouth. They are airborne or are transmitted through food or sharing of utensils. Young children in nursery school and preschool easily contract these illnesses as they tend to put toys and other objects into their mouths. Heat can be intense so that there is often high fever with rapid depletion of Yin and fluids. Because of inherent Yin deficiency and immature organs, children are especially vulnerable to Wind-Heat invasion which can be very virulent and progress quickly from superficial to deeper levels.

The Four Levels are:

- Wei Qi
- Qi
- Nutritive Qi, Ying level
- Blood.

Wei Qi Level

This is the most superficial level of attack by Wind-Heat, and correlates to the Tai Yang and beginning Shao Yang Stages of Wind-Cold invasion.

Wind-Heat injury at this level disrupts all of the Wei Qi functions of warming and nourishing the skin, of controlling the opening and closing of pores, and of protecting the body from external pathogens. The child presents with moderately elevated fever that is higher during the day. From a biochemical standpoint, the fever is due to the release of bacterial toxins that stimulates an immune response, which in Chinese medicine would be viewed as a struggle between Wei Qi and the Wind-Heat pathogen. The child presents with a confusing clinical picture, as the fever is often accompanied by an aversion to cold with some shivering, due to the impairment of the warming function of Wei Qi. There is minimal or no sweating when the pores are not regulated. As Wei Qi is associated with Lung Qi, the child is often coughing. Heat symptoms include headache, a red sore throat with exudate, and thirst. The tongue has a slightly red tip, and the pulse is an excess pulse: superficial and fast.

This level of Wind-Heat disorder correlates to Western diagnoses of sinusitis, *Streptococcus* tonsillitis, otitis media, cystitis. The treatment is usually antipyretics for fever and a course of antibiotics for the infection. Chinese treatment consists of dispersing Heat and expelling the pathogen.

Qi Level

This level represents a further penetration of the Wind-Heat pathogen to the Shao Yang and Yang Ming channels and organs, and is beginning to involve the Tai Yin structures. The virulence of the pathogen—the strength of the burglar—is quickly evident as the invasion progresses rapidly from the most superficial Yang level to the beginning of Yin level in just two stages. The child may still have some resistance and tries to expel the pathogen. Fever can be markedly elevated as more toxins are released. Fever can alternate with Cold as Heat consumes Yin fluid. The child is irritable and uncomfortable from Heat.

The symptoms can be quite variable, depending on the location of the pathogen. The cough can progress further down the respiratory tract to the bronchi and even pulmonary tissues, resulting in bacterial bronchitis and pneumonia. The evidence of Heat in the lower respiratory tract is the production of thick, purulent Phlegm. The older child complains of fullness in the chest, even burning chest pain.

Heat in the Stomach gives the clinical picture of a Yang type of abdominal pain that worsens with pressure, accompanied by nausea, vomiting, dry throat, loss of appetite. Damp Heat in the Large Intestine can manifest as foul diarrhea with mucus. When Heat is severe and becomes Fire, there may be bloody stools. As Heat dries up fluid and as the body becomes dehydrated with diarrhea, the child then becomes constipated.

Shao Yang Heat in children usually manifests as symptoms along the Gallbladder channel instead of the organ. These include complaint of a bitter taste and pain in the hypochondriac region along the Gallbladder distribution, and earaches.

The Western diagnoses consist of bacterial bronchitis and pneumonia, bacterial gastroenteritis, or staphylococcal food poisoning. The treatment is antibiotics specific to the type of bacterial infection. Fever is treated with antipyretics and fluid replacement may require intravenous hydration.

Chinese medicine would vigorously dissipate Heat, replenish fluid, and continue in the fight to expel the pathogen.

Nutritive Qi Level

The Wind-Heat pathogen can quickly penetrate to the Nutritive Qi level. Nutritive Qi circulates in channels and blood vessels and throughout the organs. The Shao Yin channels and organs, the Heart and Kidneys, are now also involved, so that this level is similar to the Shao Yin Stage of Wind-Cold invasion. The overall Heat symptoms continue to an even more dramatic degree: the fever is much higher and follows the Yin pattern of being elevated in the afternoon and evenings; the mouth is very dry and throat feels "raw." Heat in the Heart manifests as disturbance of Shen: severe irritability, restlessness, insomnia, and even delirium. Heat in the blood vessels manifests as erythematous, maculopapular rashes. Kidney Yin deficiency manifests as decreased urine output.

The Western diagnoses and integrated treatment program would be those discussed for Wind-Cold invasion at the Shao Yin Stage.

Blood Level

This level marks the deepest penetration by the Wind-Heat pathogen, and correlates to the Jue Yin, or Terminal Yin, stage of illness. The child is gravely ill. The fever is markedly elevated. With near depletion of Yin fluid, Heat has transformed into Fire, manifesting as various forms of bleeding: hemorrhagic rash, bloody stools, hemoptysis, hematemesis, epistaxis. The extreme disturbance of Shen manifests as delirium or even coma. Liver Wind manifests as grand mal, tonic–clonic seizures.

The Western diagnoses include: sepsis; meningitis, especially the virulent meningococcal meningitis; encephalitis; severe opportunistic infections in immune compromised hosts such as leukemics. The child is in the pediatric intensive care unit fighting for his life. An integrated treatment program would again be the most beneficial.

The burglar metaphor clearly compares and contrasts the Western and Chinese medicine approaches. Western medicine begins by killing the burglar, whereas the Chinese advocates initially chasing the burglar away. Western medicine tends to treat symptoms—the various unpleasantness left by the burglar, Chinese medicine believes that it is necessary to get rid of the burglar from the outset. In later stages of illness, it is necessary to get out the "big gun"—the potent intravenous antibiotics—and kill the burglar. After the child survives the invasion, the much weakened child needs a great deal of tonification and strengthening in order to fully recover—the house needs a lot of repairing of broken windows and doors, holes in the walls. Since no Western medication tonifies the human system, Chinese medicine would be invaluable to strengthen and balance the child so that he would not be vulnerable to an attack by other "burglars."

Other External Pathogens

The Wind-Cold and Wind-Heat are the most common pathogens that cause illness in children. Three other external pathogens that may cause both external and internal diseases include Dampness, Dryness, and Fire.

Dampness

Dampness is a Yin pathogen and therefore usually injures Yang. Dampness may be acute or chronic. Acute exposure to Dampness, such as the child playing in the rain, sitting with a wet swimsuit on the wet poolside, usually results in rapid onset of general Damp symptomatology without any organ involvement. When exposure to Dampness is chronic, such as living in a damp basement, the child's interior contracts Dampness over time so that the Spleen and sometimes Kidney are affected. The course is more gradual with a thinner discharge than that in external Dampness. Since children are inherently Spleen deficient, and modern diet and lifestyle tend to injure the Spleen, children today are much more susceptible to Dampness (see Table 6.4).

Dampness is characteristically heavy, dirty, and sticky. The heaviness gives the sensation of "extra load" on the body, so that the child with Dampness complains of being tired. Dampness tends to settle in the Lower Energizer and lower part of the body, giving rise to a sensation of fullness in the abdomen and heaviness in the legs. It can flow upwards from the legs into the pelvic area, the Bladder, and the Intestines. When Dampness injures Spleen Yang, Spleen deficiency contributes to increasing Dampness. When Dampness prevents clear Yang from ascending to the head to brighten the sense orifices and clear the brain, there is hazy feeling of the head.

Dampness makes bodily fluids dirty and sticky, so that any Damp discharge is thick and unclear, more difficult to eliminate. When Dampness is combined with Heat, the condition correlates with Western concept of purulent discharges in bacterial infections: cloudy urine in bladder infection, purulent vaginal discharges, eczema with a secondary bacterial infection becomes impetigo that oozes thick, dirty fluid.

Dryness

Dryness is a Yang pathogen and therefore injures Blood and Yin. Dryness can be external or internal. External Dryness arises from the weather or environment, such as hot summer weather or excessive heating in the home and school during winter time that induces an artificial dry condition. Internal Dryness is due to Yin deficiency. Since children are inherently Yin deficient, they are very vulnerable to any drying conditions that can further deplete fluid. The two organs that are most vulnerable to Dryness in children are the Stomach and the Lung. Stomach needs fluid for its "rotting and ripening" of food. When children eat in a hurry, drink ice-cold drinks with meals, or do not drink an adequate amount of fluid with food, the Stomach can develop Yin deficiency. The clinical symptoms consist of dryness of lips, mouth, throat, and tongue.

TABLE 6.4	*External and internal Dampness*		
		External Dampness	**Internal Dampness**
	Onset	Acute, rapid	Gradual, chronic
	Characteristic body fluid	Heavy, dirty, sticky	Thinner than exterior
	Organ		Spleen deficiency, sometimes Kidney

The Lung in children is also vulnerable to Dryness. The respiratory tract needs a physiologic amount of fluid for lubrication. Chronic exposure to Dryness produces an irritative, dry, hacking cough. Since skin corresponds to the Lung, Dryness in the Lung can be reflected as dry, irritative skin.

Fire

Fire is an extreme form of interior Heat due to the transformation of any of the other external pathogens. Fire dries out Fluids much faster than Heat resulting in more severe Yin deficiency. Fire damages blood vessels and causes bleeding, ranging from mild epistaxis to more severe forms of internal bleeding, such as hemoptysis, hematemesis.

Dietary Disturbance

Besides the external pathogens, the other major cause of acute symptoms in children is dietary disturbance. A careful dietary history would be able to reveal the various digestive disturbances, such as food stagnation, Stomach Qi stagnation, and Stomach Yin deficiency. This is discussed in detail in Chapter 8.

Chronic Illness in Children

When the symptoms have persisted for more than a few weeks, or when they recur on a regular basis, the child has developed a chronic illness. Whereas the acute disorders are exterior conditions that can affect the Wei Qi and meridians, and enter the organs in more serious stages and levels, the chronic disorders are interior conditions that have entered the internal organs. Emotional and even spiritual symptoms accompany the energetic and physical symptoms, which are characteristic of the specific organ(s) involved.

The Five-Element Developmental Theory discussed in Chapter 5 would be very helpful in evaluating chronic disorders, because it not only helps to determine the vulnerable organ(s) according to the child's age and development, but also, more importantly, helps to determine the organ of *origin* of the chronic disorder. Treatment is more effective when the imbalance in the *root* organ of the chronic condition is corrected.

The discussion of chronic conditions will begin with the overall assessment of chronic excess or deficiency, the general pathogenic states of interior Cold, Heat, Damp and Phlegm, followed by evaluation using the developmental protocol.

Excess or Deficiency

Just as in acute illness, decide if the child has a chronic excess or deficient condition. If you cannot decide, think whether this is a problem that should not be there or it is a problem because it is missing something. For example, impulsivity and disproportionate anger should not be there, they are excess symptoms. On the other hand, dry skin is a problem because there is not enough fluid in the skin, and so there is Yin deficiency.

Interior Imbalance

The interior imbalances consist of Interior Cold, Interior Heat, Dampness and Phlegm. General symptoms would manifest as each pathogenic force affects the child as a whole, and specific symptoms would manifest as each imbalance affects a particular organ. Chapter 9 discusses in detail characteristics of each disease entity that reflect interior imbalances.

Interior Cold

Interior Cold may result from recurrent invasions by external Cold pathogens, or from chronic conditions or medications that deplete Qi and Yang. The symptoms consist of general systemic and specific organ manifestations of Cold due to contraction and vasoconstriction. The normal physiologic response to Cold is to preserve warmth to the internal organs, which can be accomplished by vasoconstriction of the skin and external tissues. These would manifest as cold skin, cold limbs, pale skin, feelings or sensations of being cold and chilled. When Cold causes vasoconstriction and contraction in the internal organs, the child would manifest pain and other symptoms specific to the organs involved. The pain is due to decreased circulation of Yang, and would characteristically come on suddenly. It is of a deficient nature, alleviated by warmth or pressure. Cold in each organ would manifest symptoms specific to the organ; e.g., Heat in the Stomach would manifest as epigastric pain with some other accompanying Stomach symptoms, such as nausea and vomiting. Cold in the Lungs would manifest as cough with chest pain, minimal white Phlegm, shortness of breath. Cold in the Large Intestine would manifest as abdominal pain and coldness, diarrhea.

Interior Heat

Interior Heat can result from recurrent invasions of external pathogenic Heat or from chronic conditions that deplete Yin and Fluid. The symptoms consist of general systemic and specific organ manifestations of Heat causing vasodilatation and hypermetabolic state. The normal physiologic response to Heat is to open the pores of the skin and dissipate Heat. This results in a flushed external appearance with red face, red eyes, warm skin, fever. Mild Heat in the blood manifests as various forms of red skin rash. Severe states of Heat that turn into Fire manifest as bleeding. Heat drying up Yin and Fluid results in dryness, such as dry mouth, dry throat, and decreased excretion of fluids, such as scanty output of urine and constipation. The pain due to excess Heat is of an excess nature, aggravated by pressure. Heat in each organ would manifest symptoms specific to the organ. Chronic Heat affecting the Heart and Liver Yin would result in disturbances of the Shen and the Ethereal Soul.

Internal Dampness and Phlegm

Dampness and Phlegm are often seen in children, especially since both are due to Spleen dysfunction, and children's inherent Spleen deficiency is increasingly aggravated by modern diet and lifestyle. There are several distinct differences between Dampness and Phlegm. While Dampness can be both internal and external, with only internal Dampness associated with Spleen dysfunction, Phlegm is always internal and is associated with Spleen, Lung and Kidney dysfunction. Dampness affects primarily the lower part of the body, organs and joints; Phlegm has a predilection for the middle and upper parts of the body and channels under the skin. Dampness gives a feeling of heaviness in the head, but does not affect the Mind; Phlegm makes the head feel heavy and dizzy and "mists" the Mind so that thinking becomes unclear. Dampness affects mostly Yang organs and the Spleen; Phlegm affects mostly Yin organs, especially the Lung in children, and the Stomach (see summary in Table 6.5).

Emotional Issues in Chronic Conditions

Chinese medicine emphasizes the importance of emotions and spiritual involvement in chronic disorders. They correspond to the organ(s) involved as shown in Table 6.6. The emotions and spiritual qualities also correspond to the respective phases of development, so that a Wood child would be in need of direction and tends to be irritable, restless, impatient.

DIAGNOSIS OF CHRONIC DISORDERS USING THE FIVE-ELEMENT DEVELOPMENTAL THEORY

The Five-Element Developmental Theory can be used to identify the vulnerable Element and the corresponding organs and channels, and the *origin* of chronic disorders so that a more comprehensive understanding of the disease can be reached. The following protocol can be used for evaluation and for devising a treatment plan:

1. Identify the organ involved in the chronic disorder according to presenting symptoms. For example, Lungs in an asthmatic child.
2. Identify the vulnerable Element/organ(s) that corresponds to the phase of development, e.g., Water/Kidney in the young child, Wood/Liver in the school-aged child. A young asthmatic needs to have Kidney tonification,

TABLE 6.5	*Dampness and Phlegm*	
	Dampness	**Phlegm**
Interior/exterior dysfunction	Interior, exterior	Interior only
Origin	Only interior = Spleen dysfunction	Spleen dysfunction Fire on body fluids
Organ dysfunction	Spleen dysfunction	Spleen, Lungs, Kidneys
Areas of body affected	(1) Primarily lower part of body	(1) Middle and upper body
	(2) Organs/joints	(2) Channels under skin
In the head	Feeling of heaviness	Heaviness and dizziness
Affects Mind	No effect	Mists Mind
Channels	No effect	Swelling and lumps under skin
Organs affected	Mostly Yang organs and Spleen	Mostly Yin organs and Stomach
Treatment	Spleen to eliminate Damp	Stomach to resolve Phlegm

TABLE 6.6	Emotional states and spiritual involvement			
Organ	**Element**	**Physiologic**	**Pathologic**	**Spirit**
Kidney	Water	Willpower	Fear	
Liver	Wood	Direction	Anxiety, anger	Ethereal Soul (Hun)
Heart	Fire	Joy, passion	Explosive anger	Shen
Spleen	Earth	Thinking	Worry, obsession	
Lung	Metal	Organization	Sadness, depression	Corporeal Soul (Po)

whereas a school-aged asthmatic needs to have treatment for Liver imbalance, either Liver stagnation or Liver Yin deficiency (Liver–Lung related in destructive cycle).

3. Identify and treat the *origin* of the disorder according to the developmental age of onset.

For physical conditions, identify the vulnerable organ at the time when symptoms first appeared. For example, a 12-year-old child who had bronchiolitis at 3 months of age has Kidney imbalance as the origin for the asthma, so that he would need to have Kidney tonification, treatment of Liver imbalance, in addition to the treatment for Lung symptoms.

This explains the progressive difficulty in treating older children with chronic disorders that originated at an earlier age. More Elements and organs are involved, so that treatment and management becomes more complex.

For emotional conditions, identify the vulnerable Element during the time of trauma. For example, a recalcitrant teenager was abused in the second grade. His Fire symptoms are rooted in the Wood phase of development, in the injury to the Liver Yin.

4. Treating children entails well child care, prophylactic preventive care. Balancing the corresponding vulnerable Element helps to maintain well-being and prevent development of chronic disorders.

FAMILY INTERACTION IN CHRONIC DISORDERS

Childhood disorders often reflect family dynamics. With the advent of family therapy in the 1960s, dysfunctional family interactions are often found to play a significant role in a child's chronic illness. Pediatricians are well aware of instances when children manifest symptoms during family stress; e.g., an asthmatic child has an acute attack when parents are arguing. When there is suspicion that parental interactions contribute to the child's symptomatology, the Five-Element Developmental Theory can be used to further elucidate possible conflict between family members.

A family corresponds to the Five Elements as follows: The father is generally regarded as Heaven, the Emperor, the Heart, the Fire; and mother is Mother Earth. The child is the tree, the Wood. Father provides the guidance and mother the nourishment. In modern society where both parents work and share in childcare, both parents are "Emperors" and "Mother Earth." In single-parent households, one parent takes on both roles. In an ideal household where both parents are well-balanced, perfect beings, the child grows into a perfect tree. In an imperfect world, both parents carry "baggage" from their development into rearing children. Children may manifest more symptoms when they are at the developmental phase which had been a problem for one of their parents. For example, an asthmatic child diagnosed at age 3 begins to have more acute attacks as he enters the Wood phase of development, especially when he is around his father. More detailed history about the father reveals that the father was severely traumatized emotionally around age 7. The father's irritability and anger reflects his being "stuck" at his own Wood phase of development, which in turn makes him clash with the son as the child manifests more Wood characteristics. The Western approach would send everyone for family therapy. Chinese medicine can treat the "whole" child by balancing the child's Wood vulnerabilities, and possibly by also treating the parents, such as with herbs that can mitigate the father's Wood anger.

REFERENCES

1. Maciocia G. (1989) *The Foundations of Chinese Medicine, A Comprehensive Treatise for Acupuncturists and Herbalists.* Edinburgh, Churchill Livingstone.
2. Flaws B. (1997) *A Handbook of TCM Pediatrics, A Practitioner's Guide to the Care and Treatment of Common Childhood Diseases.* Colorado, Blue Poppy Press.
3. Nelson W.E. *et al.* (eds)(1996) *Nelson's Textbook of Pediatrics*, 15th edition. Philidelphia, W.B. Saunders, Co.

7 Pediatric Acupuncture Modalities and Treatment Protocols

Acupuncture is very effective for treatment of a wide spectrum of pediatric conditions. Children usually respond quickly because the majority of their illnesses are acute and tend to be more superficial, and because they usually have not had years of emotional issues to complicate their illnesses. The younger the child, the easier it is to bring about Qi balance with acupuncture. Various treatment modalities are well accepted by children and simple treatment protocols can be applied in the majority of pediatric conditions.

THE PRACTITIONER'S QI

The Qi state of the acupuncturist is of utmost importance in the treatment of pediatric patients. Children, even babies, are very intuitive and sensitive to physical and emotional states of people around them. In Western medicine, patients are more compliant if they feel connected with the physician. Whereas a Western physician can prescribe a medication over the phone, Chinese medicine is more hands-on healing. At the time of treatment, the acupuncturist and the child share a Qi field. When the practitioner is in a good state of Qi balance, positive Qi would be directed to the child to make the treatments more effective.

Therefore, it would be advisable for the practitioner to routinely engage in Qi enhancing practices, such as Qigong, or Tai Chi, meditation. Here is a very simple exercise to activate Qi prior to treating children.

First, place your palms together to line up the Luogong point, HT-8. Then vigorously rub the palms together. The palms should become warm within seconds. Then rub the whole hands together, working Qi into the fingertips. This, combined with thinking healthy, healing thoughts, would enhance the efficacy of the treatment.

TREATMENT MODALITIES

Children of all ages can tolerate needle acupuncture treatment. However, for those who have needle phobia, many noninvasive modalities are effective and well accepted: electrical stimulation, magnets, laser, and acupressure.

Needle Acupuncture

Supplies

- 32, 34 gauge needles, $1/2$ inch and 1 inch are usually sufficient; in very obese teenagers, consider using $1 1/2$ to 2 inch needles.
- Shorter needles are easier to control as children tend to wiggle and move around so that there is less risk of accidentally poking them with the needle. Thinner needles bend easily and may be more painful to insert, especially in muscular children.
- Ion pumping cords: these cords are semi-conductors with alligator clamps at the ends—usually black and red—and a diode that conducts unidirectional electro-ionic energy flow from the black terminal to the red terminal. This potentiates movement of Qi and is readily accepted by children since they do not feel anything from the stimulation.

Technique

Babies have very fine skin with more subcutaneous fat. This actually makes insertion of the needle more difficult because there is less firmness to anchor the needle. It would be helpful to grasp and tent the skin and subcutaneous tissue and insert the needle quickly. Figure 7.1 shows a baby having needle acupuncture on ST-36.

- Birth to age 5: 0.5–1 inch 34, 32 gauge. Short needles are easier to insert and have less risk of catching on clothes. One inch needles may be used for very muscular or obese children.
- Age 5–12 years: 32 gauge, 1 inch needles. Some children have tough skin, and thinner needles bend easily and can be more painful to insert.
- Age > 12 years: adult needles.

Tonification of a point: twirl the needle clockwise (with the child as the clock) to tonify a point.

Sedation of a point: twirl the needle counterclockwise to sedate a point.

Tonification of a meridian: use the Five-Element points on the arms and legs. Place the black (north) pole on a point closer to the beginning of the meridian (i.e. a lower number point) and the red (south) pole on a higher number. For example, to tonify the Kidney, needle KI-3 and KI-10. Connect with the ion pumping cord by placing the black clamp on KI-3 and the red clamp on KI-10, so that energy flows from KI-3 to KI-10, the normal direction of flow in the Kidney channel. Time for tonificaton: 8–10 minutes.

Sedation of a meridian: opposite of tonification: place black clamp on higher number point and red clamp on lower number point. For example, to sedate the Large Intestine, needle LI-5 and LI-11, connect the ion pumping cord by placing the black clamp on LI-11 needle and red clamp on LI-5 needle, so that the stimulation is directed opposite to normal flow of the meridian.

Time for sedation: 15–20 minutes.

Penetration: it is not necessary to penetrate very deeply, especially in infants and young children whose Wei Qi flows very superficially. 0.5 to 1.0 mm to $1/4$ inch would suffice in most cases. If using ion pumping cord, need to insert the needle far enough so that the clamp is not too heavy, which may bend or even

FIGURE 7.1 *Baby having needle acupuncture on ST-36. The child is looking at the acupuncturist and the needle and showing no fear. (Reproduced with permission.)*

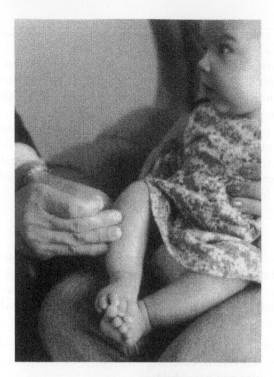

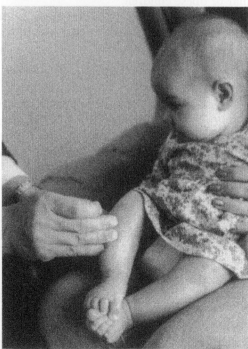

pull out the needle. The clamp can also be secured by taping the cord or the clamp on the skin.

Number of points: too many points left for too long a period of time can sedate a young child.

- *Babies under 12–24 months of age*: usually there is nonretention of needles. The needles are inserted, twirled clockwise a few times for point tonification and counterclockwise for point sedation, and then the needle is withdrawn. Children between 12 months to 24 months who can be held to sit still on parents' laps can have very brief retention of needles for a few seconds to a minute.
- *Infants and toddlers less than 2 years of age*: up to 4 points for a Five-Element treatment each side; if more than one treatment needs to be given, e.g. expel pathogen, dispel Cold treatment, it would be better to do one treatment at a time. Let the child rest a few minutes and reassess.
- *Children 2–6 years of age*: 4–6 points on each side. Needles can be retained for 2–3 minutes as tolerated for tonification. Some younger children would resist being held still during needle retention.
- *Children 7–12 years of age*: up to 6–8 points on each side. Needles can be retained for 4–5 minutes, as tolerated for tonification.
- *Children 12–18 years of age*: 8 points on each side. Needles can be retained for 5–7 minutes as tolerated for tonification.

Advantages of needle acupuncture: strong treatment modality, can treat multiple points at the same time.

Disadvantages: invasive, painful, poor acceptance by young children.

Electrical Stimulator

Supplies

The point finder is a simple hand-held instrument that "buzzes" when it locates an active acupuncture point and can give brief stimulation of low frequency.

Electrical stimulators that can be adjusted for various frequencies are larger instruments and usually expensive. The ear points have different frequencies, usually 5 Hz for points that correlate to abdominal organs, 10 Hz for ear points that correlate to the extremities and trunk. The body points can be treated with 10 Hz.

Treatment

Tonification: 6 seconds on ear points; 12 seconds on body points.

Sedation: 12 seconds on ear points; 24 seconds on body points.

Advantages: noninvasive, no needles, better acceptance by children than needles.

Disadvantages: sometimes can have uncomfortable sensation, such as a sharp pinching or stinging sensation; time consuming—can treat only one point at a time.

FIGURE 7.2   *Two different electrical stimulators. A has more sophisticated adjustments for intensity and frequency. B is a pole finder with limited adjustment for intensity and sensitivity, but not frequency. C and D show a child being treated with the electrical stimulator, which can treat only one point at a time. (Reproduced with permission.)*

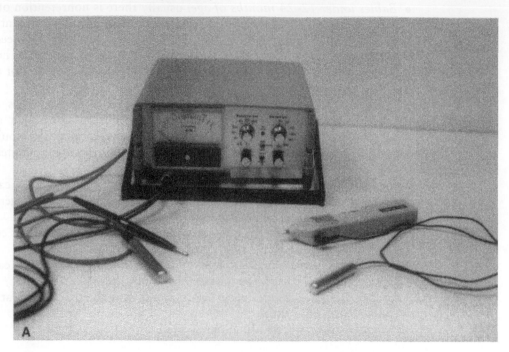

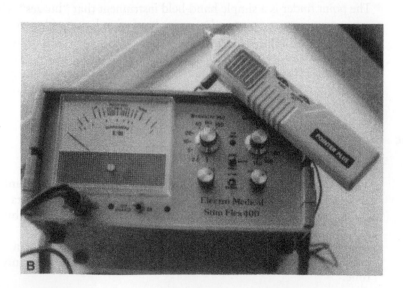

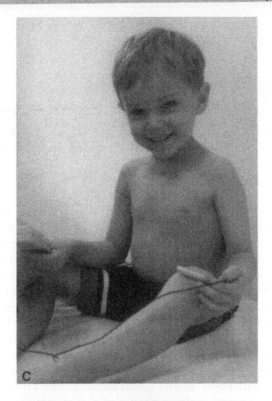

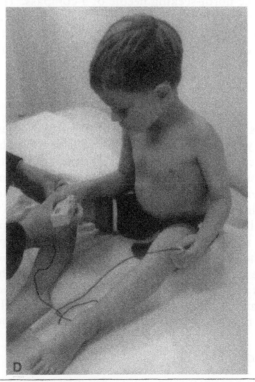

Magnets

Supplies

800 to 10 000 gauss magnets.

- Pole identifier.
- Ion pumping cords: the same ones as used for needles; the red and black clamps readily attach to the magnets (see Figure 7.3).

Principle for Magnet Use

The precise mechanism of action of magnets is yet undefined. It is now known that Qi has electromagnetic properties. Since acupuncture points are sites of electrical instability, and the meridians are located in the connective tissues with electro-ionic physiology, magnets most likely achieve an electro-physiologic effect by inducing small electromagnetic currents at the acupoint. These currents are then propagated unidirectionally along the Qi channels. It is postulated that between paired magnets, Qi flows in the connective tissue energetic pathways from the bionorth (−) pole to the biosouth (+) pole, which mimics the universal electromagnetic energy that flows from north to south.[1] The designation of bionorth (−) and biosouth (+) is based on the earth's geographic North and South Poles. The bionorth (−) side of the magnet will point to the geographic South Pole (the Antarctic) and will attract the north-seeking needle of a compass. The biosouth (+) side of the magnet will be repelled by the north-seeking needle of a compass and will point to the geographic North Pole (the Arctic). It should be noted that this is opposite to the definition used by the National Bureau of Standards (NBS).

Technique

Magnets can be applied to individual points, or can be used in a circuit connected by ion pumping cords. Most pole identifiers have the biosouth side of its reference magnet exposed so that it attracts the bionorth (−) pole of the magnet being tested and repels the biosouth (+) side of the magnet being tested. (A pole identifier with the bionorth side exposed would do the opposite: attract the biosouth (+) pole of the magnet being tested.) The 10 000 gauss magnets are small individual magnets without adhesive tapes so that they need to be secured to the skin with small round band-aid type tapes, surgical or paper tape. The 800 gauss magnets are usually sold attached to small round tapes with the protruding end usually being the bionorth (−) pole. Some 800 gauss magnets are gold colored for biosouth pole and silver colored for bionorth pole. These can be given to parents for home treatment. Figure 7.4 shows the placement of magnets on a child and connection of the ion pumping cord.

Treatment of Individual Acupoints

- *Simple tonification of one acupoint*: place the biosouth pole of the magnet facing downward on the skin, with the bionorth pole of the magnet facing outward. This would direct Universal Qi to flow into the child and therefore tonifies.

FIGURE 7.3   *A 800 gauss magnets that come with tapes. The top part of picture shows the side of magnets that come into contact with the skin: left, silver, is for sedation; right, gold, is for tonification. The lower part of picture shows the tapes as they would appear on the skin. B The 10 000 gauss magnet does not come with tape and can be attached to a blank tape with either the (−) north pole or the (+) south pole facing the skin. A pole identifier is shown on the lower left hand corner. The top surface of the identifier is bionorth, which indicates that the south pole of the magnet would attach to the pole identifier and the north pole of the magnet would be repelled. C Ion pumping cords showing (−) clamp as black/north pole, (+) clamp as red/south pole, with the diode directing flow from (−) to (+).*

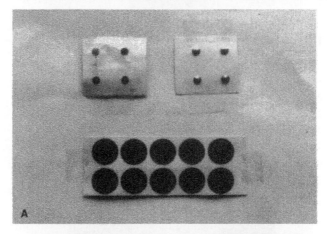

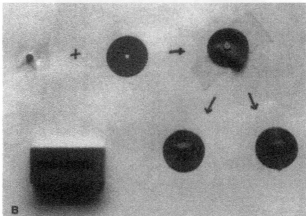

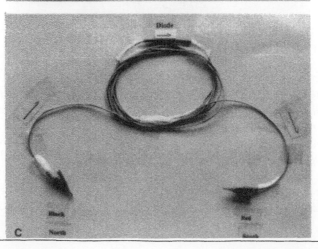

FIGURE 7.4   *Placement of magnets on a child. A Magnets placed on individual acupoints. B Magnets placed on the 10 Shu points for tonification of the immune system. Additional magnets can be attached on the outside of the tapes for augmentation of power. 10 000 gauss magnets are applied in this case. (Reproduced with permission.)*

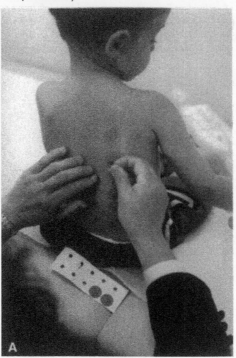

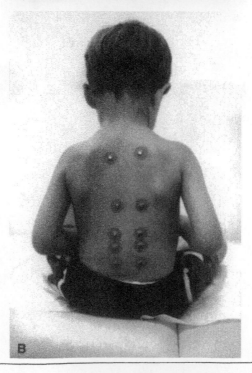

FIGURE 7.5   *A baby having Kidney tonification with magnets, with (−) magnet on KI-3 and (+) magnet on KI-10, and the ion pumping cord is attached with black clamp on KI-3 and red clamp on KI-10. (Reproduced with permission.)*

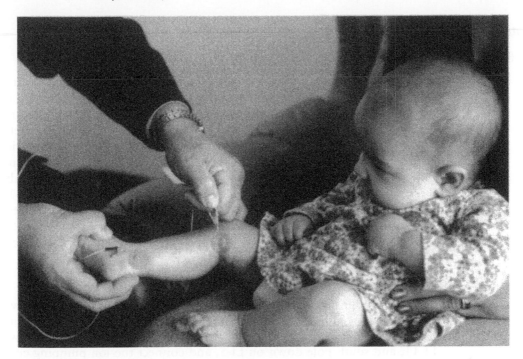

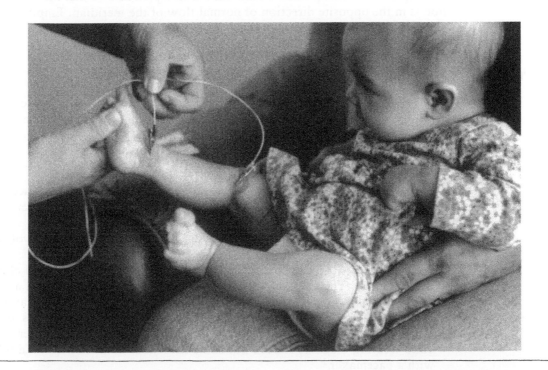

- *Simple sedation of one acupoint*: place the bionorth pole of the magnet on the skin, with the biosouth pole facing outward. This directs Qi flow away from the body and is therefore dispersing or sedating.

Treatment of a Meridian

Tonification of a Meridian

Use the Five-Element points on the arms and legs. Place the bionorth pole facing downward on a lower number point and the biosouth pole facing downward on a higher number point. Connect the ion pumping cord by placing the black (−) alligator clip/clamp on the lower number magnet and the red (+) clamp on the higher number magnet (the clamp automatically attaches to the magnet). For example, to tonify the Kidney, place the north pole facing downward on KI-3 and south pole on KI-10, connect with the ion pumping cord with the black clamp on KI-3 and red clamp on KI-10 so that there is increased energy flow from KI-3 to KI-10, the normal direction of flow in the Kidney channel. Empirically, children can be tonified in 20–30 minutes.

Sedation of a Meridian

This is the opposite of tonification: place the bionorth pole facing down on higher number point and the biosouth pole facing down on lower number point. For example, to sedate the Large Intestine, place the north pole down on LI-11, and south pole down on LI-5, and connect the ion pumping cord by placing the black clamp on LI-11 and the red clamp on LI-5 so that the stimulation is in the opposite direction of normal flow of the meridian. Empirically, children can be sedated in approximately 30 minutes.

Current FDA Position

The FDA has not approved magnets for therapeutic (acupuncture) use. On a local level, the Board of Medicine or the regulating acupuncture board in several states in the US have approved application of magnets on acupoints; however, the FDA has warned that no medical claims can be made with magnet treatment.

- *Advantages*: easy to use, noninvasive, non-painful, children readily accept modality; can treat multiple points at the same time, and can treat entire meridians. Parents can apply 800 gauss magnets for home treatment.
- *Disadvantages*: longer time than needles needed for treatment; magnets often get lost at home.
- *Cautions*: parents must be extremely cautious when there are small children at home. The magnets can come off of the adhesive tapes, and accidental ingestion can occur. There is one case report of a child having developed an intestinal fistula as a result of magnet ingestion.[2] It is also important to avoid magnet contact with credit cards and computers. A child wearing magnets should not come into close contact with an adult with a pacemaker.[1]

Laser

Supplies

Currently 1–5 mW red beam lasers are readily available commercially. Red beam laser pointer pens have very low energy, usually < 5 mW. Lasers > 5 mW are more difficult to obtain, although there are a few vendors.

Continuous wave and pulsed wave red-beam and infrared-beam lasers are also available commercially but they can cost over $1000, especially if the mW power output is greater than 100 mW.

Principle for Laser Use

Lasers were first invented in 1960, and laser acupuncture and low level laser therapy (LLLT) have been researched and practiced extensively in China, Russia, Spain, Germany, Austria, Hungary, and Czechoslovakia for over 30 years,[3] and are slowly being accepted in the United States. Laser acupuncture has been used for numerous childhood conditions in China, and a few Western scientific studies have demonstrated laser efficacy in reducing postoperative vomiting after strabismus surgery[4] and in minimizing spasticity in cerebral palsy.[5] The author has conducted a pilot study funded by the National Institutes of Health on children with attention deficit disorder using laser acupuncture.[6]

The two major parameters of laser are power output of the laser (as measured in milliwatts) and wavelength of the laser light (as measured in nanometers). Energy densities used for treatment of an acupuncture point (or

| FIGURE 7.6 | Readily available lasers: 5 mW laser pen (left) and <2 mW laser pointer pen (right). These can treat only one point at a time. |

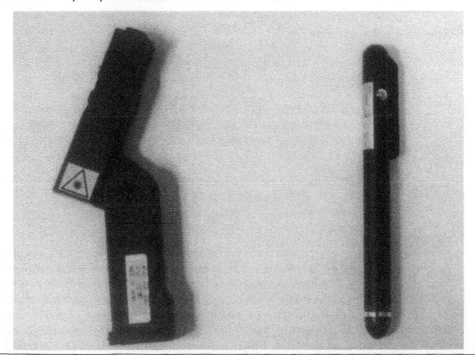

specific area) are expressed in terms of a unit of work energy, or joule, and expressed as joules per cm^2 (J/cm^2). Laser acupuncture or low-level laser therapy (LLLT) usually use lasers which range in power output from 5 to 500 mW, Class IIIb lasers. (These lasers have very low power, compared to the lasers that are greater than 100 W used as a cutting instrument in surgery. More than 500 mW would begin to burn the skin.) While ambient room light consists of many different wavelengths and is scattered, laser light is monochromatic and coherent, and can therefore concentrate and focus on one point, and can begin to penetrate the skin and tissues. The therapeutic range of wavelengths for laser acupuncture is between 600 and 1000 nm.[7] The lower wavelengths would be blocked by hemoglobin; and the higher wavelengths, by water, so that desirable energy penetration could not be achieved.[3] Naeser at Boston University School of Medicine recommends using primarily red-beam (600–700 nm) and infrared-beam (780–1000 nm) lasers. The red-beam laser has only a shallow penetration, around 0.8–1 mm, on acupuncture points located on the hand, foot (not the heel), face, and sometimes the ear. The red beam laser is therefore appropriate for treatment of the shallow Jing-well points on the fingers and toes. The infrared lasers have deeper penetration, approximately 2.5 cm in depth, and are more appropriate for treatment of deeper acupuncture points, such as those located on the back and the limbs. Pulsed lasers are more complex devices that have multiple settings for delivering various numbers of pulsed beams per second for specific indications. The mechanism of laser is photobiostimulation, most likely due to the emission of photons when excited electrons return to the original orbit. This "triggers" biochemical, electrochemical, and structural changes at the cellular level (especially with increases in ATP), which may in turn improve cellular function and alter the outcome of disease.[8] The calculation for laser energy is a function of the power output of the laser, the size of the aperture, and the time it is used.

Calculation of Joules of Energy[3]

$$1 \text{ Joule } = \frac{1 \text{ Watt}}{1 \text{ second}}$$

A standard 5 mW laser (0.005 W) with a 0.5 cm (centimeter) diameter aperture on the probe tip would generate a beam spot size of 0.196 cm^2. The time needed to emit 1 J/cm^2 (energy density) is computed according to the following formula:

(Average output power in Watts × seconds)/beam area in cm^2 = 1 J/cm^2
[(0.005 W) × (x seconds)] / 0.196 cm^2 = 1 J/cm^2
so, x = 0.196/0.005 seconds
        = 39.2 seconds.

Therefore, placing a 5 mW laser with a 0.5 cm diameter aperture on an acupuncture point requires 39.2 seconds to emit 1 J/cm^2. In adults, acupuncture points are often treated with 4–8 J/cm^2, taking 156.8–313.6 seconds, or about 2.5–5 minutes per point. Some investigators posit that an anti-inflammatory effect occurs with a minimum of 4 J/cm^2. This energy density, e.g., is often used to promote wound healing in nonhealing wounds.[9] Currently, there are 200 mW near infrared-beam lasers available which emit 1 J/cm^2 every 1 or 2 seconds, depending on the beam aperture. These more powerful lasers greatly decrease the necessary treatment time to reach 4 J/cm^2, an energy density often used as a starting point to treat acupuncture points.

Currently, energy density recommendations for laser treatment of children is not yet defined. Naeser[10] and the author recommend the following:

- Children > age 12 years, adult doses are probably appropriate.
- Children > age 6 years, $^1/_3$ adult dose.
- Babies: usually only 5–10 seconds per point, with a 5 mW red-beam laser with 0.5 cm diameter aperture.
- Microsystem points, e.g., ears—probably half the stimulation of body point.

Current FDA Position

The FDA considers low level laser therapy to be an investigational modality, therefore no medical claims of cures are permitted. (Until 1995, acupuncture needles were considered investigational.) The National Institutes of Health is interested in the efficacy of laser acupuncture and has funded the author's research in laser acupuncture treatment of attention deficit hyperactivity disorder.

Advantages

Easy to use, noninvasive, non-painful, well accepted by children.

Disadvantages

Limited commercial supply; can treat only one point at a time unless the practitioner has more than one laser. Low energy laser acupuncture can be time consuming; however, the treatment times are dramatically shortened with lasers which have a more powerful output.

Contraindications

Avoid shining the laser light beam directly into eyes, as laser can cause retinal damage; do not use in children taking cytotoxic drugs; do not use on bony growth end plates in growing children; do not shine the laser on warts or any rapidly growing skin lesions, such as cancerous growths; do not apply on fontanelles of infants.[10]

For more information on laser acupuncture, see: www.Acupuncture.com/Acup/laser.htm.

Acupressure

Applying pressure to an acupuncture point is a very effective treatment for children.

Technique

Acupressure on a point can be applied by using the thumb or the tips of second and third fingers. The palm or the four fingers together can massage a larger area. For tonification apply acupressure or massage in a circular, clockwise direction—with the child as the clock. The child's left side is 3:00 o'clock, right side is 9:00 o'clock. The pressure should be firm but not painful. Massage a minimum of 50 strokes per point or area.

Advantages

Acupressure is easy to apply; parents and even children themselves can learn to apply acupressure for home treatment. Parents and children feel empowered that they themselves are doing something to maintain health instead of relying on medications.

Disadvantages

Acupressure is usually not as strong as other treatment modalities. It is time consuming, one can only massage one or two points at the same time.

MICROSYSTEMS IN PEDIATRICS

Acupuncture is based on a natural Taoist philosophy that man is a microcosm and Nature is the macrocosm. Within the human body there are many microsystems, each one with either somatotopic mapping of the body or mapping of the meridians. The ear microsystem is the most familiar and most frequently used by general acupuncturists.

Ear Microsystem

Theoretical Principle

The human body is mapped somatotopically as an inverted fetus, with the head and face on the ear lobe. The French have now developed an elaborate four-phase system which is too complex for application here. The ear points used are phase I simple somatotopic mapping of various organs on the ear.[11]

Supplies

Small needles are used or small silver or gold colored pellets with adhesive tapes that can be applied to the microsystem ear points.

Advantages

- Easy access of points
- Non-needling well accepted by children
- Pellets can stay on ears for days to prolong treatment effect
- The somatotopic mapping is in great detail. This is especially helpful for accessing different parts of the central nervous system for treatment of, e.g., seizure disorder and attention deficit disorder.

Disadvantages

Needling is more powerful but painful and not well tolerated even by older children. Older children usually do not like parents to massage their ears, and the point locations are very specific so that even parents can only massage general areas and not specific points. Children can be taught to massage general areas of the ear, e.g. the ear lobe.

PREVENTIVE PEDIATRIC ACUPUNCTURE

Preventive medicine is the key in both Eastern and Western pediatrics. The two components in both disciplines are health maintenance and preventive treatment.

Health Maintenance

Health maintenance in Western medicine consists of regular well child checkups with physical examination; nutrition assessment that includes appropriate supplements such as with vitamins; and prevention of childhood illnesses with immunization. Chinese pediatrics is comparable in its concern for maintaining well being with the following five basic components:

- Dietary recommendations
- Recommendations for proper lifestyle
- Regular acupuncture treatment to tonify the immune system and to keep the organs in balance
- Self-help Qigong breathing exercises
- Daily home maintenance regimen for parents.

Dietary Recommendations

Chinese diet focuses on a balance of the five flavors and appropriate manners of eating. This is discussed in detail in chapter 8.

Proper Lifestyle

Today, a stressful lifestyle has become the norm for both adults and children. All pediatric practitioners need to advise children that optimal health means a balance of rest with activity, study with physical exercise.

Regular Acupuncture Treatment

Tonification of the Immune System

While immunization is a major tenet of Western pediatrics, acupuncture has been shown to increase immunity and modulate inflammatory response. Children of all ages—especially infants—can benefit from periodic acupuncture treatment. This is similar to Western well child checkups to ensure that the organs are balanced and to tonify the immune system. The following simple protocol uses points that would strengthen both humoral and cellular immunity.

- ST-36—the major immunity point
- LI-4 if used together with ST-36 in children.

Shu points associated with Wei Qi production and movement:

- BL-13 Lung Shu
- BL-18 Liver Shu
- BL-20 Spleen Shu
- BL-21 Stomach Shu
- BL-23 Kidney Shu.

Treatment consists of needle insertion, and twirling clockwise to tonify the points.

- Magnets: south pole on the skin, north pole facing outward to tonify each individual point
- Laser: follow the treatment protocol for body points according to age of the child.

Keeping the Organs in Balance

Periodic routine acupuncture visits would enable the practitioner to treat early stages of organ imbalance. Routine tonification of the master points of the three Energizers: CV-17, -12, -6 would help to strengthen children and maintain health.

Qigong for Children

While Western medicine provides daily supplements as part of essential well being, Chinese medicine has various techniques—such as Tai Chi, meditation, Qigong—that children can learn to strengthen themselves mentally and physically. These skills enable children to be more self-reliant for handling physical discomfort, reducing stress and calming the mind so that they would be less likely to turn to drugs and alcohol.

The term Qigong is derived from two Chinese words, Qi and Gong, which can be roughly defined as "Qi work" or "breathing skills." Qigong has a verbal history of 10 000 years, and written history of approximately 4000 years. A myriad of Qigong exercises have been developed over the past several thousand years. Currently, there are over 10 000 styles of Qigong being practiced worldwide. The two very basic Qigong exercises are abdominal and microcosmic breathing.[12]

Abdominal Breathing

This occurs naturally in infancy, and children can relearn it much more easily than adults. Breathe in through the nose, with the mouth closed, the tip of the tongue touching the roof of the mouth behind the top front teeth. Breathe in deeply to expand the chest and continue breathing into the abdomen. Hold the breath in the abdomen for 1–3 seconds, then breathe out slowly through the open mouth. Parents can help the child "visualize" abdominal breathing by placing one hand on the child's abdomen and asking the child to breathe deeply by "pushing" the hand out. As the child exhales, parents can gently press on the abdomen to help push out more air so that the next breath can be a deeper one. After some practice, children often naturally breathe abdominally. This is especially helpful at a time of stress or when the child needs to calm down.

Microcosmic Breathing

This is an extension of abdominal breathing. The child breathes into the abdomen as above. As the child exhales slowly with his mouth open, tell the child to imagine that the breath is traveling down the abdomen around the sacrum and up the middle of the spine to the top of the head and out through the mouth. This circulates Qi through the Conception Vessel meridian during inspiration, and connects around GV-1 up the Governor Vessel meridian along the midline of the back to the top of the head and down to GV-24 and out through the mouth. Since the Conception Vessel is the major Yin channel and the Governor Vessel is the major Yang channel, microcosmic breathing fills the two channels with Qi. This is especially powerful for bringing Qi to the brain.

Qigong can also be used to actively engage children in their treatment. During the treatment, the practitioner can say to the child, "Take a deep breath, and when I put the needle in (or magnet on), make your breath go right over here." There is a Chinese Qigong saying: "Where the thought goes, Qi goes." The mere suggestion of "putting" the breath there would enable the child to bring Qi to the acupoint, and potentiate the efficacy of treatment.

Children can also be taught to activate their Luogong point. This would be especially helpful when they are taught to do acupressure. Older children should be taught acupressure so that they can "treat" themselves regularly. Even children at 2–3 years of age can begin to learn to massage themselves "to feel better."

Daily Home Regimen for Parents

Parents are usually diligent in making sure that their children take vitamins or prescribed medications. They are even more eager to learn basic massage and acupressure skills because they feel empowered that they are actively contributing to their child's health instead of administering a pill. They can learn simple massages and acupressure that take only minutes a day. Three basic general acumassages are abdominal massage, back Shu point massage, and meridian massage. Parents can do just one or all three sets, daily or several times a week, depending on their availability. Each massage should take no more than 2–3 minutes. For children with specific conditions, parents can learn a few specific points for acupressure.

First, teach the parents to warm up their hands by activating the Luogong points. They also need to be in a healing frame of mind so they are advised not to massage their children when they are angry or stressed.

Abdominal Massage

The abdomen is a microcosm where the Five Elements are situated in a circle with the umbilicus as the center. Regular massage of the abdomen can harmonize the Five Elements. This is also the Middle Energizer where digestive Qi needs to flow smoothly. Parents can massage with their palms or the four fingers bunched together. Massage around the umbilicus 50 times in the clockwise and 50 times in the counterclockwise direction. (The child is the clock so that the child's face is 12 o'clock, the left side is 3 o'clock, and the right side is 9 o'clock.) When the child has diarrhea, massage only in the counterclockwise direction. In cases of constipation, massage only clockwise direction. The massage is best done with firm pressure. However, if the child dislikes firm pressure, even gentle touching would be beneficial.

Back Shu Point Massage

Regular massage of the Bladder Shu points can harmonize Qi flow to all the organs, especially the Yin organs. The massage begins at the shoulder level downward along the Bladder meridian on both sides to the buttocks. Parents need to lift up their hands and begin the massage again at the shoulder level and massage downward in the direction of the flow of the Bladder meridian. This can be done 30–50 times, once or twice a day. Since the back Shu points are part of the immune treatment protocol, this massage theoretically can tonify the child's immunity.

Massage of the Meridians

Parents can also be taught to massage the major meridian direction of Qi flow: up the inside of the legs to the abdomen for the three leg Yin channels; up the abdomen to the armpit, then down the inside of the arms to the fingertips for the three arm Yin channels. Follow the channels as they curve around the fingers, and massage upward along the outside of the child's arms for the three arm Yang channels, then down the back and down the dorsum of the legs to massage the three leg Yang channels. This can be done 10 times each day.

Specific Acupoint Massage

When children are ill, especially when they have chronic conditions, parental home treatment is a must to help prolong treatment effects. Parents can be taught specific acupoints applicable to the child's condition. These are discussed with disease entities in Chapter 10.

Preventive Treatment

Western medicine has prophylactic treatment to prevent recurrence of illnesses, such as treating chronic serous otitis with daily antibiotics to prevent recurrence of acute otitis media. Chinese medicine has a similar perspective in following the ancient tenet of "winter disease, summer cure." Treating children when the disease is not active is the most effective way to prevent recurrence. This theory

FIGURE 7.7 *Baby having A abdominal massage and B back Shu point massage. (Reproduced with permission.)*

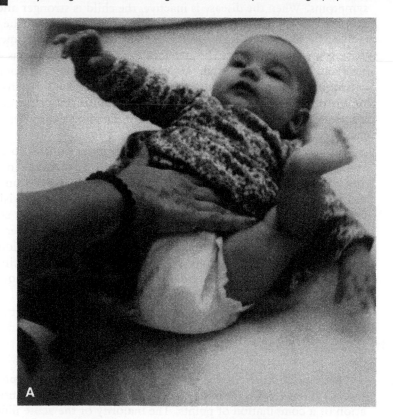

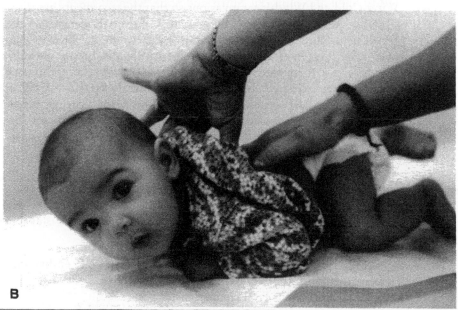

posits that during a flare-up, treatment is directed toward controlling the acute symptoms. When the disease is inactive, the child is stronger and treatment can be directed toward eradicating the root of the problem. The most common example is the treatment of asthmatics during the summertime when children are not having symptoms. During an acute attack, treatment is directed toward reversing rebellious Lung Qi. When children are not symptomatic, treatment can be directed toward Lung tonification. This is also consistent with the important TCM theory of balancing Yin and Yang in treatment. Using Yang points for Yin diseases and Yin points for Yang diseases are very powerful treatments to bring the body into balance.

The Five-Element Developmental Theory can also help to prophylactically strengthen children. For example, a child in the Water phase of development is vulnerable for Kidney imbalances therefore would benefit from regular Kidney tonification treatments as part of "well child acupuncture visits." The Water child is also gradually becoming more vulnerable to the next stage of developmental disorders—Liver Yin deficiencies. Tonification of Liver Yin would help prepare the child for the next phase of development. In addition, since children are usually prone to developing respiratory and gastrointestinal symptoms in the fall and winter seasons, preventive pediatrics consists of tonification of Spleen and Lung during the spring and summer.

PEDIATRIC ACUPUNCTURE TREATMENT

The best acupuncture treatment of children consists of deciphering treatment priority and careful selection of a few key points based on knowledgeable creation of a combination of points. The majority of the acute illnesses are due to Wind-Cold and Wind-Heat invasions so that the treatments are directed toward expelling Wind and either Cold or Heat. Other pathogens such as Damp and Dryness can also be easily dispelled in the early stages. Since acupuncture has been shown to be effective in tonifying and regulating the immune system, a basic immune treatment can be added to the treatment of pathogenic invasions that have not progressed to the critical stages or levels. Chronic illnesses in children usually consist of excess internal Heat or Cold, or organ deficiency. Five-Element four-point protocols are simple yet powerful treatments for dispersing Heat and Cold and for organ tonification.

General Selection of Points for Symptomatic Treatment

The hierarchy of descending potency of acupuncture points is as follows:

- Gate points: LI-4, LR-3
- Curious meridian points: present since the four-cell embryonic stage, can exert global effect for children with more severe illnesses
- Principal meridians Five-Element master points
- Distal points
- Local points.

The acupuncture points are shown in the Appendix in Figures A.15–A.31.

Local and Distal Points

The local and distal points are considered the weakest combination of points for treatment but are easiest to select. Children generally respond well to these regimens for symptomatic relief of mild, acute illnesses. The local points are those acupuncture points close to the location of symptoms, and distal points are usually located distally along the same meridian or along the connecting principal meridian. Examples are:

- Upper respiratory tract symptoms:
  - Rhinorrhea
    - Choose local points LI-20 and a distal point along the Yang Ming principal channel, such as ST-45
    - Treat bilaterally
  - Watery eyes
    - Choose GB-1, BL-2, ST-2 as local points. These points are best treated in children with acupressure; choose distal points along the three Yang meridians, such as GB-34 and BL-60
- Ear pain
  - Choose local points GB-2, SI-19, TE-21, and GB-34 as a distal point
  - NB: GB-34 and BL-60 are the most frequently used distal points for head and upper body symptoms.

Selection of General "Big" Points

These are major points that exert specific effects globally.

- ST-36, everything, especially for immune tonification; tonifies Yin Qi, Yuan (Original) Qi, Nutritive Qi, Stomach Qi
- LI-4 is a strong point for immune tonification when used in combination with ST-36
  - it is a strong dispersing point for headaches or any excess symptoms of the head and face
  - *it should be used with caution in a deficient child*
- GV-16, Wind Palace—to expel both internal and external Wind
- GB-20, Wind Pool—to expel external Wind
- LI-11 clears Heat anywhere
- GV-14—fever of any origin
- ST-40 resolves Dampness or Phlegm anywhere
- KI-7—expels Cold; can be augmented with supportive means, e.g. hot steam
- CV-17, CV-6—tonify Qi globally;
  - CV-17 is the intersection of Pericardium, Heart, Liver, Spleen, Triple Energizer and Small Intestine, tonifies Qi
  - CV-6 is good for tonifying chronic Qi deficiency
- CV-12, intersection of Spleen, Stomach, Triple Energizer and Lung, tonifies Middle Energizer
- GV-20 and Sishenchong—stimulate brain, clear mental cloudiness due to any cause
- BL Shu points for tonification of Yin organs
  - BL-13 Lung
  - BL-15 Heart

- BL-18 Liver
- BL-20 Spleen
- BL-23 Kidney
- CV-8: strong point to warm Cold abdomen/Middle Energizer with placement of warming herbs or ginger (acupuncture needling is contraindicated)
- BL-60, Mountain of Kunlun, is the strongest movement point on Tai Yang. Nicknamed the "universal garbage dump" by the UCLA medical acupuncture course, it is frequently used as a distal point to pull energy inferiorly from proximal points on any Yang channel
- Yintang, CV-7—relieves geopathic stress: electromotive force, X-rays, computers, light
- GV-26 for emergencies; add KI-1 if emergency involves CNS, e.g. seizure, head trauma
- Si Feng—special points for children (M-UE-9) on the palmar surface, in the transverse creases, of MCP, PIP, DIP, middle four fingers; treat nutritional impairment, food stagnation; has a very strong dispersing action, do not use in extremely deficient conditions.

General Treatment Protocols

Tonification and Regulation of Immune Response

- ST-36 is the major point for immune system
- LI-4 must be in combination with ST-36 for children
- Bladder Shu points: BL-13, -18, -19, -20, -23.

Treatment is by needle insertion and twirling clockwise to tonify the points.

Magnets are used by placing the biosouth (+) pole on the skin, and the bionorth (–) pole facing outward (Figure 7.8). If using ion pumping cords, connect with black (–) clamp on BL-13, and red (+) clamp on BL-23 to potentiate flow through the Bladder Shu points.

Tonification

Tonification Protocols

Simple tonification of Yin or Yang of an organ/meridian is shown in Table 7.1. The simple two-point tonification and sedation of a meridian is as follows. Tonification and sedation of an entire channel can be carried out with a simple two-point protocol, using the Five-Element command points on the arms and legs. The principle of this technique is based on the electrophysiology of acupuncture.

Although the precise nature of Qi is not determined, it is well known now that Qi has electromagnetic flow, and that acupuncture points are areas of decreased electrical resistance and therefore increased electrical conductance. Insertion of a needle into one acupuncture point can create a local electro-ionic disturbance. Tonification techniques such as twirling the needle in a clockwise direction or inserting the needle in the direction of flow of the meridian in essence are maneuvers that induce a small flow of energy from Earth's electromagnetic field. Needles inserted at two separate points create an agitated

FIGURE 7.8 *Left. Bionorth (–) magnet is placed on LI-20, connected with ion pumping cord to biosouth (+) magnet placed on BL-60 as treatment for rhinorrhea. Right. Four-point magnet treatment for dispersing Lung Heat: bionorth (–) on LU-10, HT-7; biosouth (+) on LU-5, KI-10.*

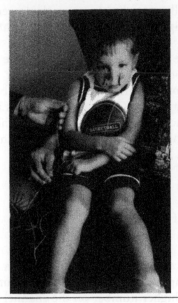 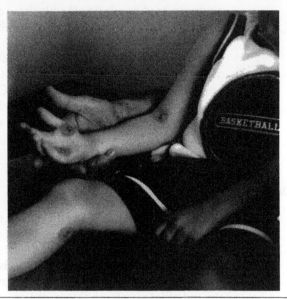

TABLE 7.1 *Simple tonification of Yin or Yang of an organ/meridian*

	Yin	**Yang**
Lung	LU-9—tonifies LU Yin	LU-9—tonifies LU Qi
		LU-7 stimulates descent and dispersion of LU Qi
		Circulates Wei Qi, releases exteriorly
Spleen	SP-6—tonifies Blood and Yin	SP-3—tonifies Spleen
Stomach	CV-12, SP-6—tonifies ST Yin	ST-36—tonifies both ST Qi and ST Yin
Heart	HT-7—tonifies Heart Blood	HT-5—tonifies Heart Qi
Kidney	KI-3—tonifies KI Yin, Essence	KI-3—tonifies KI Yang
	KI-6—nourishes KI Yin	KI-7—tonifies KI Yang
Liver	LR-3 nourishes LR Blood and Yin	LR-3, LR-13 moves LR Qi

electro-ionic energy flow from the needle that induces a net negative charge to the needle with positive charge until equilibration occurs. The flow can be potentiated by stimulating the needles electrically—which even teenagers find unpleasant and some young children find frightening—or by connecting the needles with an ionic pumping cord.

Tonification

Needle Technique

Insert needle into two command points on a channel, connect the ion pumping cord by placing the black alligator clamp (bionorth) on the a lower number and the red alligator clamp (biosouth) on a higher number along the channel to stimulate energy in the direction of flow of the meridian.

Magnets

Place the bionorth pole facing downward on a lower number point and the biosouth pole facing downward on a higher number point. Connect the ion pumping cord by placing the black (−) alligator clip/clamp on the lower number magnet and the red (+) clamp on the higher number magnet (the clamp automatically attaches to the magnet).

For example, to tonify Kidney, needle or place the magnet with the bionorth pole facing downward on KI-3, and needle or place the magnet with the biosouth pole facing down on KI-10. Connect the ion pumping cord by placing the black clamp on KI-3 and the red clamp on KI-10 so that there is increased energy flow from KI-3 to KI-10, the normal direction of flow in the Kidney channel. Empirically, children can be tonified with needles in 5–10 minutes, and with magnets and ion pumping cords in 20–30 minutes.

Sedation

Sedation of a meridian is the opposite of tonification.

Needle Technique

Insert needle into two command points on a channel, connect the ion pumping cord by placing the black alligator clamp (bionorth) on the higher number and the red alligator clamp (biosouth) on a higher number on the channel to stimulate energy flow in the *opposite* direction as the meridian.

Magnets

Place the bionorth pole facing downward on a higher number point and the biosouth pole facing downward on a lower number point. Connect the ion pumping cord by placing the black (−) alligator clip/clamp on the higher number magnet and the red (+) clamp on the lower number magnet (the clamp automatically attaches to the magnet).

For example, to sedate the Large Intestine, needle or place the bionorth pole facing down on LI-11, and south pole down on LI-5, and connect the ion pumping cord by placing the black clamp on LI-11 and the red clamp on LI-5 so that the stimulation of flow is in the opposite direction of normal flow of the meridian. Empirically, children can be sedated with needles in approximately 15–20 minutes, and with magnets in approximately 30 minutes.

Five-Element Four-Point Protocol for Tonification and Sedation of an Organ

Very powerful tonification and sedation of organs follows the nurturing and controlling relationships of the Five Elements. To strengthen a deficient organ, a tonification protocol tonifies the "mother" and sedates the "grandmother" using corresponding points on the organ meridian and the respective horary points on the "mother" and "grandmother" meridians. For example, to strengthen the Spleen, the Yin Earth organ, the "mother" of the Earth point on the Spleen channel is SP-2, the Fire point. The "grandmother" point on the Spleen channel is SP-1, the Wood point. Then go to the corresponding Fire and Liver channels and choose the horary points: the Fire point on the Fire channel is HT-8 and the Wood point on the Liver channel is LR-1. A Five-Element four-point tonification of Spleen would therefore consist of tonifying SP-2, HT-8, and sedating SP-1, and LR-1. To weaken an excess organ, the protocol would tonify the "grandmother" and sedate the "son." For example, to weaken an excessive Gallbladder, the Yang Wood organ, tonify GB-44, the "grandmother" Metal point on the Gallbladder channel, and sedate GB-38, the "son" Fire point on the Gallbladder channel. Then go to the corresponding Metal and Fire channels and choose the horary points: tonify LR-1, the Metal point on the Liver channel, and sedate SI-5, the Fire point on the Small Intestine channel.

In general, use Yin organs to tonify or sedate the respective Yin organs, and Yang organs to tonify or sedate the respective Yang organs. Therefore, strengthening the Spleen would involve the Yin organs, Heart and Liver; whereas sedating the Gallbladder would involve the Yang organs, Large Intestine and Small Intestine.

- Needling technique: twirl the needle clockwise to tonify a point, and counterclockwise to sedate a point
- Magnet: apply the biosouth (+) pole of the magnet facing downward on the skin to tonify a point, and place the bionorth (–) pole facing downward on the skin to sedate a point.

Table 7.2 lists the Five-Element points on all the meridians, Table 7.3 the horary points and Table 7.4 lists the four-point tonification protocols and Table 7.5 the sedation protocols for each organ. The Heart is usually used for the Fire organ instead of Pericardium. Table 7.6 summarizes the tonification protocol and Table 7.7 summarizes the sedation protocol.

TABLE 7.2 Five-Element points on all meridians

	Yin organs						Yang organs				
	Wood	Fire	Earth	Metal	Water		Metal	Water	Wood	Fire	Earth
LU	11	10	9	8	5	LI	1	2	3	5	11
SP	1	2	3	5	9	ST	45	44	43	41	36
HT	9	8	7	4	3	SI	1	2	3	5	8
KI	1	2	3	7	10	BL	67	66	65	60	40
PC	9	8	7	5	3	TE	1	2	3	6	10
LR	1	2	3	4	8	GB	44	43	41	38	34

TABLE 7.3 Five-Element horary points

	Wood	Fire	Earth	Metal	Water		Metal	Water	Wood	Fire	Earth
LU					8	LI	1				
SP			3			ST					36
HT		8				SI				5	
KI					10	BL		66			
PC		8				TE				6	
LR	1					GB			41		

TABLE 7.4　Four-point tonification protocol

Yin organs

	Wood	Fire	Earth	Metal	Water	LU	SP	HT	KI	PC	LR
LU		−LU-10	**LU-9**				**SP-3**	−HT-8			
SP	−SP-1	**SP-2**						**HT-8**			−LR-1
HT	**HT-9**				−HT-3				−KI-10		**LR-1**
KI			−KI-3	**KI-7**		**LU-8**	−SP-3				
PC	**PC-9**				−PC-3				−KI-10		**LR-1**
LR				−LR-4	**LR-8**	−LU-8			**KI-10**		

Yang organs

	Metal	Water	Wood	Fire	Earth	LI	ST	SI	BL	TE	GB
LI				−LI-5	**LI-11**		**ST-36**	−SI-5			
ST			−ST-43	**ST-41**				**SI-5**			−GB-41
SI		−SI-2	**SI-3**						−BL-66		**GB-41**
BL	**BL-67**				−BL-40	**LI-1**	−ST-36				
TE		−TE-2	**TE-3**						−BL-66		**GB-41**
GB	−GB-44	**GB-43**				−LI-1			**BL-66**		

Bold indicates tonification.

−, sedate.

TABLE 7.5 Four-point sedation protocol

Yin organs

	Wood	Fire	Earth	Metal	Water	LU	SP	HT	KI	PC	LR
LU		**LU-10**			–LU-5			**HT-8**	–KI-10		
SP	**SP-1**			–SP-5		–LU-8					**LR-1**
HT			–HT-7		**HT-3**		–SP-3		**KI-10**		
KI	–KI-1		**KI-3**				**SP-3**				–LR-1
PC			–PC-7		**PC-3**		–SP-3		**KI-10**		
LR		–LR-2		**LR-4**		**LU-8**		–HT-8			

Yang organs

	Metal	Water	Wood	Fire	Earth	LI	ST	SI	BL	TE	GB
LI		–LI-2		**LI-5**				**SI-5**	–BL-66		
ST	–ST-45		**ST-43**			–LI-1					**GB-41**
SI		**SI-2**			–SI-8		–ST-36		**BL-66**		
BL			–BL-65		**BL-40**		**ST-36**				–GB-41
TE		**TE-2**			–TE-10		–ST-36		**BL-66**		
GB	**GB-44**			–GB-38		**LI-1**		–SI-5			

Bold indicates tonification.
–, sedation.

| TABLE 7.6 | Summary of tonification protocol | | | |

	Tonify		Sedate	
LU	LU-9	SP-3	LU-10	HT-8
SP	SP-2	HT-8	SP-1	LR-1
HT	HT-9	LR-1	HT-3	KI-10
KI	KI-7	LU-8	KI-3	SP-3
PC	PC-9	LR-1	PC-3	KI-10
LR	LR-8	KI-10	LR-4	LU-8
LI	LI-11	ST-36	LI-5	SI-5
ST	ST-41	SI-5	ST-43	GB-41
SI	SI-3	GB-41	SI-2	BL-66
BL	BL-67	LI-1	BL-40	ST-36
TE	TE-3	GB-41	TE-2	BL-66
GB	GB-43	BL-66	GB-44	LI-1

| TABLE 7.7 | Summary of sedation protocol | | | |

	Tonify		Sedate	
LU	LU-10	HT-8	LU-5	KI-10
SP	SP-1	LR-1	SP-5	LU-8
HT	HT-3	KI-10	HT-7	SP-3
KI	KI-3	SP-3	KI-1	LR-1
PC	PC-3	KI-10	PC-7	SP-3
LR	LR-4	LU-8	LR-2	HT-8
LI	LI-5	SI-5	LI-2	BL-66
ST	ST-43	GB-41	ST-45	LI-1
SI	SI-2	BL-66	SI-8	ST-36
BL	BL-40	ST-36	BL-65	GB-41
TE	TE-2	BL-66	TE-10	ST-36
GB	GB-44	LI-1	GB-38	SI-5

Five-Element Four-Point Protocol for Dispersing Cold and Heat

A simple but powerful Five-Element four-point protocol can be used to disperse both internal and external Cold and Heat as summarized in Table 7.8. To disperse Heat from an organ, tonify the Water point and sedate the Fire point of the organ, then tonify the Water point on the Water meridians, Kidney or Bladder channels (the horary points) and sedate the Fire point on the Fire meridians, Heart and Small Intestine channels. To disperse Cold, do exactly the opposite: tonify the Fire point and sedate the Water point of the organ channel, and tonify the Fire point on the Heart or Small Intestine channels, and sedate the Water point on the Kidney or Bladder channels. Use corresponding Yin channels for Yin organs, and Yang channels for Yang organs.

For example, to disperse Heat from the Stomach: tonify ST-44, the Water point on Stomach meridian, and sedate ST-41, the Fire point on the Stomach meridian. Then go to the horary points on the Yang Water and Fire channels: tonify BL-66, the Water point on the Yang Water Bladder channel, and sedate SI-5, the Fire point on the Yang Fire Small Intestine channel. The opposite treat-

TABLE 7.8	Summary of dispersing Heat and Cold			
Organ	**Tonify Water point**	**Sedate Fire point**	**Tonify Horary Water**	**Sedate Horary Fire**
Dispersing Heat Yin organs				
LU	**LU-5**	LU-10	**KI-10**	HT-8
SP	**SP-9**	SP-2	**KI-10**	HT-8
HT	**HT-3**	HT-8	**KI-10**	PC-8
KI	**KI-10**	KI-2	**KI-10**	HT-8
PC	**PC-3**	PC-8	**KI-10**	HT-8
LR	**LR-8**	LR-2	**KI-10**	HT-8
Yang organs				
LI	**LI-2**	LI-5	**BL-66**	SI- 5
ST	**ST-44**	ST-41	**BL-66**	SI-5
SI	**SI-2**	SI-5	**BL-66**	TE-6
BL	**BL-66**	BL-60	**BL-66**	SI-5
TE	**TE-2**	TE-6	**BL-66**	SI-5
GB	**GB-4E**	GB-38	**BL-66**	SI-5
	Sedate Water point	**Tonify Fire point**	**Sedate Horary Water**	**Tonify Horary Fire**
Dispersing Cold Yin organs				
LU	LU-5	**LU-10**	KI-10	**HT-8**
SP	SP-9	**SP-2**	KI-10	**HT-8**
HT	HT-3	**HT-8**	KI-10	**PC-8**
KI	KI-10	**KI-2**	KI-10	**HT-8**
PC	PC-3	**PC-8**	KI-10	**HT-8**
LR	LR-2	**LR-8**	KI-10	**HT-8**
Yang organs				
LI	LI-2	**LI-5**	BL-66	**SI-5**
ST	ST-44	**ST-41**	BL-66	**SI-5**
SI	SI-2	**SI-5**	BL-66	**TE-6**
BL	BL-66	**BL-60**	BL-66	**SI-5**
TE	TE-2	**TE-6**	BL-66	**SI-5**
GB	GB-4E	**GB-38**	BL-66	**SI-5**

Bold indicates tonification.

ment would be the effect for dispersing Cold. For example, if there is internal Cold in the Lungs, tonify LU-10, the Fire point on the Lung channel, and sedate LU-5, the Water point on the Lung channel. Then go to the Yin Water and Fire channels, and tonify HT-8, the Fire point on the Yin Fire Heart channel and sedate KI-1, the Water point on the Yin Water Kidney channel. The Five-Element Heat/Fire and Cold/Water points are shown in Table 7.9.

TABLE 7.9		Five-Element Heat/Fire and Cold/Water points								
	Wood	Fire	Earth	Metal	Water		Metal	Water	Wood	Fire	Earth
LU	11	10	9	8	5	LI	1	2	3	5	11
SP	1	2	3	5	9	ST	45	44	43	41	36
HT	9	8	7	4	3	SI	1	2	3	5	8
KI	1	2	3	7	10	BL	67	66	65	60	40
PC	9	8	7	5	3	TE	1	2	3	6	10
LR	1	2	3	4	8	GB	44	43	41	38	34

Specific Treatment Protocols

The principle of treatment is to expel the pathogen, bring the body into a state of balance, and tonify the child after the acute illness.

Wind Invasions

Two major points to expel Wind:

- GB-20 Fengchi, Windpool
- GV-16 Fengfu, Palace of Wind.

Wind-Cold Invasion

Treatment is according to the stage of invasion.

Tai Yang Stage

- LU-7, LI-4, BL-12—TCM recommended points for expelling Wind-Cold
- LI-4 + KI-7 to cause sweating
- LI-20 local point for nasal congestion, can connect with an ion pumping cord to a distal point, e.g., a Stomach point or the universal dumping point, BL-60
- Tonify Wei Qi with complete immune protocol or use minimally with BL-13, BL-20, BL-23.

Shao Yang Stage

- LU-7, LI-4, BL-12
- LI-4 + KI-7
- GV-14 if there is fever
- Use two-point tonification protocol to prophylactically tonify the Stomach and Large Intestine channels to prevent progression of invasion into the Yang Ming stage
- After the Shao Yang symptoms have abated, tonify the immune system.

Yang Ming Stage

- Lots of extra fluids to prevent dehydration
- GV-14 and cooling measures for fever

- LI-11 overall clearing of Heat
- Use the Five-Element four-point protocol to disperse Heat in the Yang Ming channels: Large Intestine or Stomach or both
- Use two-point tonification protocol to prophylactically tonify the Spleen and Lung channels to prevent progression of invasion into the next stage
- After the Yang Ming and any Shao Yang symptoms have abated, tonify the immune system.

Tai Yin Stage

Vigorously dispel Cold from the Lung or Spleen with the Five-Element four-point protocol.

- KI-3, KI-7 tonify Yang, warms the child
- LU-7, BL-13 for cough
- LU-5 resolves Lung Phlegm, restores descending of Lung Qi
- Use two-point tonification protocol to prophylactically tonify the Shao Yin organs: e.g., HT-3 (–) to HT-7 (+); KI-3 (–) to KI-10 (+)
- After the child recovers, tonify the immune system and the Lung.

Shao Yin Stage

There is internal Cold in the Shao Yin channels and organs and the child is gravely ill. Intensive Western treatment with intravenous antibiotics and medications, close monitor of vital signs, are necessary. Acupuncture treatment can be directed toward expelling Cold from the Heart and Kidney. The treatment now is toward strengthening the child by diminishing internal Cold as the child is too weak at this point to expel the pathogen.

It is necessary to vigorously tonify the Liver Blood and Yin by using the Five-Element four-point tonification protocol, which is stronger than the two-point simple tonification of the meridian.

After the child recovers, tonify the immune system and all the internal organs that have been injured in the invasion.

Jue Yin Stage

The child is critically ill and needs emergency/intensive Western treatment and monitoring. There is a great swing between the extremes of Cold and Heat symptoms, and acupuncture treatments for dissipating Cold and Heat must be carried out with great care as to not overly cool or warm the child. Acupuncture can be used as an adjunctive, symptomatic treatment for symptoms such as vomiting. After the child recovers, long-term tonification treatments are needed to restore balance to all the internal organs.

Wind-Heat Invasion

Wei Qi Level

- Expel Wind with GB-20, GV-16
- LI-4 + KI-7 to cause sweating

- GV-14 for fever
- LI-11 to clear Heat
- KI-3 to balance alternative fever and chills
- Tonify immune system
- Local points, e.g. CV-22 for pharyngitis.

Since Wind-Heat invasions spread quickly, it is important at this beginning level to tonify the subsequent organs to prevent further penetration of the pathogen. Use a simple two-point technique to tonify Shao Yang and Yang Ming channels.

Qi Level

Vigorously treat fever with GV-14, LI-11, and disperse Heat from whichever channel that is manifesting clinical symptoms. For example, cough with fever and yellow phlegm indicates Lung Heat, so the treatment is the Five-Element four-point protocol to disperse Lung Heat. Abdominal pain with vomiting and dry throat indicates Stomach Heat, and the treatment is the Five-Element four-point protocol to disperse Stomach Heat. Replenish fluids to prevent dehydration.

Vigorously tonify the next level to prevent further progression of invasion. For example, if the invasion is in the Yang Ming channel and organ, use the Five-Element four-point tonification protocol to tonify the Lung. If there are already Lung symptoms, use the Five-Element four-point tonification protocol to tonify the Heart and the Kidney. Since Wind-Heat is much more virulent than Wind-Cold, the four-point protocol is stronger than the two-point simple tonification of the meridians.

After expelling the pathogen, continue vigorously tonifying the various organs and channels, and tonify the immune system.

Nutritive Qi Level

Treatment is the same as the Shao Yin stage of Wind-Cold invasion.

Blood Level

Treatment is the same as the Jue Yin stage of Wind-Cold invasion.

Dampness

- ST-40 is a major point for resolving Dampness
- SP-9 is another major point, especially for Dampness in the Lower Energizer
- Dampness often combines with Heat, and treatment of Damp Heat can be directed toward resolving Dampness and dispersing Heat from specific organ/channels.

REFERENCES

1. Colbert A. (2001) Magnet researcher. Personal communications.
2. Honzumi M., Shigemori C., Ito H., Mohri Y., Urata H. & Yamamoto T. (1995) An intestinal fistula in a 3 year old child caused by the ingestion of magnets: report of a case. *Surgery Today* 25(60): 552–553.
3. Liu S. (2001) Laser acupuncture primer. *California Journal of Oriental Medicine* 12(1): 23–29.
4. Schlager A., Offer T. & Baldissera I. (1998) Laser stimulation of point P6 reduces postoperative vomiting in children undergoing strabismus surgery. *British Journal of Anesthesia* 81: 529–532.
5. Asagai Y., Kianai H., Miura Y. & Ohshiro T. (1994) Application of low reactive-level laser therapy (LLLT) in the functional training of cerebral palsy patients. *Laser Therapy* 6: 195–202.
6. Loo M., Naeser M.A., Hinshaw S. & Bay R.B. Laser acupuncture treatment for ADHD. NIH grant #1 RO3 MH56009–01.
7. Naeser M.A. & Wei X.B. (1994) *Laser Acupuncture, An Introductory Textbook for Treatment of Pain, Paralysis Spasticity, and Other Disorders.* Boston Chinese Medicine, Boston.
8. Makela R. & Makela A. (1999) *Laser Acupuncture.* Earthpulse Flashpoints, Finland.
9. Mester E., Mester A.F. & Mester A. (1985) The biomedical effects of laser application. *Lasers in Surgery and Medicine* 5: 31–39.
10. Naeser M.A. (2001) Personal communication.
11. Oleson T. (1996) *Auriculotherapy Manual: Chinese and Western Systems of Ear Acupuncture.* Los Angeles, Health Care Alternatives.
12. Chow E.P.Y. & McGee C.T. (1996) *Miracle Healing from China. Qigong.* Coeur d'Alene, ID, Medipress.

8 | Dietary Management

The Western pediatrician monitors the diet closely during the first year of life as part of well child evaluations, taking care to note whether the baby is breast fed or formula fed, the number of ounces (grams) at each feeding, age at introduction of solids, etc. After that, adequacy of diet is interpreted in terms of the child's growth parameters: height and weight plotted on growth curves according to sex and age of the child. A child with average height and weight is usually considered healthy, with failure to thrive and obesity bracketing the two extremes of the weight spectrum.

In older children, the pediatrician advises a balanced diet consisting of foods from five major nutrient groups: carbohydrates, fats, proteins, vitamins, and minerals. Food values are measured in terms of precise number of calories they yield: 4 calories per gram of carbohydrate or protein, 9 calories per gram of fat. (1 kilogram-calorie, equivalent to 1000 gram calories, is the amount of energy that can raise 1 kg of water by 1°C.)

Proteins are needed for growth of tissues and for maintaining physiologic balance. Carbohydrates, which become glucose or sugar, provide the bulk of the energy in our daily diet. Fats are useful as stored energy, a sort of reserve tank, when carbohydrates are depleted. The Food and Nutrition Board gives recommendations of daily dietary and calorie allowances according to a person's age and sex. Freshness, time of harvest, flavor (except for sweet taste), the effect of food on organ systems or body temperature are not taken into consideration in this calorie-based dietary system. Indeed, children who fail to thrive are often given synthetically prepared, bland tasting, high caloric canned foods to boost their weight. Excess sweets and junk foods are usually discouraged.

In some instances, a nutritionist is consulted for calorie counting as in obesity or for special diet as in diabetes. However, in spite of all the biochemical explanations, modern science is still baffled by most conditions associated with food, such as obesity and eating disorders.

Chinese pediatricians place much more emphasis on the diet throughout childhood. They are concerned not only with what children eat, but when, where, and how they eat. Although it is unclear where the phrase "we are what we eat" originated, it well reflects the Chinese emphasis of food in relationship to health and disease. The Chinese love of food is evidenced by their renowned cuisine, whereby a person may have a different dish each day without duplication for at least one year. There is a saying that goes something like this: If something new were invented today, the Germans would try to analyze it, the Americans would want to find a way to send it to the Moon, and the Chinese would try to eat it. It is, therefore, no surprise that health and disease are considered to be intimately related to the diet. As a matter of fact, since foods have medicinal values, there are some Chinese physicians who consider all illnesses arise from inadequate and inappropriate eating.

Dietary management in children focuses primarily on the types of food which have global effects and those that have organ specific effects; and on the manner of eating food. Any disturbance after food is consumed should also be taken into consideration.

TYPES OF FOOD

Food for Overall Health Management

Maintenance Diet: Fresh, Natural, Organic

Except for the difference in taste, the Western caloric system is not concerned with freshness, so that a frozen packet of broccoli has the same calories as an equal amount of fresh broccoli.

Freshness is very important in the Chinese diet, since Qi comes from living things: plants and animals. Eating vegetables as soon as they are harvested and eating animals as soon as they are slaughtered would provide the maximum Qi from the food. The Chinese traditionally go to the market at dawn for freshly picked vegetables and for live fish still swimming in the tanks. The food Qi, Gu Qi, combines with the Qi in the air we breathe, to form Nutritive Qi that circulates in our body. From this standpoint, there is no Nutritive Qi value in packaged and frozen foods. Vegetables grown organically without pesticides and animals naturally fed are preferred to minimize chemical contamination in foods.

The diet needs to have a balance of five flavors for maintaining organ harmony: pungent/spicy, salty, sour, and bitter and natural sweet taste. This is discussed in greater detail in the section on flavors.

Food Tonics

Foods can be used as tonics for overall states of deficiency. There are four general categories of food tonics: Yin tonics, Yang tonics, Qi tonics, Blood tonics. The management is straightforward: when there is Yin deficiency, give the child Yin tonics and decrease foods that are Yang tonics; vice versa with Yang deficiency. When the child has Qi or Blood deficiency, give Qi and Blood tonics, respectively.

Yin Tonics

Children are constitutionally Yin deficient, which is easily aggravated by recurrent illnesses with Heat that consumes Yin. Eating Yin tonic foods regularly can diminish the injurious effects of Heat illnesses. Some foods that tonify the Yin are: abalone, apples, asparagus, bananas, barley, beets, blackberries, cantaloupes, clams, coconut milk, crab, cuttlefish, dates, duck, eggs (chicken), figs, grapes, honey, kidney beans, lemons, mandarin oranges, mangoes, microalgae (especially *Chlorella* and *Spirulina*), millet, mussels, oysters, peas, pears, pineapples, pomegranates, pork, rice, sardines, sea cucumber, seaweed, shrimp, star fruit, string beans, tomatoes, tofu, walnuts, watermelons, wheat, wheat germ, and yams. By adding more liquid to these foods to make soups or stews, the Yin quality is increased and the healing property is enhanced.

Yang Tonics

Children tend to be overall Yang excessive and Yin deficient, but have "young Yang and young Yin." However, sometimes Yang tonics would be appreciated in specific deficiencies, such as Spleen, which is often both Yin and Yang deficient. The Yang tonics can be given in small amounts in order not to aggravate the usual Yin deficiency state: chestnuts, cinnamon, cloves, dill seeds, lobster, pistachio nuts, raspberries, and strawberries.

Qi Tonics

Children have tender Qi that can easily become deficient due to physical or emotional stress, chronic illness, improper diet, too much studying or exercise. The symptoms are milder than Yang deficiency and may occur gradually over several weeks or months: fatigue, a lower-than-normal voice, a general feeling of weakness, a poor appetite, abdominal swelling, chronically soft stools, and frequent colds or infections. The Qi tonics can alleviate general Qi deficiency: beef, bird's nest, cherries, chicken, coconut, dates (red and black), eel, gingko, ginseng, goose, grapes, herring, honey, licorice, logan (dragon eye dried fruit), octopus, pigeon (egg and meat), potatoes (sweet and white), rabbit, rice, sugar (rock), shark's fin, shitake mushrooms, squash, string beans (white), sturgeon, and tofu.

Blood Tonics

Because Qi is the driving force for blood, a Qi deficiency is often accompanied by a Blood deficiency. The latter might be aggravated by any bleeding condition, such as nosebleeds, or menstruation in teenage girls. The most common Western diagnosis of this kind of deficiency is anemia, and its symptoms include dizziness, palpitations, nervousness, a pale complexion, numbness in the hands and feet, and, in teenage girls, a lightening of the menstrual flow. When Shen is affected, there may also be an inability to concentrate, insomnia, and forgetfulness. The Blood tonics can help: beef, eggs (chicken), grapes, ham, lichi nuts, liver (beef and pork), longan, milk (human breast), octopus, oysters, sea cucumber, and spinach.[1]

Contraindications to Tonics

There are two contraindications to giving tonics. Tonics are contraindicated during an active infection, which is equivalent to "trapping the burglar" described in Chapter 6. After the acute infection is cleared—the burglar is chased out—then tonify the child.

Tonics are contraindicated in digestive disorders, because the tonic may not be digested or absorbed. It is better to first treat the underlying gastrointestinal problem, and then give appropriate tonics to give the child an overall boost.

Thermoregulatory Properties of Foods

Western medicine emphasizes overall body temperature as a reflection of health. Normal temperature is 98.6°F (37°C) orally. Hyperthermia, fever, usually signifies infection; while hypothermia may indicate exposure to cold weather or chronic conditions, even cancer. Foods are not attributed with any direct effect on body temperature.

Chinese medicine recognizes that foods have powerful thermoregulatory properties that influence Qi and fluid movements. These properties constitute the major herbal, medicinal value in foods. The thermoregulatory properties have the following characteristics:

- *Hot*: Yang foods that direct Qi and fluid upward and outward to the skin; e.g., beets, brussel sprouts, cinnamon, lamb, peaches, pepper (black, white, cayenne)
- *Warm*: similar to hot foods, but milder effect; e.g., asparagus, chicken, peanuts, red wine, squash
- *Neutral*: most foods fall into this category: e.g., chard, lettuce, sweet potato, taro root, brown rice, rye, almond, peanut, fish
- *Cool*: Yin foods that direct energy and fluid downward and inward, so that the upper part of the body and the skin are cold; e.g., barley, eggplant, pork, strawberries, tofu
- *Cold*: similar to cool foods, but with a stronger effect: e.g., apples, celery, cottage cheese, mussels, salt.

The various foods are listed in Table 8.1.

The cultivation and physical characteristics of plants affect their thermoregulatory properties; the more cooling foods are ones that grow quickly, such as lettuce and radishes; chemically fertilized (which grow more quickly); and foods with "cooler" colors, such as blue, green, and purple, whereas foods that are red, orange, and yellow are more warming.

Food preparation and cooking can affect thermoregulatory properties. Any process that breaks up food, such as chopping or cutting, would release more Qi and Heat. Moderate cooking loses relatively few nutrients and breaks down food structures so that more nutrients are made available. Cooking for a long time on low heat is more warming than cooking for a short time on high heat. Among cooking methods, the usual order from most warming to least is: deep-frying or tempura, baking, stir-frying, sautéing, pressure cooking, simmering, steaming, and waterless cooking to below the boiling point. Cooking with electricity produces the lowest amount of warmth and is therefore not recommended for weak people. Microwave cooking damages the molecular structure of food and diminishes Qi. Raw foods require more Qi for digestion and is therefore cooling.

A well-balanced diet is one that consists of the right amount of hot, warm, neutral, cool, and cold foods. Too many hot or warm foods and too few cool or cold foods can lead to excess Heat (or excess Yang) symptoms such as dry mouth, constipation, thirst, red face, aversion to heat, sweaty palms, red rashes, a faster heart rate, nervousness, and so on. Children with excess Heat should be given fewer hot or warm foods and more cool or cold foods; more liquids; while reducing their stress.

Excess Cold (excess Yin) symptoms may be chill sensations, copious urine, watery stools, increased fear, white complexion, aversion to cold, difficulty in moving, and so on. These children should be given more hot or warm foods and fewer cool or cold foods, and no raw or microwaved foods.

Phlegm/Damp-producing foods are very important in children, since they are injurious to the Spleen, which is constitutionally deficient in children.

TABLE 8.1	Thermoenergetic properties of foods				
	Cold	**Cool**	**Neutral**	**Warm**	**Hot**
Vegetables	Chinese cabbage, bean sprout, seaweed, snow pea, water chestnut, white mushroom	Beet, carrot, corn, cucumber, turnip, zucchini, broccoli, cabbage, celery, potato, eggplant, pumpkin, spinach, watercress, alfalfa sprout, asparagus, cauliflower, bamboo shoot, bok choy, button mushroom, endive, lettuce, romaine lettuce, soy bean sprout, summer squash, winter melon, winter squash	Chard, lettuce, Shitake mushroom, sweet potato, taro root, yam	Bell pepper, Chinese chive, green bean, kale, leek, mustard, green onion, parsley, parsnip	Garlic, scallion, ginger
Fruits	Banana, cantaloupe, grapefruit, pear, watermelon	Apple, apricot, fig, lemon, orange, peach, persimmon, strawberry, tomato	Chinese date, mango, olive, papaya	Cherry, grape, coconut, plum, dried papaya, lychee, pineapple, raspberry, tangerine	
Grains		Millet, pearl barley, white rice, wheat	Buckwheat, brown rice, corn meal, rice bran, rye	Oats, sweet rice, wheat bran, wheat germ	
Seeds, Beans	Pumpkin seed	Mung bean, soy bean, tofu, winter melon seed	Almond, black sesame seed, filbert, kidney bean, peanut, pea, sunflower seed	Black bean, brown sesame seed, chestnut, lentil, pine nut, walnut	
Animal products	Pork	Chicken egg, clam, crab	Fish (ocean), gelatin, dairy products, oyster	Beef, chicken, fish (freshwater), shrimp, turkey	Lamb
Miscellaneous	Salt, vitamin C, white sugar	Tea	Barley malt, rice malt, black fungus, honey, white fungus	Brown sugar, coffee, molasses, rice vinegar, wine	

Dampness and Phlegm obstruct Qi flow in the channels, and also prevent the Spleen from carrying out the digestive functions of transforming and transporting Qi. Spleen deficiency and Damp can in turn be responsible for respiratory congestion and Phlegm formation.

- *Phlegm-producing foods*: milk and milk products, sugar, honey, peanuts, almonds, or pork
- *Foods that thin Phlegm*: mushrooms, papaya, potatoes, pumpkin, radishes, strawberries, string beans.

FOOD FOR SPECIFIC ORGAN MANAGEMENT ACCORDING TO THE FIVE ELEMENTS

The Five-Element correspondence of flavors and seasonal variation can be used both for organ health maintenance and for overcoming a specific organ weakness (Table 8.2).

Flavors

Chinese medicine posits that each of the major flavors of food has a specific effect on Qi flow, on body fluids, and on the Five-Element Yin–Yang organ couplets.

Ideally, a child should have a diet with a balance of the five basic flavors. A diet with either a deficiency or excess of a flavor would weaken the corresponding organs. However, the age of the child and the developmental phase, would also contribute to the vulnerability of the organ/system and therefore to a specific flavor. For example, a child in the Wood phase of development would be more vulnerable to the sour taste.

In general, naturally occurring flavor is always preferable to artificial flavoring, so that the sweetness in fruits and vegetables are healthy for children, whereas cakes, candies, and cookies with added sugar are not. However, artificial flavoring can be added in moderate amounts to balance a deficiency; e.g., extra salt can be added if there is a deficiency of salty foods in the diet.

Sour-Liver (Wood)

Sour is a Yin flavor and tends to cause contraction, which has an astringent effect on body fluids and energy. It enters the Liver and helps with digesting

TABLE 8.2	The Five Elements: organ, flavor and seasonal correspondences		
Element	**Taste**	**Organs**	**Time of year**
Wood	Sour	Liver, Gallbladder	Spring
Fire	Bitter	Heart/Pericardium, Small Intestine/Triple Energizer	Summer
Earth	Sweet	Spleen/Pancreas, Stomach	Late Summer
Metal	Pungent/spicy	Lung, Large Intestine	Fall
Water	Salty	Kidney, Bladder	Winter

rich, greasy, fatty, and high-cholesterol foods. The taste derives from a great variety of acids, including citric, tannic, and ascorbic (vitamin C). It is the least common taste in the Western diet. The most purely sour flavors occur in black and green teas and blackberry leaves. Other sour foods are hawthorn berries, lemons, limes, pickles, sauerkraut, sour apples (crabapples), and sour plums.

Most children are Liver Yang excessed and Liver Yin deficient. Yin tonic foods would help the child achieve a better internal Liver balance of Yin and Yang. Many junk foods that children prefer tend to be greasy, fried foods such as French fries, chips, fried chicken, which are injurious to the Liver. A healthy balance of sour, spicy and sweet foods would harmonize the Metal–Wood, Wood–Earth Ke cycle relationship, and equal amounts of salty, sour, and bitter foods would prevent excess or deficiency in the Water–Wood–Fire nurturing cycle.

Bitter-Heart (Fire)

Bitter is a Yin flavor, a cooling one that moves Qi downward in the body. A moderate amount of bitter foods can reduce excess Fire conditions such as loudness, a red complexion, and aggressiveness, but too much can sometimes bring about the opposite effect. The bitter flavor can also reduce fever, clear heat (e.g., from eating too many rich foods), bring about dryness.

Bitter foods include most medications as well as alfalfa, bitter melon, chamomile, dandelion leaf or root, *Echinacea*, hops, romaine lettuce, rye, and valerian.

Most children find a bitter taste too harsh. Mary Poppin's formula of "a spoonful of sugar makes the medicine go down" would work only if the "sugar" is a naturally occurring sweet food. The powerfully bitter taste of medicine may cause Fire deficiency. Heart deficiency, being the Mother of Spleen, may result in the Spleen/Earth deficiency. Naturally sweetened foods may strengthen the Spleen, whereas artificial sugar would further weaken the Spleen, and disrupt the digestion of the medication.

A small amount of naturally occurring bitter foods would help to balance the Heart, especially in the teenager during the Fire phase of development. While children rarely manifest cardiac symptoms, a bitter taste used sparingly can help in Spleen deficiency symptoms such as digestive problems, fatigue, or even poor concentration for memorizing facts.

In children who tend to be cold, weak, or dry, or have excess Lung symptoms, bitter taste should be used cautiously as Fire controls and therefore weakens Metal/Lung. From a Chinese medicine standpoint, it is therefore paradoxical to give bitter tasting medications to children with asthma or recurrent pneumonia.

Sweet-Spleen/Pancreas (Earth)

Sweet is the most common flavor in children's diet. It is a Yang flavor that generally has a warming effect and moves Qi upward and outward through the skin. It builds tissues and fluids—the Yin of the body—and, therefore, also strengthens Yin deficiencies.

The sweet flavor naturally predominates in most people's diet because most foods in nature have this taste: grains, vegetables, nuts, seeds, and fruits. A reasonable predominance is compatible with human physiology, since the Spleen and the Stomach are Earth organs and have a predilection for sweetness. However, children today eat an overabundance of candies, cakes, cookies, and sodas—foods with artificial sweeteners which are very detrimental to the digestive organs. Even the snacks that are considered "healthy" actually contain excess sweeteners. There is biochemical support for naturally occurring sweet foods being healthier than synthetic sweet foods. Both have the formula $C_6H_{12}O_6$. However, the biochemical structure of fructose—the sugar in most fruits and some vegetables—is a ketone, a very reactive organic compound of the general structure R–C=O–R', in which R and R' represent organic radicals and C=O is the ketone radical. Under ordinary conditions, ketones oxidize quickly to water and carbon dioxide and are important intermediaries in cell metabolism. Carbohydrate breaks down into simple monosaccharide glucose, the main nutrient for the brain and major source of energy. Artificial sweeteners, especially confectioners' sugar, is high in calories, more difficult to digest, and has less nutritional value.

The most important naturally occurring sweet foods are all of the grains. These carbohydrates break down into glucose. Other examples are:

- Fruits: apples, apricots, cherries, dates, figs, papayas
- Vegetables: beets, button mushrooms, carrots, chard, cucumbers, eggplants, peas, potatoes, shitake mushrooms, squash, sweet potatoes, yams
- Nuts and seeds: almonds, chestnuts, coconuts, sesame seeds and oil, pine nuts, sunflower seeds, walnuts
- Natural sweeteners: molasses, rice syrup, and honey. It is important to note that since honey is often given for congestion as it dries up mucus, it should be used with caution in deficient children since honey can continue to exert a drying effect and injure the Yin.

Because Earth nurtures Metal, naturally sweet foods can assist the Lungs, especially during a state of deficiency. They're also good for children who tend to become deficient: dry, cold, nervous, thin, or weak. Aggressive, angry, or impatient children—the Wood Yang excess ones—can benefit from the retarding effect of the sweet flavor. In this kind of situation, extra consumption of wheat, rice, and oats often helps.

Both Western and Chinese physicians would advise the overweight child to decrease their intake of sweet foods. The Western physician comes from the perspective that sweets are high in calories. The Chinese physician recommendation is based on the fact that the overweight children—as well as children who tend to have mucus—are Spleen deficient, and excess sweets cause further deficiency. It is also important that children learn to chew carbohydrates and other sweet foods thoroughly. The salivary enzymes in the mouth breakdown the foods and alleviate the burden to the Stomach and Spleen.

Milk and milk products are advocated in the West as an important constituent in children's diet. According to Chinese medicine, these are Phlegm-producing foods that are injurious to the Spleen, which prefers dryness. The combination of artificially sweetened foods and Phlegm-producing foods predispose children to a weak Spleen and Spleen deficiency.

Pungent/Spicy-Lung (Metal)

This flavor has Yang qualities. It warms the body, assists the circulation of Qi and Blood, stimulates the digestive process, disperses mucus, and enters the Lungs. Cough and mucus-producing respiratory conditions, such as URI, bronchitis, asthma, can deteriorate when there is a deficiency of spicy flavors in the child. Examples of pungent/spicy foods include: garlic, mint, scallion, chamomile, which induce diaphoresis and therefore are beneficial for expelling pathogens in the early stages of invasion. These and other spicy foods, such as basil, cayenne, cinnamon, garlic, ginger root, onions, pepper, cannot be given to children during fever. The more cooling ones, such as peppermint, white pepper, or radish leaves, can be given during fever. The medicinal potency of pungent/spicy foods can be diminished by cooking.

To tonify the Lungs, the child needs to eat almost equal amounts of naturally sweet foods (Earth nurtures Metal) and pungent/spicy foods, with proportionately fewer bitter foods (Fire destroys Metal). Because Metal nurtures Water, cautious consumption of pungent/spicy foods (avoiding excess) can help children who manifest Kidney Yang deficiency with symptoms of coldness, such as cold extremities. Pungent/spicy foods should also be consumed sparingly in dry and heat conditions. Spices should also be decreased in children on medication to prevent further injury to the Liver, since Metal controls Wood, and medications often weaken the Liver.

Salt-Kidney (Water)

Salt is the second most common flavor in a child's diet, present in excess amount in many junk foods that children like: chips, pretzels, and French fries.

Salt is a Yin flavor and tends to cool, moisten, and detoxify the body. In a balanced amount, it can increase appetite and improve digestion. It is beneficial in conditions of dryness (e.g., gargling with salt water is advisable for a sore throat; and brushing the teeth with fine salt, for mild gum inflammations).

Major salty foods are salt itself and seaweed (such as kelp). Other salty foods are miso, pickles, and soy sauce. Barley and millet are primarily sweet foods, but they also have salty qualities.

To tonify Kidneys, the child should consume equal amounts of salt and pungent/spicy foods (Metal nurtures Water), with proportionately fewer sweet foods (Earth destroys Water). In any Kidney disorder, such as congenital kidney disease, salt intake should be restricted. Because Water controls Fire, excess salt can also have an adverse effect on the Heart, which is important in the teenage Fire developmental stage.

Food and Seasons

The Western diet places little emphasis on foods' relation to the seasons. With the convenience of preserved and frozen foods, eating foods that are in season is no longer a necessity. Chinese medicine adopts a different point of view. Man is part of Nature, a microcosm within a macrocosm. Giving children foods that are in season would enable them to be more in tune with the rhythm of Nature, with the natural progression of the Five Elements.

Wood-Spring

Spring represents youth, renewal, and growth, like a young tree relying on nutrients from the earth and ascending into the sky. A good spring diet reflects all of these characteristics: naturally sweet foods of Earth; green, leafy vegetables; sprouts and seeds; and raw or tender, young vegetables, such as baby carrots and small beets.

Decrease foods that are taxing on the Wood-Liver: fat, greasy foods; chemicals (medications are predominantly metabolized in the Liver); alcohol and processed foods. Children in the Wood phase of development are especially vulnerable, so that young drinkers sustain much greater insult to the Liver than teenagers and adults. Some Chinese dietary experts believe that "spring fever" is caused by ingesting seasonally inappropriate foods that are poorly digested and metabolized and convert into Heat and, therefore, a sense of "fever."[2]

Cooking in the spring should include some pungent/spicy herbs and seeds: basil, bay leaf, caraway, dill, fennel, marjoram, and rosemary. Food should be cooked for a shorter time at a higher temperature: stir-frying, sautéing with just a small amount of oil (to avoid Liver harm), and steaming or simmering lightly. Since spring is Wood, growth, movement, children should be physically active.

Fire-Summer

Summer is the most Yang of all the seasons. Children should engage in a lot of outdoor activities, sit in the shade to cool off naturally, and drink lots of water to prevent dehydration. They should eat brightly colored fruits and vegetables that are in season, and eat light meals, such as salads with sprouts, alfalfa, and cucumber; vegetables like tofu; fruits like watermelon, apples, and lemon; and drinks like lemonade, apple juice. They should avoid heavy foods such as meat, eggs, and an overabundance of grains, nuts, and seeds. Food should be prepared as quickly as possible using high heat.

Pungent/spicy foods in modest amounts can sometimes be beneficial because they trigger sweating: e.g., cayenne, ginger (fresh, not dried), horseradish, and pepper (black as well as red and green hot peppers). The principle here is to bring the body into harmony with the temperature of the environment. Sweating disperses body heat through the pores, so that the skin temperature more closely approximates to the hot summer temperature and, accordingly, the body feels more comfortable. This is why countries in the tropics frequently have very spicy cuisines. Moderation is important: when children eat excessive amount of hot, spicy foods in the summer, they can lose too much internal Heat as they enter the colder months in fall and winter.

Contrary to modern Western practice, ice-cold drinks or foods are not recommended even during the hottest summer days. Putting such foods into the Stomach causes contraction and slows down the digestive process. In addition, the pores contract so that they don't sweat, resulting ultimately in a more uncomfortable, "feverish" feeling. The same sort of shock occurs when children move quickly from the hot, outside air into a very cold, air-conditioned room. One of the worst drinks for children is the icee, which contains ice, sugar, and food coloring—the latter two often contain an organic aldehyde radical which has the same effect as alcohol.

Earth-Late Summer

This is time of harvest and transition from Yang (growth) to Yin (rest). Children need to slow down and do things in moderation. During this Earth season, encourage the pediatric patients to engage in calming activities to become more centered.

Children need to eat more "earthy-colored," naturally sweet foods such as carrots, yellow corn, and yellow squash; round-shaped foods for centering are apricots, cabbage, cantaloupe, chestnuts, filberts, garbanzo beans, millet, peas, rice, soybeans. Foods should be cooked with mild spices and at moderate temperatures.

Metal-Fall

It is ironic that children begin school in fall, a time when they should start to pull inward and slow down in preparation for winter. However, Metal corresponds to organization, an important skill that children learn in school such as organizing their time, their studies; and for older children, their plans for college and the future.

Since Metal corresponds to the Lungs, and the external orifice for the Lung is the nose, the fragrance and smell from cooking food slowly on lower heat can stimulate children's appetite. This is the season when respiratory illnesses such as URI and asthma are prevalent. Infants and young children in the Metal/Metal to Water transition phase of development are especially vulnerable. Since dryness is injurious to Lungs, children can benefit from eating foods that tend to moisten the body: almonds, apples, barley, barley malt, clams, crabs, dairy products, eggs, fungus (black and white), herring (cooked), honey, millet, mussels, oysters, peanuts, pears, persimmons, pine nuts, pork, rice syrup, seaweeds, sesame seeds, spinach, and soybean products, including soy milk and tofu.

Water-Winter

Winter is the most Yin of all the seasons. At this time of the year, children need more rest as the days grow shorter. Just like hibernating animals, they need to keep the inside of their body warm, while contracting the pores to keep their skin cool so that they harmonize with the outside environment. Children can afford to gain a little weight as it is the season to store up food that can be burned off the following summer.

In winter, warm, hearty soups with a little added salt are the perfect meals. Too much water in the soup can weaken the organ systems. Cooking should be at a low temperature for a long time. Unless salt is not advisable for medical reasons (like a Kidney disorder), salt intake can be increased. Counterbalance the salty foods with some bitter foods to nourish the Heart and preserve joyfulness. Good Kidney-nourishing foods are barley, millet, miso, seaweeds, salt, and soy sauce. Since winter is cold, children should eat more naturally warming foods.

MANNER OF EATING

Other than concerns for possible indigestion when children eat too fast, Western medicine in general disregards manner of eating as calories do not change regardless of how they are consumed. Chinese medicine posits that even with the most nutritious and freshest foods, the manner of eating can cause significant Qi disturbance.

Healthy eating encompasses more than just consuming food. Meals should be pleasant experiences so that children enjoy eating and value food. The major cuisines in the world take great care in the presentation of food to make meals pleasing to the eye which would in turn stimulate appetite. A glob of mashed potatoes and macaroni may fill up a hungry little stomach but would do little to encourage enjoyment of eating.

The manner of eating entails an adequate amount of time spent eating, times of meals, eating habits, appetite variations, and the emotional state while eating.

Adequate Amount of Time for Eating

Today's fast-paced life often translates into meals on the go. Children eat on the way home from school, to the soccer game—often swallowing before thoroughly chewing the food. With parents' busy work schedule, fewer and fewer families spend time eating together. Children resort to heating up leftovers or packaged foods in the microwave, and eating while doing homework, reading, or watching TV.

Western pediatricians advise children that eating too fast can lead to indigestion. Digestion begins with chewing, which stimulates the secretion of salivary enzymes that initiate the digestive process. The Chinese also recognize the value of saliva, and call it the "golden, precious fluid" that imparts warmth to food.

The partially digested food is then sent down to the Stomach, which "rots and ripens" food. This correlates to the Western concept of further breakdown of food by stomach acid and enzymes. When children swallow food without chewing properly, the Stomach receives a large amount of food that has not been appropriately broken down by salivary enzymes. It becomes overloaded, resulting in Qi and food stagnation. The Stomach is overwhelmed and overworked, leading to Stomach Qi deficiency. The next step of digestion involves Spleen Qi, which transforms food into Nutritive Qi and transports Qi to the rest of the body. When the child routinely eats while studying, Spleen Qi is needed also for thinking and learning information, which can lead to Spleen Qi deficiency. This may occur even with "mindless" activities like watching TV.

Time of Meals

Western medicine generally recommends that children eat three healthy meals a day, with breakfast in the morning, lunch around the noon hour, and dinner in the evening. Chinese medicine follows the 2-hour horary cycle when each organ operates at its maximum Qi. Stomach Qi is at the maximum between 7 a.m. and 9 a.m., while Spleen Qi is maximum between 9 a.m. and 11 a.m. They are at the minimum between 7 p.m. to 9 p.m. and 9 p.m. to 11 p.m., respectively. Therefore, the most physiologic schedule is eating a good breakfast, an early lunch, and a light dinner before 7 p.m. It would also be sensible to avoid eating big meals in the evening, and to eat no food after 9 p.m.

The busy schedule of the school-age children often necessitate physiologically detrimental eating style. They frequently skip breakfast, especially those children who begin school early in the morning around 7 a.m. When Stomach Qi is not called to duty, it gradually becomes deficient. Children then often eat dinner after sports, music lessons, and other extracurricular activities—at 7 p.m. or even after 9 p.m.—the period of lowest Stomach and Spleen Qi function. Then there are those children who routinely would eat a snack such as cookies or ice cream before bedtime. All of these can lead to Stomach Qi and Yin deficiency.

Eating Habits

Children often develop poor eating habits that can cause Stomach and Spleen deficiency, food stagnation, or even physical symptoms of abdominal pain.

Some children nibble all day long instead of eating regular meals. Digestive functions would be erratic throughout the day, resulting in food stagnation and possibly also Stomach Qi stagnation.

Radical Changes in Dietary Habits

When there are sudden changes in dietary habits—which are frequently associated with divorce and moving house, when the family routine is disrupted—children may experience abdominal pain, especially in the epigastric region, and other Stomach complaints.

The extreme dietary habits occur in eating disorders, when there is excessive fasting or binge eating followed by self-induced vomiting. Both the Spleen and Stomach are stressed and become deficient.

Appetite Variations

Pediatricians are frequently confronted by parents who complain about their children's picky eating habits and appetite problems. When the growth parameters are within the normal range, parents are usually reassured that there is nothing of concern. Chinese medicine offers some explanation:

- Children who are picky eaters or who have poor appetite generally are Spleen Qi deficient
- When the appetite is good, but the bowel movements are irregular, there is strong Stomach Qi but deficient Spleen Qi
- Irregular appetite usually suggests some lingering pathogenic factor.

Emotional State While Eating

Western medicine sometimes attributes indigestion symptoms to stress during meals. The Chinese posit that eating should be a pleasant experience. The smell of food, pleasant conversations and/or music, even the sound of food preparation or clanging of utensils are appetite stimulants for moving digestive Qi. On the other hand, unpleasant emotions should not be part of any meal. Emotions often cause Heat to flare up—such as Liver Fire rising—as well as decreasing digestive functions, and can lead to Stomach Qi stagnation with Heat.

DISTURBANCES ASSOCIATED WITH EATING

- *Vomiting a little after feeding*: this is indicative of Stomach Yang deficiency, water in the Stomach, or in infants, indicates mother's milk may be too watery
- *Vomits a lot of partly digested food*: at any age, this means either stagnation or Spleen Cold from deficiency
- *Phlegm accumulation*: the child may simply vomit water, being unable to bring up the thick phlegm
- *Dry heaves*: the other end of the spectrum from Phlegm stagnation is dry heaves, which may be dehydration from fluid loss or Yin deficiency
- *Abdominal distention after meals*: this usually means Qi stagnation and Spleen Qi deficiency.

Table 8.3 summarizes manner of eating with energetic disturbances.

TABLE 8.3	Summary of eating and energetic imbalances					
	Food stagnation	ST Qi stagnation	ST Qi deficiency	ST Yang deficiency	ST Yin deficiency	SP Qi deficiency
Manner of eating						
Eat on the run, eat fast	X	X	X			
Eat while studying/reading	X	X				X
Eat while watching TV	X	X				X
Not chewing properly	X	X	X			
Not allowing digestion time			X			
Wrong time for eating						
Skip breakfast			X			
Eat dinner late			X		X	
Poor eating habits						
Nibbling	X	X				
Sudden change in habits (abdominal pain)	X	X				
Extreme—eating disorders			X			X
Appetite						
Poor appetite, picky eater						X
Irregular appetite (lingering pathogenic factor)						
Good appetite, irregular BM (Stomach strong)						X
Disturbance after eating						
Vomit a little				X		
Vomits partially digested food	X		X			
Dry heaves					X	
Abdominal distention		X				X
Eating while emotionally upset	+Heat					

TABLE 8.4 *Types of food*

Type of food	Injury to specific organ
Excess artificially sweetened	Spleen/Pancreas
Excess salt	Kidney
Greasy, fried	Liver
Phlegm-producing	Spleen
Thermoregulatory "Cold"	Spleen

DIETARY RECOMMENDATIONS FOR CHILDREN

Diet for Health Maintenance

- Give children fresh, nutritious foods that have a balance of five flavors
- Keep a regular eating schedule as much as possible
- Eat foods appropriate to the seasons as much as possible
- Avoid junk/greasy, artificially sweetened, artificially colored foods
- Avoid excess energetically Hot or Cold foods
- Institute healthy manner and habits for eating.

Diet as Treatment

- Food as medicine works slowly, therefore they do not produce quick and instantaneous changes
- Treat general conditions and deficiency states with tonics
- Tonics are contraindicated:
  - during the course of an active infection
  - when there is a digestive problem, as the child may throw it up, or not absorb it. First correct the digestive problem, then give appropriate tonics
- Supplement acupuncture treatment of Cold and Heat conditions with thermoregulatory foods
- Decrease the common foods that many children today prefer. Table 8.4 lists the five types of food and the corresponding injuries to organs
- Treat specific organ imbalance with corresponding flavors:
  - increase that flavor if there is deficiency, and
  - decrease the flavor if the child is consuming excess amount
- Discontinue detrimental manners of eating
- Explore individual and family reason for excess emotions during meals and treat underlying emotional problems
- Also consider involving child and/or family in therapy.

REFERENCES

1. Cao J. *et al.* (1990) *Essentials of Traditional Chinese Pediatrics.* Beijing, Foreign Language Press.

2. Pitchford P. (1993) *Healing with Whole Foods, Oriental Traditions and Modern Nutrition.* Berkeley, North Atlantic Books.

9 Childhood Infections and Immunizations: Update and Controversies

Immunization is a significant, integral part of conventional pediatrics. It is the cornerstone of preventive, well child care. It is also a major social and political issue, as many states in the US and countries worldwide require proper vaccinations for admission to schools. There is growing concern and controversy regarding the appropriateness of vaccinating children, particularly infants. The benefits and risks of immunization have created an upheaval for both pediatric practitioners and for parents. Many parents are raising questions about their necessity and potential side-effects, and some are seeking alternatives to traditional vaccines. It is of paramount importance for practitioners of both Western and Chinese medicine to be informed of the different perspectives so that they can be better prepared to answer parents' questions. This chapter discusses both Western and Chinese medicine perspectives about childhood immunization, and provides current immunization recommendations. It must be emphasized that the purpose of this chapter is to provide information. The author makes no recommendations. The difficult decision of whether or not to vaccinate is up to each individual parent, who needs to be as well informed as possible on the pros and cons of each vaccination, and weigh the risks and benefits of allowing the child to contract a particular childhood disease versus the risks and benefits of vaccination. Ultimately it is the parents who must live with the outcome of their decision.

WESTERN MEDICINE AND IMMUNIZATION

Scientific Principle of Vaccination

The Western medicine basis for immunization is to produce the same sort of active immunity as contraction of the disease itself. Natural disease induces a response from the person's own immune system that produces antigen-specific antibodies and cellular immunity. The active immunity can last many years or even a lifetime. The advantage to vaccination is the production of the same active immunity without the discomfort of the disease process and its potential complications. Passive immunity is protection produced by an animal or another human, and transferred to the immunized subject by injection. This type is not permanent, lasting weeks, months, or years.

There are two basic types of vaccines: live attenuated and inactivated vaccines. Live attenuated vaccines are produced by modifying a disease-producing "wild" virus or bacteria in a laboratory so that it retains the immunogenic effect without causing illness. Inactivated vaccines can be composed of either whole viruses or bacteria, or fractions of subunits, toxoids, conjugates which are composed of pure cell-wall polysaccharides from bacteria.[1]

Efficacy of Vaccines

In 1870 Louis Pasteur created the first live attenuated bacterial vaccine. Modern vaccination began with licensing of measles and trivalent oral polio vaccines in 1963. Since then, statistics in support of vaccinating childhood diseases are impressive. The eradication of smallpox is a testimonial to the power and efficacy of vaccination: In 1966, the United Nations World Health Organization (WHO) launched worldwide smallpox vaccination. At that time, about 10 to 15 million cases of the disease occurred each year, with more than 2 million deaths. In 1979, 2 years after the last indigenous case of smallpox was reported in 1977, WHO declared that smallpox had been eradicated from the world.[1] Although no other disease has been met with as successful eradication, the evidence is still overwhelming in support of vaccine efficacy.

Measles

Descriptions of measles dates as far back as the seventh century AD. In the tenth century AD, it was "more dreaded than smallpox."[1]

The measles virus is a paramyxovirus. It is 100 to 200 nm in diameter, with a core of single-stranded RNA. It causes systemic infection, with the respiratory epithelium of the nasopharynx as the primary site. The incubation period from exposure to prodrome averages 10–12 days, and from exposure to onset of rash averaging 14 days (range is 7–18 days). The prodrome lasts 2–4 days (range 1–7 days), characterized by fever, which can peak stepwise to as high as 103 to 105° F (39.4–40.5 °C), followed by upper respiratory symptoms of cough, rhinitis, and/or conjunctivitis. Pathognomonic for measles are Koplik's spots, blue–white spots on the buccal membrane, and these occur 1–2 days before the rash and persists until 1–2 days after disappearance of the rash. The measles rash is a maculopapular rash that begins as discrete lesions and then becomes confluent. It starts at the hairline, moves to the face and upper neck, and then proceeds downward to the hands and feet. It usually lasts 5–6 days.

Approximately 30% of measles cases have complications, the most common being diarrhea, followed by otitis media, and pneumonia, the leading cause of death due to measles. Encephalitis occurs in 0.1% of reported cases. Subacute sclerosing panencephalitis (SSPE) is a rare degenerative central nervous system disease thought to be due to persistent measles virus infection of the brain. It can occur 1 month to 27 years after the onset of the acute infection, with an average of 7 years. The onset is insidious, with progressive deterioration of behavior and intellect, ataxia, myoclonic seizures, and eventually death. SSPE has been extremely rare since early 1980s.

Diagnosis is primarily clinical. Positive serum IgM antibody combined with clinical presentation is diagnostic. Laboratory isolation of measles virus from specimens, such as nasopharyngeal aspirate, urine, throat swabs, is reserved for epidemiologic surveillance to help determine the geographic origin of the virus.

Before the measles vaccine, there were approximately 500 000 cases and 500 deaths reported annually with epidemic cycles every 2–3 years. The actual number of cases was estimated at 3–4 million annually. More than 50% of persons had had measles by age 6 and more than 90% by age 15. The highest incidence was in 5–9-year-olds, who generally accounted for more than 50% of the reported cases. After measles vaccination began in 1963, the incidence of measles decreased by more than 98%, and 2–3-year epidemic cycles no longer occurred. In 1978 a measles elimination program set a goal to eliminate indigenous measles by October 1 1982. Although the goal was not met, only 1497 cases (0.6 cases per 100 000) were reported in 1983, the lowest annual total ever reported up to that time. From 1985 through 1988, 42% of cases occurred in persons who were vaccinated on or after their first birthdays; 68% in school-aged children (5–19 years). The occurrence of measles among previously vaccinated children led to the recommendation for a second dose in this age group. Intensive efforts to vaccinate rapidly brought down the incidence of measles in 1993–1999. Since 1993, the largest outbreaks of measles occurred in populations that refused vaccination.[1]

Current measles vaccine is a live, attenuated strain, usually given in combination with mumps and rubella vaccines (MMR). The vaccine produces an inapparent or mild, noncommunicable infection. Antibodies develop in approximately 95% of children vaccinated at 12 months of age and 98% of children vaccinated at 15 months of age. Mumps vaccine is a live attenuated mumps virus vaccine that produces an antibody response in 97% of children. The duration of the vaccine-induced immunity is believed to be at least 25 years, most often lifelong. The first dose is recommended for children after 12 months of age, and a second dose is given between 4–6 years old. Both doses are given at the same time as measles and rubella as MMR vaccine.

Mumps

Mumps was described by Hippocrates in the fifth century BC. It is a paramyxovirus that has a single-stranded RNA genome. It is transmitted via respiratory droplets. It replicates in the nasopharynx and regional lymph nodes. The incubation period is 14–18 days. Nonspecific prodromal symptoms include myalgia, anorexia, malaise, headache, and low-grade fever. The most common clinical manifestation is parotitis, inflammation of the salivary gland, which occurs in 30–40% of infected persons. The single or bilateral parotitis usually subsides by 1 week to 10 days. Up to 20% of mumps infections are asymptomatic, with 40–50% having very mild, nonspecific symptoms or primarily respiratory symptoms.

Mumps complications can be CNS involvement: aseptic meningitis is common, occurring asymptomatically (findings of inflammatory cells in the cerebrospinal fluid) in 50–60% of infected persons, with up to 15% manifesting symptoms of meningitis, such as headache and stiff neck. Encephalitis is rare, occurring at less than 2 per 100 000 cases. Orchitis (testicular inflammation), is the most common complication in postpubertal males, with a 20–50% incidence. Orchitis may occur before, simultaneously with, or after the onset of parotitis. Symptoms consist of pain and swelling. Approximately 50% have some degree of testicular atrophy, but sterility is rare. Oophoritis (ovarian inflammation) occurs in 5% of postpubertal females but does not impair fertility. Pancreatitis is infrequent with transient and reversible hyperglycemia. Deafness caused by mumps is one of the leading causes of acquired sensorineural deafness in childhood, with the estimated incidence of approximately 1 per 20 000. Hearing loss is unilateral in approximately 80% of cases. Onset is sudden and results in permanent hearing impairment.

Diagnosis is usually clinical, especially in the presence of parotitis. The mumps virus can be isolated from saliva, urine, and cerebrospinal fluid. The specimen should be collected within the first 5 days of illness. Serology tests with enzyme immunoassay (EIA) and radical hemolysis antibody tests are more reliable and diagnostic than complement fixation (CF) and hemagglutination inhibition (HI) antibody tests.

Prior to 1967 when the mumps vaccine was licensed, the disease primarily occured in 5–9-year-olds. In the 1980s, there was a shift towards older children. Since 1989, there has been a steady decline after institution of the second mumps vaccine.[1] Mumps vaccine is also a live attenuated strain with similar antibody response and duration as the measles vaccine.

Rubella

Rubella was initially considered to be a variant of measles until 1814, when it was described as a separate disease in the German medical literature. The rubella virus was first isolated in 1962. It is a togavirus, an enveloped RNA virus with a single antigenic type. Rubella is transmitted via the respiratory route, and replicates in the nasopharynx and regional lymph nodes. A viremia occurs 5–7 days after exposure with spread of the virus throughout the body. It is during viremia that the transplacental infection of the fetus occurs in congenital rubella syndrome.

The incubation period varies from 12 to 23 days. Symptoms are usually mild, with 30–50% of cases being subclinical or inapparent. In children, prodrome is rare and rash is usually the first manifestation. In older children, there is often a 1–5 day prodrome with low grade fever, malaise, swollen glands, and upper respiratory symptoms preceding the rash. The maculopapular rubella rash begins on the face, progresses from head to foot, and lasts about 3 days. It is occasionally pruritic and does not coalesce as measles rash. Lymphadenopathy may begin 1 week before the rash and last several weeks, with postauricular, posterior cervical, and suboccipital nodes the most commonly involved. Adults often have accompanying arthralgia and arthritis. Uncommon complications occur more frequently in adults than in children, except for thrombocytopenic hemorrhagic manifestations which occur more often in children, with an incidence 1 per 3000 cases.

Diagnosis is clinical, substantiated by laboratory confirmation using serology testing demonstrating significant rise in rubella IgG or presence of IgM antibodies. Viral isolation is reserved as an epidemiologic tool.

The most disastrous consequence is the congenital rubella syndrome (CRS). All organs can be affected, resulting in multiple manifestations that include microcephaly, mental retardation, deafness, cataracts, cardiac defects, bone alterations, and liver and spleen damage. The primary purpose for vaccination against rubella is the prevention of CRS. Infants with CRS can shed large quantities of virus from body secretions for up to 1 year and can therefore transmit the disease to anyone caring for them who is susceptible, especially a pregnant woman.

Rubella epidemics used to occur every 6–9 years. The last major US epidemic occurred in 1964 resulting in 12.5 million cases of rubella infection, about 20 000 newborns with CRS, and estimated cost of $840 million, approximately $200 000 per lifetime cost per case. Rubella vaccine, a live attenuated virus which is not communicable, was first licensed in 1969. No large epidemics have occurred since that time. Smaller outbreaks have occurred since 1969 in non-vaccinated populations, e.g., congregations of people who refused vaccination for religious and philosophical reasons.[1]

Pertussis

In the twentieth century, pertussis has been one of the most common childhood diseases and a major cause of childhood mortality in the US. Prior to the availability of pertussis vaccine in the 1940s, over one million cases of pertussis were reported, an average of 175 000 per year (approximately 150 cases per 100 000 population). Since widespread use of the vaccine began, incidence has decreased more than 98%, to an average of about 3700 cases per year since 1980. In unimmunized populations in the world, pertussis continues to cause approximately 300 000 deaths per year.[1]

Diphtheria

Prior to immunization with diphtheria toxoid, diphtheria was a major cause of morbidity and mortality in children. In England and Wales during the 1930s, diphtheria was among the top three causes of death for children under age 15 years.[1] Diphtheria toxoid became routinely used in the 1940s. From 1980 through 1999, only 49 cases of diphtheria were reported in the US. Only one case per year was reported in 1998 and 1999.

Diphtheria toxoid is not available as a single antigen; it is given in combination with tetanus toxoid and pertussis vaccine in children, which contains three to four times as much diphtheria toxoid as adult combination of diphtheria –tetanus toxoid.[1]

Tetanus

Prior to the 1940s, 500–600 cases of tetanus were reported annually (approximately 0.4 cases per 100 000 population). After the introduction of tetanus toxoid, tetanus incidence fell dramatically and steadily. Since the mid 1970s, 50–100 cases have been reported each year, with the occurrence primarily in older persons until the latter 1990s, when an increase occurred in younger drug users. Almost all of the reported cases are in persons who have either never been vaccinated or who have not had a booster in 10 years.

Polio

The first outbreaks of polio were reported in Europe and the US in the early nineteenth century. Subsequently, epidemics of polio were reported with increasing severity from the northern hemisphere every summer and fall. Polio reached a peak in the US in 1952, with over 21 000 paralytic cases. Inactivated (Salk) polio vaccine, IPV, was licensed in 1955 and used extensively from then until the 1960s, when trivalent oral polio vaccine (OPV) became the vaccine of choice in the US and most other countries of the world in 1963. OPV contains live attenuated strains of all three serotypes of poliovirus. These live attenuated viruses replicate in the intestinal mucosa and lymphoid cells, and in lymph nodes that drain the intestine. Vaccine viruses are excreted in the stool of the vaccinated person for up to 6 weeks after a dose. After introduction of OPV vaccine in 1963, the incidence of polio fell dramatically. The last case of wild-virus polio was reported in the US in 1979.[1]

However, one case of vaccine-associated paralytic polio (VAPP) occurred for every 2–3 million doses of OPV administered, which resulted in 8 to 10 cases of VAPP each year in the US. Since 1980, VAPP has accounted for 95% of all cases of paralytic polio reported in the US.[1] In 1996 the Advisory Committee on Immunization Practices (ACIP) recommended a sequential schedule of IPV followed by OPV, but the risk of VAPP continued. Beginning in 2000, the ACIP recommends exclusive use of IPV.[1]

Although polio elimination was certified in the Americas in 1994, and there is worldwide polio immunization, the risk of polio still exists in many parts of the world, such as India,[2] Laos,[3] the eastern Mediterranean and Africa.[1] The Centers for Disease Control, CDC, reported an outbreak of polio in the Dominican Republic and Haiti as recently as the winter of 2000.[1]

Haemophilus influenzae

Haemophilus influenzae was first described in 1892. Before the introduction of effective vaccines, *H. influenzae* was the leading cause of bacterial meningitis and other invasive bacterial disease among children under age 5 years. In the early 1980s, it was estimated that 20 000 cases (40–50 cases per 100 000 population) occurred annually in the US. Two-thirds of cases were among young children less than 18 months of age. Ninety-five percent of invasive diseases were caused by *H. influenzae* type b (Hib) virus. After the institution of Hib vaccine in the late 1980s, Hib disease declined dramatically by more than 99% compared to the prevaccine era.[1] In a 1990 survey of 29 309 children vaccinated between 18 and 60 months of age, Hib vaccine was found to be very safe and effective: only 2% developed local and systemic reactions; 0.15% required hospitalization; one 30-month-old child developed Hib meningitis and one 29-month-old child died.[4] In 1996–1997, only 144 confirmed cases of Hib invasive disease were reported.[1] A similar decline was seen in other countries.[5]

The pure polysaccharide vaccine (HbPV) licensed in 1985 had low efficacy in children under 18 months of age. In 1987, the first Hib conjugate vaccine (PRP-D, ProHIBIT), which was the chemical binding of a polysaccharide to a protein "carrier," greatly improved immunogenicity, especially in young children.[1] The conventional medical community feels that the Hib conjugate will likely eliminate Hib disease in infancy.[6]

Pneumococcus

Streptococcus pneumoniae is a gram-positive bacterium with 90 known serotypes. The polysaccharide capsule is the primary pathogenic virulence factor.

It continued to cause widespread illnesses and deaths even with the advent of penicillin in the 1940s. Pneumococci are common inhabitants of the respiratory tract, with approximately 27 to 58% of students as asymptomatic carriers. Clinically, pneumococcal infection tends to have an abrupt onset with fever and shaking chills. The cough is productive with purulent sputum, and may be accompanied by chest pain, tachypnea, shortness of breath, and hypoxia. Pneumococci cause an estimated 150 000 to 570 000 of infections each year. The major invasive pneumococcal diseases include acute otitis media, pneumonia, bacteria, and meningitis. Pneumococcus is the leading cause of bacterial meningitis among children under 5 years of age, with approximately 10 cases per 100 000 children under 1 year of age.[1,7]

The first pneumococcal vaccine was licensed in the US in 1977. The first conjugated vaccine was licensed in 2000. This vaccine was demonstrated to have more than 90% efficacy against the seven most invasive serotypes that account for about 80% of serious illnesses in children under age 6 years.[7]

Hepatitis B

Epidemic jaundice was first described by Hippocrates in the fifth century BC. The first recorded cases of hepatitis B were thought to be those associated with smallpox vaccination in 1883. In the twentieth century, serum hepatitis was observed following use of contaminated needles. Hepatitis B surface antigen (HBsAg) was first described in 1965. Approximately 10% of all acute hepatitis virus (HBV) infections progress to chronic infection. As many as 90% of infants who acquire HBV infection from their mothers at birth become carriers. Thirty to 50% of children who become infected with HBV between 1 and 5 years of age become carriers.[1]

In the 1980s, populations of the US and Canada exhibited increasing incidence of hepatitis B. Hepatitis B vaccines have been avilable in the US since 1981. From 1981 to 1991, vaccination programs targeted at high-risk populations did not impact on overall disease incidence. In 1991, a comprehensive hepatitis B prevention program in the US included prenatal testing of pregnant women for HBsAg to identify newborns who require immunoprophylaxis for the prevention of perinatal infection and added hepatitis B to its universal, routine infant immunization schedule.[1] Canada implemented hepatitis B immunization programs for preadolescents (9 through 13 years of age). Hepatitis B coverage of infants rose from 8% in 1992 to 82% in 1996 in the US. In Canada, hepatitis B vaccine among preadolescents was greater than 90% coverage in 1996.[8]

Early hepatitis B vaccine was a plasma-derived vaccine, which was not well accepted, possibly because of fear of transmission of live HBV. Since 1986, recombinant hepatitis B vaccine has been used, which is produced by inserting a plasmid containing the gene for HBsAg into common baker's yeast. The yeast cells then produce HBsAg, which is harvested and purified. It contains over 95% HBsAg, and HBV infection cannot result from use of the recombinant vaccine.[1]

Each year it is estimated that 200 000 people, mostly young adults, get infected with hepatitis B virus. More than 11 000 people have to stay in the hospital because of hepatitis B, and 4000 to 5000 people die from chronic hepatitis B.[9] Hepatitis B vaccine is given as three intramusclar doses, which is 80–100% effective in preventing infection.[1]

Varicella (Chickenpox)

Chickenpox occurs virtually in everyone. The majority of cases are mild and self-limiting. However, complications include secondary bacterial infection, pneumonia (rare in children) and central nervous system manifestions ranging from aseptic meningitis to encephalitis.[1] Each year there are 11 000 hospitalizations and 120 deaths. Varicella vaccine, a live attenuated viral vaccine, was licensed for general use in Japan and Korea in 1988, and in the US in 1995. Initially given to immune compromised persons, it was added routinely to the pediatric immunization schedule in many states for all children between 12 to 18 months of age in 2001.[10]

Current Statistics

At the present time, vaccine-preventable disease rates are at their lowest level ever. In 1999 there were reports of only 86 cases of measles, 238 cases of rubella, 1 case of diphtheria, 33 cases of tetanus, and no wild polio in the US.[1]

Vaccine Safety

Vaccine safety is monitored closely. Adverse events are reported to the Vaccine Adverse Event Reporting System (VAERS), administered by the Centers for Disease Control (CDC) and the Food and Drug Administration (FDA). Approximately 10 000 adverse cases are reported each year. Data are shared internationally by independent scientific experts on the Joint Committee on Vaccination and Immunization and committees of the Medicines Control Agency. Surveillance results in product withdrawal when there is clear evidence of a safety issue.[11]

Current Recommended Immunization Schedule

Currently, the immunization schedule recommends routine administration of childhood vaccines through 18 years of age. It is endorsed by the American Academy of Pediatrics (AAP), the American Academy of Family Physicians (AAFP), and the Advisory Committee on Immunization Practices (ACIP).[12]

DTaP (Combined Diphtheria, Tetanus Toxoids, and Acellular Pertussis Vaccine)

- 5 doses of DTaP given at 2 months, 4 months, 6 months, 15–18 months, and 4–6 years
- Td (tetanus and diphtheria toxoids) is recommended at 11–12 years of age if at least 5 years have elapsed since the last dose of DPT, DTaP, or DT
- Subsequent routine Td boosters are recommended every 10 years.

IPV (Inactive Polio Vaccine)

Four doses of IPV—given at 2 months, 4 months, 6–18 months, and 4–6 years.

Hib (Haemophilus influenzae Type b Conjugate Vaccines)

- One to four doses—number of doses needed depends on age when series is started
- Generally given at 2 months, 4 months, 6 months, and fourth dose between 12 and 15 months.

Hepatitis B (Hep B)

Three doses of Hep B vaccine:

- HBsAg-negative mothers—infants born to HBsAg-negative mothers should receive
  - first dose of HepB vaccine by age 2 months
  - second dose at least one month after the first dose
  - third dose at least 4 months after the first dose, 2 months after second dose, but not before age 6 months
- HBsAg-positive mothers—infants born to HBsAg-positive mothers should receive
  - Hep B vaccine and HBIG, hepatitis B immunoglobulin within 12 hours of birth
  - second dose recommended at 1–2 months of age
  - third dose at 6 months of age
- Mothers whose HBsAg status is unknown—these infants should receive Hep B within 12 hours of birth.

All children and adolescents who have not been immunized against hepatitis B should begin the series during any visit.

MMR (Combined Measles, Mumps and Rubella Vaccine)

Two doses of MMR are given

- First dose now recommended at age 12–15 months
- Second dose at 4–6 years of age to cover those children who failed to respond to the first dose to produce immunity.

PCV 7, Heptavalent Conjugate Pneumococcal Vaccine

Pneumococcal conjugate vaccine was licensed in 2000 for routine use. Four doses are given at 2 months, 4 months, 6 months, and 12–15 months.

Varicella Vaccine

In 2001, new guidelines were instituted for varicella vaccination in many states. In California, beginning on July 1 2001, varicella vaccine is required by law for children aged 18 months and older entering child care; children entering kindergarten for the first time, and older children under age 18 years who are from out of state or out of country, transferring to a California school for the first time with no documented history of the chickenpox disease or the varicella vaccine.[13]

Future of Vaccination

There are plans to expand immunizations in the near future to include herpes simplex virus, cytomegalovirus, group B streptococci, parainfluenza, adenoviruses, and other viruses.[14]

General Contraindications for Vaccination

General contraindications include: moderate or severe acute illnesses with or without a fever; previous anaphylactic (severe allergic) reaction to the vaccine; high fever, neurological symptoms such as convulsions, encephalopathy, decreased level of consciousness. MMR and varicella vaccine are contraindicated in immune compromised children. Local redness and swelling, mild acute illness, low grade temperature, concomittant administration of antibiotics, convalescent phase of illness, recent exposure to an infectious disease, or allergies to penicillin or nonspecific allergies, and stable neurologic conditions such as cerebral palsy are not considered contraindications and vaccinations may still be given.[1]

Administration Statistics

In 1996, approximately 98% of American children received their basic series of immunizations at the time of school entry, and 67% of 2-year-olds were immunized according to schedule.[15] However, in 1998, only 79% of children 19–35 months received a complete series of vaccines. The low-income and minority children are at greater risk for under-immunization,[1] since vaccines are expensive. For example, the California public health department lists the *per dose* costs of vaccines as follows:

- DTaP $18.50
- Hib $18.12
- MMR $28.19
- Hep B $29.73
- IPV $15.42
- Varicella $44.56
- Pneumococcal conjugate $58.00

Recently, the concern about potential adverse effects associated with vaccines has resulted in some parental reluctance for vaccination.

Adverse Effects Associated with Vaccination

Several serious pediatric conditions are controversially attributed to vaccination: immune compromise, neurologic sequelae, autism, and Crohn's disease.

Vaccination and the Immune System

Within the medical community, concern is expressed about what vaccination may do to an immature immune system, especially that in neonates.[16]

Controversial debates are ongoing regarding the possible connection between vaccination and autoimmune illnesses, such as the association between measles and anti-hepatitis B virus (HBV) vaccines with multiple sclerosis (MS). Patients who received these vaccines have presented with clinical autoimmune symptoms and have been found to have antibodies in the brain. Tetanus toxoid, influenza vaccines, polio vaccine and others have been related to autoimmune phenomena ranging from autoantibodies production to full-blown illness, such as rheumatoid arthritis (RA) and Guillain–Barré syndrome. Recent evidence suggests that autism may be related to the immune system.[17]

At this time, only one published study of a controlled animal experiment examined the possible causal relation between vaccines and autoimune findings: healthy puppies immunized with a variety of commonly given vaccines were found to produce a variety of autoantibodies. However, none developed frank autoimmune illness. The mechanism(s) of autoimmune reactions following immunization has not yet been elucidated. One possibility is molecular similarity between some viral antigen (or other component of the vaccine) and a self-antigen. This similarity may be the trigger to the autoimmune reaction.[18]

Pertussis Vaccine and Neurologic Sequelae

Prior to 1991, whole-cell pertussis vaccine was used. It was composed of a suspension of formalin-inactivated *Bordetella pertussis* cells. Up to half of the doses were associated with local reactions such as redness, swelling and pain at the injection site. Fever and other mild systemic symptoms were also common. Convulsions occurred in one case to 1750 doses administered, and acute encephalopathy occurred rarely at 10.5 cases per million doses administered. Sudden infant death syndrome (SIDS) and infantile spasms have also been suggested to be associated with DPT vaccination.[1] In the 1970s, reports linking pertussis vaccine with infant brain damage[19] attracted media attention, which in turn caused a great deal of parental and professional anxiety. The immunization rate fell from 80% to 30%. Between 1976 and 1988, three major pertussis epidemics occurred in the US, resulting in over 300 000 hospitalizations and at least 70 deaths.[11] In countries such as Sweden, Japan, UK, Ireland, Italy, and Australia, anti-vaccine movements have targeted pertussis whole-cell vaccines.[20]

Opponents to the pertussis vaccine have argued that the risks of vaccination outweigh the benefits. In addition, the decline in pertussis incidence is due to improvements in living conditions and not to the vaccine; modern medical therapy makes pertussis disease a relatively trivial illness. Proponents for the vaccine argue that as there is not one distinct syndrome resulting from vaccination, the temporally associated adverse events probably represent the expression of an underlying condition rather than an illness caused by vaccine. That is, many congenital neurologic disorders usually manifest in the first year of life. The mild febrile and other systemic effects of pertussis vaccine may stimulate or even precipitate symptoms of underlying CNS disorders that will eventually and inevitably be expressed, such as febrile seizures and epilepsy.[1] The largest study to date conducted by the National Institute of Child Health and Human Development at the National Institutes of Health (NIH) revealed that SIDS was actually less likely to occur in recently vaccinated infants. Another large study showed that permanent neurologic sequelae due to pertussis vaccine is so rare as to be unquantifiable.[21]

Nevertheless, concerns about brain damage led to the development of acellular pertussis vaccine (DTaP) that contains purified, inactivated components of *B. pertussis* cells. This form is associated with a lower frequency of adverse events and is more effective in preventing pertussis disease. It was first licensed for the fourth and fifth doses of the pertussis series in 1991, and for the primary series in 1996. Several studies conducted in Europe and Africa revealed that DTaP vaccines licensed in the US have efficacy ranging from 71 to 84%. Currently, only acellular pertussis vaccine is used.[1]

No encephalopathy has so far been reported. Adverse reactions consist of local reactions, low grade fever, rare occurrence of moderate to severe systemic reactions, such as higher than 105 °F (40.5 °C) fever, seizures, persistent crying for over 3 h, and hypotonic hyporesponsive episodes (HHE). HHE is the sudden onset of hypotonia, hyporesponsiveness, and pallor or cyanosis that occurs within 48 h usually after pertussis vaccine administered to children under age 2 years. It occurred in approximately one out of every 1750 DTP vaccinations. The largest published report of 40 000 cases concluded that HHE does occur after the administration of DTaP and other nonpertussis containing vaccines, but that it is generally benign, self-limited, and nonrecurrent.[22]

The connection of encephalopathy with pertussis vaccine was biologically more plausible than the proposed link between pertussis, measles vaccines and autism.[11]

Autism

Pertussis, Measles Vaccine and Autism

The incidence of autism has increased from 1 in 10 000 in 1978 to 1 in 300 in 1999 in some US communities. A study of 60 autistic children suggests that a possible cause of autism may be due to a pertussis toxin found in the DPT vaccine. The toxin separates the G-alpha protein from retinoid receptors, which are critical for vision, sensory perception, language processing and attention—characteristic problems of autism. Those children most at risk have at least one parent with a pre-existing G-alpha protein defect, presenting clinically with night blindness, pseudohypoparathyroidism or adenoma of the thyroid or pituitary gland. Natural vitamin A may reconnect the retinoid receptors.[23]

Measles Vaccine's Relation to Autism and Crohn's Disease

In recent years, there is increasing discussion centering on the controversy concerning the association of the MMR vaccine with autism and Crohn's disease.

MMR and Autism

A British study of 12 autistic children revealed lymphoid nodular hyperplasia throughout the gastrointestinal tract. This finding led to the hypothesis that essential vitamins and nutrients are malabsorbed, whereas nonpermeable peptides, "undegraded toxins," are abnormally absorbed. These toxins enter the liver and the CNS, resulting in changes that manifest as autism. In eight children, parents reported developmental regression characteristic of autism started shortly after the children received MMR vaccine.[24,25] Other studies in Ireland revealed the findings of measles virus in the gastrointestinal tract of 96% of autistic children, compared to 6.6% in normal children. All of the autistic children had had measles vaccination.[26] Numerous editorials, epidemiologic reports, and the World Health Organization have negated any association between MMR and autism, and attributed the link as mere coincidence, since autism usually presents at 12–18 months of age, when the MMR vaccine is given.[27–34]

Measles Vaccine and Crohn's Disease

Following the 1994 national measles–rubella vaccination campaign for a second MMR given to school-aged children, there has been a "dramatic escalation" in pediatric Crohn's disease.[35] Dr. John O'Leary in Ireland found measles virus in 75% of children with Crohn's disease.[26] Two Swedish studies suggest a high risk of Crohn's disease in those exposed to measles *in utero*.[36,37] Other reports suggest the possibility that vaccination with live, attenuated measles vaccine could confer the same risk for inflammatory bowel disease as those exposed to measles *in utero*.[38,39]

These are refuted by the World Health Organization[40] and by numerous studies that reveal no causal link between second measles vaccine and Crohn's disease.[41–45] The association may be attributed to artifact, chance, or even biased methodology.[46]

Decline in MMR Vaccination

The controversies have instigated media attention, leading to a decline in MMR vaccination.[47] In the UK, vaccination fell 1% nationally, and fell 2% or more in 1/5 of the districts after adverse publicity in the press linked MMR vaccine to Crohn's disease.[48] Even nurses admit to being concerned about vaccine safety and would not give their *own* children a second dose of MMR.[49] Physicians, nurses, and health practitioners are often confronted by anxious parents, who have also taken their concern to the politicians. In April 2000, Congressman Dan Burton (R-Ind), who has two grandchildren with onset of autistic symptoms shortly after having the MMR vaccine, chaired a congressional hearing on this subject. The controversy no doubt will continue for the foreseeable future.

CHINESE MEDICINE AND VACCINATION

Historical Perspective

The Chinese were among the first to vaccinate, beginning with smallpox vaccine. Infections in Chinese medicine are considered to be external evil or pathogenic Qi that cause Qi imbalance in people who are vulnerable. There are epidemic external evil Qi that are so powerful that they can cause illness in even the healthiest, the most well-balanced individuals. Smallpox is one such pathogen. The Chinese took fluid with pox virus from the pox lesions of the relatively healthy people who were afflicted—those who had a very mild course, had only a few pox—dried the fluid into powder form, and instilled it into the noses of people who had not yet contracted the disease to induce immunity. This method was called pox planting, described in *Forgotten Tradition of Ancient Chinese Medicine*, translated by Paul Unschuld.

Chinese Medicine Theory Regarding Immunization

Level of Illness: Natural versus Vaccine Induced

As Chapter 6 pointed out, Chinese medicine posits that Wind-Heat infections progress according to the Four Levels: Defensive Wei Qi level, Qi level, Nutritive Qi level, and Blood level. The majority of the infections in children occur at the more superficial levels: Defensive Wei Qi and Qi levels. When the infections enter the Blood level, they are much more severe. Injected vaccinations must enter the Blood level to be effective and to induce a serum antibody response. This is not troublesome from a biochemical standpoint, because vaccinations that are derived from attenuated or killed viruses can induce an immune response but are no longer considered to have infectious abilities.

From a bioenergetic Chinese medicine standpoint, however, they still carry the *energy* of the virus and can cause lingering infections—that is, the energy of the attenuated or killed viruses can continue to cause Qi changes in the child. In addition, since the vaccine is injected into the blood, the Qi of the infectious agent is therefore introduced into the deepest Blood level. The classic intranasal vaccine enters the body via the nose, the external orifice for the Lung, the organ that controls Wei Qi. This simulates the natural disease process that occurs at the more superficial levels. The vaccination stimulates the Defensive Qi and Qi circulation, and strengthens children so that they are stronger to expel the external pathogen from the system—to drive out the burglar from the house—instead of allowing the infection to penetrate deeper into the body.

Effects of Vaccine Combination

Chinese medicine also posits that the body can usually effectively handle only one process at a given time. When two separate processes occur at the same time, the human system could become overwhelmed, especially the tender system of an infant or a young child. Therefore, although multiple vaccines given at the same time are less traumatic for children and save nursing time, they can easily overwhelm an immature immune system and make the child weak and deficient. In addition, while a local reaction, mild acute illness, low grade temperature, concomittant administration of antibiotics, or allergic reactions are not contraindications to vaccination, Chinese medicine would regard each of these "mild" symptomatology as a separate "process" that would be taxing on the immune system especially in the presence of a vaccine stimulus. According to many TCM practitioners, these vaccinated children in fact have a compromised immune system and are then predisposed to developing various immune disorders in later years, ranging from allergies, hypothyroidism, lupus, to even cancer.[50]

The Necessity for Natural Occurrence of Childhood Illnesses

In addition, TCM posits that the majority of childhood diseases are due to "womb toxin," i.e. residual effects of infections contracted by the mother and passed to the child in the womb. It is a natural process for the child to "expel" these toxins through childhood illnesses. If this normal outlet for accumulated toxins is blocked, the toxins can remain in the body and give rise to problems or diseases at a later age. This is in direct contradiction to Western medical practice, especially with the administration of the first MMR vaccine. Conventional medicine delays giving the MMR vaccine from age 12 months to age 15 months because of the concern that the presence of maternal antibodies would interfere with the child's own formation of antibodies to the vaccines. By waiting until 15 months of age, the maternal antibodies are no longer detectable so that the child can form his own antibodies. From the Chinese medicine viewpoint, the energy or Qi of the maternal illness still lingers even when serum antibody is no longer present, and the only way the child can expel the "womb toxin" is by having the disease naturally, which is prevented by vaccination.[51–54]

Limitation of Knowledge and Time-tested Endurance in Modern Vaccine

Western medicine emphasizes the importance of vaccine safety, but at the same time admits to limitations in knowledge of vaccine safety. In 1967, the lack of scientific documentation on the hazards of immunization prompted Sir Graham Wilson, former director of the Public Health Laboratory Service in the UK, to compile the first vaccine safety review. The National Childhood Vaccine Injury Act of 1986 established the Committee from the Institute of Medicine to review the adverse consequences of childhood vaccines. This group found severe limitations in the knowledge and research capability on vaccine safety, and identified limitations that include inadequate understanding of biologic mechanisms underlying adverse events; insufficient or inconsistent information from case reports; inadequate size or length of follow-up of many population-based epidemiologic studies.[1] Chinese medicine assesses safety based on thousands of years of practice, and tends to be skeptical about any "new" methods that have not endured the test of time—time in terms of at least centuries and not mere years or decades.

The Classical Chinese Recommendations for Vaccination

The traditional Chinese recommendations for vaccination are as follows:

1. Vaccinations should be given intranasally, to induce Wei Qi defense.
2. Only one type of vaccine should be administered at a given time because the human body can physiologically deal with only one illness or problem at a time.
3. Vaccination should not be given to someone who is already ill.
4. The universal condition should be taken into consideration during vaccination, since Nature influences our well-being. For example, vaccines should not be given at times of unfavorable and unstable climatic Qi, such as during a storm.

At this time, because of dense population in suburban and urban communities, China adopts the Western vaccination policy because of the concern that when unvaccinated children contract natural diseases, they have the potential to cause an epidemic in the general population.[47,55]

Other alternative practices, such as homeopathy and chiropractic, also recommend against vaccination. The homeopaths posit that the homeopathic vaccines are much more effective and safer than conventional vaccine. The chiropractics feel that it is safer for children to contract childhood illnesses, and spinal manipulation can help with side-effects.[56]

The Chinese Treatment for Childhood Illnesses

According to Chinese medicine, childhood illnesses are caused by fetal toxin or "womb heat" that the mother harbored and passed onto the baby prenatally or at conception. They may lay dormant until they are provoked by an external pathogen, and then express to the surface of the body as rashes or blisters. When these rashes or blisters are fully expressed, the child no longer harbors these toxins and the body heals naturally. There are case histories in the Chinese medical literature where chronic health problems develop later in life associated with incompletely expressed or expelled fetal toxins.[51–54] There are Chinese practitioners who in fact recommend purposely exposing children to childhood infections when they are still young, since symptoms are usually worse in older children and in adults. In earlier times, people had measles and chickenpox parties so that their children would get these diseases.[53,55]

In those cases where the parents decide not to vaccinate, the author recommends the following management.

Immune Tonification

Begin tonification of the immune system at birth or in early infancy. Whereas the cornerstone of Western pediatrics is prophylactic immunization, Chinese pediatrics can prophylactically tonify the child to minimize the severity of illnesses. When there is acute expression of illness, tonify the immune system after the illness has resolved.

- ST-36, LI-4
- BL-13, -18, -20, -21, -23.

Expel Heat

During the illness, dispersing Heat can prevent Heat from lingering and drying up Yin.

- LI-11, GV-14, general dispersion of Heat, treat fever.

Disperse Lung Heat—Lung controls Wei Qi and corresponds with the skin, and there are usually upper respiratory tract symptoms and possible complications with pneumonia.
Four-point protocol is:

- Tonify LU-5, KI-10; sedate LU-10, HT-8
- LU-5 tonifies Lung Yin
- KI-6, SP-6 tonifies Yin.

Tonify Kidney

Tonification of the Kidney would provide overall tonification, and to strengthen the marrow, the brain, to prevent CNS complications such as encephalitis.

In the event of occurrence of complications, such as pneumonia or encephalitis, it would be best to integrate conventional treatment with acupuncture.

Decision About Immunization

The decision of whether or not to immunize a child is a very difficult one for both parents and practitioners. The advantages of vaccination are difficult to refute, while the temporal relationship between immunization and side-effects and the controversies surrounding potential risks are disconcerting. It is the responsibility of each practitioner to inform parents of the most up-to-date pros and cons of vaccination, to be as objective as possible, put aside their own belief systems, and be supportive and understanding of whichever decision the parents make. Parents need to become as informed as possible, consider all the pros and cons, weigh the risks and benefits, and realize that ultimately they must live with the outcome of their decision.

REFERENCES

1. Public Health Foundation (2001) *Epidemiology and Prevention of Vaccine-Preventable Diseases. The Pink Book*, 6th edition. Waldorf, MD, Public Health Foundation.
2. Banerjee K. *et al.* (2000) Surveillance for polio eradication: current status and lessons learnt—India 1999. *Journal of Indian Medical Association* 98(1), 6–9.
3. Kuroiwa C. *et al.* (2000) Risk of poliomyelitis importation and re-emergence in Laos. *Lancet* 356(9240), 1487–8.
4. Vadheim C.M., Greenberg D.P., Marcy S.M.K., Froeschle J. & Ward J.I. (1990) Safety evaluation of PRP-D *Haemophilus influenzae* type b conjugate vaccine in children immunized at 18 months of age and older: follow-up study of 30,000 children. *Pediatric Infectious Diseases Journal* 9(8), 555–61.
5. Campbell H. & Carter H. (1993) Rational use of *Haemophilus influenzae* type b vaccine. *Drugs* 46(3), 378–83.
6. Heath P.T. (1998) *Haemophilus influenzae* type b conjugate vaccines: a review of efficacy data. *Pediatric Infectious Diseases Journal* 17(9 Suppl), S117–22.
7. Zimmerman R.K. & Burns I.T. (2000) Child vaccination, part 1: routine vaccines. *Journal of Family Practice* 49(9 Suppl), S22–3.
8. Scheifele D. (1998) Universal childhood hepatitis B vaccination: infants vs. preadolescents, the Canadian perspective. *Pediatric Infectious Diseases Journal* 17(7 Suppl), S35–7.
9. US Department of Health and Human Services, Centers for Disease Control and Prevention. *Vaccine Information Statement. Hepatitis B.* 8/23/2000.
10. US Department of Health and Human Services, Centers for Disease Control and Prevention. *Vaccine Information Statement. Varicella.* February 2001.
11. Nicoll A., Elliman D., & Ross E. MMR vaccination and autism 1998. Déjà vu—pertussis and brain damage 1974? *British Medical Journal* 316(7133), 715–16.
12. Advisory Committee on Immunization Practices (1999) Combination vaccines for childhood immunization: recommendations of the Advisory Committee on Immunization Practices (ACIP), *Pediatrics* 103(5 Pt 1), 1064–77.
13. California Department of Health Services, Immunization Branch. New childcare and school entry varicella IZ requirement. January 25, 2001.
14. Eskola J. (1994) Epidemiological views into possible components of pediatric combined vaccines in 2015. *Biologicals* 22(4), 323–7.
15. Kimmel S.R., Madlon-Kay D., Burns I.T. & Admire J.B. (1996) Breaking the barriers to childhood immunization. *American Family Physician* 53(5), 1648–66.
16. Ugazio A.G. & Plebani A. (1993) Vaccinations in childhood: when and why. *Recent Progress in Medicine* 84(12), 864–72.

17. Megson M.N. (2000) Is autism a G-alpha protein defect reversible with natural vitamin A? *Medical Hypotheses* 54(6), 979–83.
18. Shoenfeld Y. & Aron-Maor A. (2000) Vaccination and autoimmunity-"vaccinosis": a dangerous liaison? *Journal of Autoimmunity* 14(1), 1–10.
19. Kulenkampff M., Schwartzman J.S. & Wilson J. (1974) Neurological complications of pertussis inoculation. *Archives of Diseases of Children* 49, 46–9.
20. Gangarosa E.J. *et al.* (1998) Impact of anti-vaccine movements on pertussis control: the untold story. *Lancet* 351 (9099), 356–61.
21. Miller D., Madge N., Diamond J., Wadsworth J. & Ross E. (1993) Pertussis immunization and serious acute neurological illness in children. *British Medical Journal* 307, 1171–6.
22. DuVernoy T.S. & Braun N.M. (2000) Hypotonic–hyporesponsive episodes reported to the Vaccine Adverse Event Reporting System (VAERS), 1996–1998. *Pediatrics* 106(4), E52.
23. Megson M.N. (2000) Is autism a G-alpha protein defect reversible with natural vitamin A? *Medical Hypotheses* 54(6), 979–83.
24. Wakefield A.J., Murch S.H., Linnell A.A.J. *et al.* (1998) Ileal–lymphoid-nodular hyperplasia, non-specific colitis and pervasive developmental disorder in children. *Lancet* 351, 637–41.
25. Passwell J.H. (1999) MMR vaccination, Crohn's disease, and autism: a real or imagined "stomach ache/headache?" *Israel Medical Association Journal* 1(3), 176–7.
26. www.letstalkhealth.com
27. Chen R.T. & Destefano F. (1998) Vaccine adverse events: causal or coincidental? *Lancet* 351, 611–12.
28. DeStefano F. & Chen R.T. (2000) Autism and measles, mumps, and rubella vaccine: No epidemiological evidence for a causal association. *Journal of Pediatrics* 136(1), 125–6.
29. DeStefano F. & Chen R.T. (1999) Negative association between MMR and autism. *Lancet* 353(9169), 1987–8.
30. Tettenborn M.A. (1998) Autism, inflammatory bowel disease, and MMR vaccine. *Lancet* 351(9112), 1357.
31. Amin J. & Wong M. (1999) Measles-mumps-rubella immunisation, autism, and inflammatory bowel disease: update. *Communicable Diseases Intelligence* 2398, 222.

32. Birmingham K. & Cimons M. (1998) Reactions to MMR immunization scare. *Natural Medicine* 4(5 suppl), 478–9.
33. Fombonne E. (1999) Are measles infections or measles immunizations linked to autism? *Journal of Autism and Developmental Disorders* 29(4), 349–50.
34. Miller D., Wadsworth J., Diamond J. & Ross E. (1997) Measles vaccination and neurological events. *Lancet* 349, 730–1.
35. Wakefield A.J. (1997) *National Vaccine Information Center's First International Public Conference on Vaccination.* Alexandria, Virginia, September 13–15, 1997.
36. Ekbom A., Wakefield A.J., Zack M. & Adami H.O. (1994) Perinatal measles infection and subsequent Crohn's disease. *Lancet* 344, 508–10.
37. Ekbom A., Daszak P., Kraaz W. & Wakefield A.J. (1996) Crohn's disease after in-utero measles virus exposure. *Lancet* 348, 515–7.
38. Thompson N.P., Montgomery S.M., Pounder R.E. & Wakefield A.J. (1995) Is measles vaccination a risk factor for inflammatory bowel disease? *Lancet* 345, 1071–4.
39. Calman K.C. (1995) Measles vaccination as a risk factor for inflammatory bowel disease. *Lancet* 345, 1362–4.
40. World Health Organization (1998) Expanded programme on immunization (EPI)—association between measles infection and the occurrence of chronic inflammatory bowel disease. *Weekly Epidemiological Record* 73, 33–40.
41. Nielsen L.L.W., Nielsen N.M., Melbye M., Sodermann M., Jacobsen M. & Aaby P. (1998) Exposure to measles *in utero* and Crohn's disease: a Danish register study. *British Medical Journal* 316, 196–7.
42. Hermon-Taylor J., Ford S., Sumar N., Millar D., Doran T. & Tizard M. (1995) Measles virus and Crohn's disease. *Lancet* 345, 922–3.
43. Jones P., Fine P. & Piracha S. (1997) Crohn's disease and measles. *Lancet* 349, 473.
44. Feeney M., Clegg A., Winwood P. & Snook J. (1997) A case control study of measles vaccination and inflammatory bowel disease. *Lancet* 350, 764–6.
45. Miller E. & Waight P. (1998) Measles, measles vaccination, and Crohn's disease. *British Medical Journal* 316, 1745.
46. Metcalf J. (1998) Is measles infection associated with Crohn's disease? The current evidence does not prove a causal link. *British Medical Journal* 316, 166.

47. Begg N., Ramsay M., White J. & Bozoky Z. (1998) Media dents confidence in MMR vaccine. *British Medical Journal* 316, 561.

48. *Communicable Disease Report* (1998) 8, 41.

49. Roberts N. (1998) Why are practice nurses scared of MMR2? *General Practice Medicine* January 23.

50. Rosenberg, Z. (1999) Lectures and personal communications re: Immunizations. Pacific College of Oriental Medicine, San Diego, CA.

51. Cao J. *et al.* (1990) *Essentials of Traditional Chinese Pediatrics*. Beijing, Foreign Language Press.

52. Diagnosis and Treatment of Gynecology and Pediatrics, in *China Zhenjiuology, A Series of Teaching Videotapes,* Coproduced by Chinese Medical Audio-Video Organization and Meditalent Enterprises Ltd.

53. Flaws B. (1997) *A Handbook of TCM Pediatrics, A Practitioner's Guide to the Care and Treatment of Common Childhood Diseases*. Denver, Co, Blue Poppy Press.

54. Scott J. (1991) *Acupuncture in the Treatment of Children*. London, Eastland Press.

55. Loo M. (1999) Personal observations and staff communications, Shanghai Xin-Hua Hospital and Beijing University Hospital.

56. Loo M. (1999) Alternative therapies in children. In: Spencer *et al. Complementary/Alternative Medicine, An Evidence-Based Approach*. St Louis, MO, Mosby.

10 Common Pediatric Conditions—East and West

INTRODUCTION

Childhood illnesses are simple yet complex: Simple because the majority of pediatric disorders are acute, fairly straight forward conditions; complex because children have different physiology and pathophysiology at different ages and at different stages of development. Western medicine is simple yet complex: simple because the majority of treatment consists of prescribing medications; complex because it requires understanding of a massive amount of concrete and technical knowledge about the physical minutiae of the human body. Chinese medicine is simple yet complex: simple because it is based on very fundamental concepts and laws of nature; complex because it delves into four aspects of the human being that still "cannot be seen" and "cannot be heard," that still defy scientific proof.

An integration of the various simple complexities is no easy task. The ensuing discussions of the common pediatric conditions incorporate the latest evidence-based information for both Western and Chinese medicine. Western medicine has a myriad of valid studies that follow the strict rules of scientific principles. Research in Chinese medicine, on the other hand, has been difficult since Chinese medicine operates within a different paradigm. The scientific method is reductionistic and unifying, while Chinese medicine is holistic and individualized. Two children with the same diagnoses may be given the same medication but may receive different, more individualized acupuncture treatments.

Acupuncture research in pediatrics is further complicated by children's vulnerability to violation of their personal rights and to risk exposure. Children of the same age may have different cognitive development and different levels of comprehension required for informed consent. Children are often rendered "therapeutic orphans" because of history of abuses in pediatric research. Since the thalidomide disaster, there has been a heightened sensitivity to risks in children.

At this time, there is a paucity of data on acupuncture treatment in children. The majority of the evidence in this chapter is extrapolated from adult studies, which are often clinical reports or trials that do not meet the rigid research standards. Nevertheless, in spite of the flawed methodology that pales in comparison to its Western counterpart, the data in this chapter is the best available information on acupuncture treatment and should be valued in view of the many difficulties confronting acupuncture research that is likened to "fitting a round peg into a square hole." Sound research data is on the horizon, as the

National Institutes of Health is vigorously funding research in complementary and alternative medicine.

ABDOMINAL PAIN

Abdominal pain can be a perplexing problem for the pediatrician. It accounts for the majority of visits made by children and adolescents to pediatricians as well as gastroenterologists,[1] and is the most common complaint for pediatric hospital admission.[2] It can range from having no significant pathology to being a life-threatening, surgical emergency. The presenting symptoms are further complicated by discrepancy in the child's maturity and sensitivity to pain, and by the caretaker's subjective interpretation based on the child's behavior (especially in infants and young children). Differential diagnoses vary according to age and sex of the child, and to the timing of onset of symptoms as acute or chronic.

Western evaluation consists of a comprehensive physical examination and laboratory studies that include blood tests, urine or stool tests and X-ray studies. Recently, ultrasonography has been shown to be beneficial in evaluating children with abdominal pain.[3–10] An integrated approach can utilize Western technology to precisely identify the structural pathology, and Chinese medicine to function in a complementary fashion for identifying and treating energetic disturbances and for alleviating pain.

ACUTE ABDOMINAL PAIN

It is important for both Western and Chinese pediatric practitioners to be familiar with the common acute abdominal presentations, and to differentiate the ones that require surgery referral for either routine or emergency evaluations. Acupuncture has been recorded as a therapeutic measure for acute abdominal pain as early as the *Nei Jing*, the *Yellow Emperor's Canon of Medicine*. Although it is widely used today for adults in China,[11] its efficacy has not been adequately demonstrated in children, who are much more fragile in acute situations and who can change and clinically deteriorate much more rapidly than adults. Most likely, at least for the present, Chinese medicine can provide specific treatments for some nonemergency, pediatric conditions, and can be an adjunctive, palliative therapy for pain and other symptoms prior to and after surgery.

Acute abdominal pain in children is distinguished both in clinical manifestations and in age of presentation. Gastroenteritis and constipation are common causes of acute onset of abdominal pain at any age. Colic usually presents in infants under age 3 months. Intussusception should be suspected in slightly older infants, 6–24 months of age, who present with sudden, severe abdominal pain. Appendicitis usually affects children between 2 and 18 years of age. Abdominal pain secondary to renal disorders usually presents in the preschooler, and mittelschmerz and pelvic inflammatory disease enter the differential for a menstruating teenage girl.

Acupuncture has been shown to be effective in reducing pain and vomiting in adult patients undergoing various gastrointestinal procedures. Since the treatment is benign without side-effects, usually stimulating only a few points, this use of acupuncture can be extrapolated for pediatric patients. One clinical report used four acupuncture points: Hegu LI-4, Neiguan PC-6, Zusanli ST-36, and Gongsun SP-4 bilaterally—and demonstrated pain reduction during colonoscopy.[12] A study from Taiwan revealed electroacupuncture stimulation of PC-6 Neiguan alone was as effective as anesthetic medication in reducing postoperative emesis in patients who underwent laparoscopy.[13] Acupuncture can be used in fiberoptic gastroscopy,[14] possibly by just needling Zusanli ST-36.[15] As high as 88.2% success rate has been reported for acupuncture as analgesia for upper gastrointestinal tract endoscopy.[16] Endoscopy was found to be much easier for the practitioner and better tolerated by the patient after acupuncture analgesia was administered.[17]

NON-SURGICAL ACUTE ABDOMINAL PAIN

Colic

In babies under 3 months of age, the most common cause of "abdominal pain" is colic, described by mother as crying episodes with flexion of the legs and distended abdomen (see Colic).

Gastroenteritis

This is one of the most common presentations of acute abdominal pain in children of all ages. The predominant symptom is diarrhea, sometimes also vomiting, with accompanying generalized, nonspecific abdominal pain. The majority of cases are caused by viruses—correlates with external Cold pathogenic invasion—with rotavirus being the most prevalent. Heat pathogens correlate with bacterial agents, which include *Shigella*, *Salmonella*, *Campylobacter*, *Giardia*, and invasive *E. coli*. Most viral diarrheal illnesses last between 3 to 7 days. Children with longer symptoms should have stool cultures to identify nonviral pathogens. Treatment is directed toward the specific stage or level of invasion, with the primary focus on prevention of dehydration (see Diarrhea).

Constipation

Constipation is high on the list of causes of abdominal pain in children. In infants, recurrent episodes should lead to suspicion of Hirschsprung's disease. In breast-fed infants, periods of 7 to 10 days without stools can be normal. Abdominal pain is often accompanied by straining when attempting to defecate. This is often seen in the school-aged child who is fearful of using the public toilet. Encopresis is a condition that results when a child holds enough stool in the colon to cause abnormal stretching of the bowel resulting in decreased motility. Leakage of loose bowel contents with staining of the underwear is common (see Constipation).

Urologic Causes of Abdominal Pain

These include urinary tract infections, congenital genitourinary tract anomalies, kidney stones, and ureteropelvic junction obstruction.[18–21] Acupuncture can function both as a complementary treatment modality, such as in UTI or as an adjunctive therapy for relieving pain (see Urinary Cystitis, p. 281).

Abdominal Migraine

Abdominal migraine is a controversial syndrome[22] that may occur in a child with headaches and recurrent abdominal pains, especially with a positive family history of migraine. The abdominal component will often cease by adolescence and be replaced with more classical migrainous headaches.[23,24] Acupuncture treatment can be directed at alleviating headaches (see Headache), at relieving stress, and at diminishing abdominal pain.

Ulcer Disease

Under 6 years of age, stress ulcers are most common. Over 10 years of age, children can more verbally describe the ulcer symptoms, which usually consists of epigastric pain occurring after meals and may be accompanied by nausea and abdominal distension. The correlation of duodenal ulcerations and antral gastritis has been shown in children.[25] An Italian report of four adult patients treated with acupuncture demonstrated complete resolution of symptoms and healing of lesions demonstrated by gastroscopy.[26] There is no current data on acupuncture treatment of ulcer in children.

The suspicion of ulcer in children should be appropriately diagnosed with endoscopic evaluation and treatment coordinated with the gastroenterologist. Acupuncture may be instituted for pain relief.

Pancreatitis

Pancreatitis, or inflammation of the pancreas, is rare but may occur at any age in childhood. It may be idiopathic, with familial predisposition. The most common cause of pancreatitis in children is mumps infection. Trauma and drugs such as steroids can lead to pancreatic symptoms.[27] Ultrasonography usually shows an abnormal, nonspecific swelling of the pancreas. Adult studies indicate that a treatment protocol that integrates Chinese medicine with Western medicine reduced mortality in recently diagnosed severe pancreatitis.[28] One study indicates that body acupuncture alone was ineffective for pain relief in alcohol-induced pancreatitis,[29] but press pellets applied to auricular points Shenmen, Sympathetic, Pancreas, Abdomen and Duodenum were successful in relieving pancreatic pain in an adult.[30] Since children are receptive to noninvasive techniques, this treatment should be tried on the rare child who presents with pancreatic pain.

Chinese medicine interprets pancreatitis as Heat in the Spleen/Pancreas. A four-point Heat dispersing treatment can be used:

- Tonify SP-9, KI-10; sedate SP-2, HT-8
- Press pellets can be applied to auricular points listed above.

General Treatment of Abdominal Pain

When surgical emergencies and serious abdominal disorders are ruled out or are being treated, ST-36, CV-12 and PC-6 can be used to treat pain by harmonizing the Middle Energizer, regulating Qi, and tonifying Stomach and Spleen.

SURGICAL EMERGENCIES

It is imperative that practitioners recognize abdominal surgical emergencies. Currently, there is no data on acupuncture treatment of these entities in children.

Appendicitis

The classic clinical signs of appendicitis are fever, periumbilical pain that migrates to the right lower quadrant, producing point tenderness over McBurney's point; anorexia, vomiting, abdominal tenderness and guarding.[2] However, frequently the signs and symptoms are nonspecific, making the diagnosis difficult, especially in the younger children. Patients are often sent home with the diagnosis of gastroenteritis.[31] When the correct diagnosis is made, it is accompanied by perforation in 30 to 65% of children.[32-35] Perforation can in fact occur approximately 36 hours from the onset of pain.[33,34,36] The white blood cell count may be normal in 10% of patients and therefore is unreliable.[31] In the adolescent, gynecologic pathology and even pregnancy can mimic early appendicitis symptoms.[23] Abdominal X-ray is generally not helpful, but ultrasound is especially useful in equivocal cases of suspected appendicitis. Sensitivity is 85–90% with a specificity of 95–100% in the hands of an experienced ultrasonographer.[8] Laparoscopic surgery is being used more frequently in the pediatric population.[37]

Chinese medicine considers an extra point, Lanweixue, located approximately half-way between ST-36 and ST-37 on the right leg, as the "appendicitis" point,[38,39] It is well known for treatment of both acute and chronic appendicitis and traditionally has been considered to also have possible diagnostic value.[39] One Western study with 50 patients who had a presumptive diagnosis of appendicitis did not find the Lanweixue point to be statistically a good indicator of appendicitis,[40] whereas a clinical report from China indicates electroacupuncture administered to Lanweixue and ST-25 had a 63% cure rate for appendicitis.[41] Other reports also indicate successful acupuncture treatment for appendicitis.[42,43] Auriculoacupuncture was reported to alleviate pain in a small sample of adult patients with appendicitis.[44] Acupuncture may be considered as an anesthetic in pediatric appendectomy, since an adult clinical study revealed that acupuncture was comparable to epidural in inducing anesthesia but had less respiratory depression, hypotension, and cardiac arrhythmia, and less need for postoperative analgesic and antibiotics.[45] Another study reported acupuncture anesthesia with 96.6% success rate.[46]

At this time, because of the high sensitivity of ultrasound for diagnosing appendicitis, an integrative approach would be for the acupuncturist to immediately refer any child suspected of having the condition to a Western specialist for diagnosis. Because of the high incidence and rapidity of perforation in children, and the lack of substantiating data for acupuncture treatment in pediatric appendicitis, it would be reasonable to use acupuncture as an adjunctive therapy for pain before going to surgery or for diminishing pain and other complications after surgery. It would be advisable for the practitioner not to administer acupuncture treatment to diminish pain prior to referral as that may mask the symptoms and make clinical diagnosis more difficult.

Intussusception

Intussusception is second only to incarcerated inguinal hernias as the cause for bowel obstructions in the 2-month to 5-year-old range. The peak incidence usually occurs during 4 to 10 months of age; however, in recent years intussusception has become more prevalent in children over 2 years of age.[47] The classic triad of symptoms consists of colicky abdominal pain, vomiting, and bloody stools. Occult blood without overt blood stools may occur in up to 75% of the cases.[48] Clinical suspicion can be confirmed with either a contrast study (air or barium) or ultrasound.[49–51]

Ultrasonography is considered essential for the diagnosis of intussusception and thus should be recommended in all cases of acute abdominal pain in the population at risk for this disorder.[52] The most common location for the occurrence of pathology is at the ileocecal junction. In 95% of the cases there is no leading edge. The older the child, the more likely is the finding of a pathologic leading edge: Meckel's diverticulum (most common), lymphoma, lymphadenopathy, Henoch–Schonlein purpura.[53]

Henoch–Schonlein Purpura

This is a childhood vasculitis of unknown etiology, and is most common in children between 2 and 8 years of age. Gastrointestinal involvement occurs in approximately two-thirds of children, who usually present with abdominal pain[54] and bloody diarrhea which can lead to bouts of colicky pain and intussusception. Usually, there is a characteristic purpuric rash located on the lower extremities, buttocks, and lower arms. Arthritis and arthralgias may also develop. The abdominal pain is usually treated with systemic steroids and intussusception is managed surgically.[23]

There is so far no study on acupuncture treatment for intussusception from whatever cause. The role of acupuncture here should be adjunctive therapy to alleviate pain prior to surgery. SP-1 can be treated to stop bleeding.

Midgut Volvulus

Midgut volvulus (twisting of the intestines upon themselves) usually presents in the first few months of life. Clinical presentation consists of bilious vomiting, marked abdominal distension, and upper gastrointestinal bleeding. Plain X-ray may reveal a typical "double-bubble" sign. This is a surgical emergency, since the superior mesenteric artery is often completely or partially occluded.[23] There has been one report from China of successful treatment with acupuncture for volvulus of the stomach[55] but no reports on treatment for midgut volvulus in children.

Acupuncture can be used as palliation of symptoms before and after surgery:

- SP-1 can be used to treat acute bleeding
- PC-6 can be used to diminish vomiting.

SURGERY REFERRAL INDICATED

Some pediatric conditions should be referred for nonemergency surgical consultation. Because there is time, acupuncture may be tried with caution.

Hypertrophic Pyloric Stenosis

Pyloric stenosis is common in the first weeks of life, usually of the first-born male. The characteristic presentation is projectile vomiting after each feeding and the infant remains hungry. The incidence approaches 1 in 500 live births.[56] Surgery consists of carefully splitting the hypertrophic muscle, and is curative. There is one study which showed that electroacupuncture at just one point, Zusanli (ST-36) can regulate pylorus peristalsis, both enhancing the hypofunctioning and diminishing the hyperfunction of pyloric peristalsis.[57]

Treatment

- PC-6 can be treated to diminish vomiting prior to surgery
- ST-36 as indicated above, may be worthwhile treating while the child awaits scheduled surgery. The author has not had any experience with this.

Inguinal Hernia

Inguinal hernia repair is the most common surgical procedure in infants and children. The hernia presents as a mass that "comes and goes" in the groin or scrotum, often noticed during diaper change. One-third are diagnosed in the first 6 months of life when the risk of incarceration is highest.[58] The incidence is approximately 1–4% of children, with increased incidence in premature infants. The incidence of incarceration is approximately 10% and decreases with age, occurring rarely after 8 years of age.[58] Electroacupuncture can be used as anesthetic for herniorrhaphy.[59] There is no current data on acupuncture treatment on this condition.

Gallstones

Gallstones have a mean age of presentation of 12 years. Patients over the age of 5 years can generally localize pain to the right upper quadrant, but under 5 years, the pain is more difficult to characterize, and younger children are often asymptomatic.[60] Reports in adults indicates successful treatment of biliary colic with electroacupuncture.[40] Auriculoacupuncture has been widely used in recent years for treatment of gallstones in adults. Both needles and press pellets can be used on three to four points, such as Shenmen, Sanjiao, Gallbladder, and Sympathetic Nerve. Patients were asked to take high protein and high lipid foods in order to promote contraction of the gallbladder. Stones with a diameter less than 1 cm were the easiest to excrete.[43] It would seem worthwhile to try this treatment modality in the rare child with gallstones.

CHRONIC RECURRENT ABDOMINAL PAIN

Recurrent abdominal pain (RAP) is a broad descriptive term commonly used in pediatrics to define a heterogeneous group of patients who experience episodic attacks of abdominal pain that affect normal activity for at least 3 months.[26] It has been reported to occur in 10–15% of children between the ages of 5 and 15 years, and is considered to be one of the most encountered symptoms in childhood. Only 5% to 10% of children with RAP have an organic cause,[61–65] represented most often by constipation; inflammatory bowel disease (IBD); miscellaneous gastrointestinal causes such gastrointestinal mucosal lesions and by nephro-urologic diseases.[61–62,64,66]

Constipation, IBD, and UTI are discussed in other sections. Acid-peptic diseases are uncommon. The usual presenting symptoms are epigastric pain and/or nocturnal pain. Some children have postprandial pain and weight loss. There is often a positive family history of peptic ulcer disease. The diagnoses include esophagitis, gastritis, duodenitis, or ulcer.[67] The majority of the children with RAP have functional disorder.

Evaluation

The medical evaluation has to balance between ordering sufficient tests and avoiding an excess of diagnostic studies in order to not miss the small percentage of children with organic causes. In general, when an initial blood and urine evaluation are negative, additional studies include abdominal ultrasonography, radiography, and/or endoscopy.[64] Ultrasound is considered valuable in evaluating children with RAP.[22] Endoscopy[1,67] and even laparoscopy[68] are often considered necessary to adequately establish a diagnosis. Even when the yield may be low, the direct visualization of the abdominal structures as being normal may be helpful to the parents and the child in their understanding and acceptance of the benign nature of functional abdominal pain.[22]

FUNCTIONAL ABDOMINAL PAIN

Ninety to 95% of RAP in children are functional, which denotes a condition of unknown etiology and pathogenesis, in that specific structural, infectious, inflammatory, or biochemical cause cannot be demonstrated[69,70] Diagnosis is symptomatic, by exclusion of organic causes[70] that respond to medical treatment.[64] The management of functional disorders is more complex and difficult, and must take into account cognitive, developmental, physiologic, psychologic, and environmental aspects of the child.[71] There may be a relationship to development and maturation, as the majority of children show improvement or resolution of symptoms over time.[65]

The prevailing theories of possible pathogeneses include disturbed gastrointestinal motility, delayed intestinal transit time, and increased intensity of small intestine and colon muscle contraction provoked by a variety of physical and emotional stimuli. Biopsies have demonstrated inflammatory changes, which may be either the cause or the effect of altered intestinal motility. There appears to be a strong genetic predisposition as patients often have a family history of nonspecific abdominal illnesses, irritable bowel syndrome, and peptic ulcer or migraine headaches that are emotionally or stress related. Emotional stress from various causes, such as death or separation from a significant family member, physical illness in parents or siblings, school problems, and recent geographic moves may provoke or reinforce the pain and associated symptoms.[26]

Treatment is multifaceted, consisting of modification of responses from parents and teachers toward the symptoms, diet variations, drugs, and even psychotherapy. A sympathetic and supportive approach to the patient, parents, and teachers is important in steering the focus on the child and away from pain-oriented behavior.[70,72] Various dietary recommendations include low-fat and high-fiber diets; and restrictions: milk products, caffeinated and carbonated beverages, starches (corn, potatoes, wheat, oats), sweets. Anticholinergic medications are sometimes prescribed. Children who manifest significant emotional components are referred for psychological and psychiatric evaluations and therapy. Unfortunately, none of the remedies has been very effective. Response to treatment is especially poor in children with more than 2 years of symptoms.[73] Both parents and professionals feel baffled and frustrated, as they can clearly see that these children genuinely feel the pain, and that the symptoms interfere with school attendance and performance, peer relationships, participation in organizations and sports, and personal and family activities.

AN INTEGRATIVE APPROACH TO FUNCTIONAL ABDOMINAL PAIN

Chinese medicine can offer a valuable perspective for both diagnosis and treatment. Pathophysiology that does not have concrete anatomic and biochemical abnormality can be easily explained as energetic/Qi disturbance, with treatment directed toward rectifying the specific imbalance. An integrative approach using the Western classification of functional abdominal pain and the Chinese interpretation can elucidate and broaden the understanding of this common and difficult entity.

Western medicine classifies RAP in children into the following three clinical presentations:

1. Isolated paroxysmal abdominal pain, usually periumbilical.
2. Abdominal pain associated with dyspepsia.
3. Abdominal pain associated with an altered bowel pattern.

Isolated Paroxysmal Abdominal Pain, Usually Periumbilical

Pain typically is periumbilical in location and rarely radiates. It varies in intensity, and has inconsistent alternation of pain and pain-free periods. Pain episodes begin gradually and last less than 1 hour in 50% and less than 3 hours in 40% of patients. Continuous pain is described in fewer than 10% of children. The child usually is unable to describe the pain. There is typically no relationship to meals, a particular food, activity, and bowel habits. The pain commonly occurs in the evening, affects the child's ability to fall asleep but rarely awakens the child from sleep. Parents describe the patient as miserable and listless during most episodes of pain. During severe attacks, the child may exhibit a variety of behaviors as manifestations of intensity of pain: doubling over, grimacing, crying, or clenching and pushing on the abdomen. Commonly associated symptoms include headache, pallor, nausea, dizziness, and fatigue, at least one of which is observed in 50–70% of cases. Temperature is usually normal.

This presentation is common in adolescents and is called irritable bowel syndrome. Besides periumbilical pain and the associated symptoms, the teenager may also complain of irregular bowel movements and pain relief with defecation, sense of urgency, and feeling of bloating or abdominal distention.

Chinese medicine would term this type of RAP as Spleen Yang and Qi deficiency, with resultant Cold accumulation. The pain tends to occur during the Yin period of the day, when Yang and Qi normally diminishes. It can be severe as Cold contracts the Qi channels and Blood vessels, resulting in decreased Qi and Blood supply to the muscles and tissues. In Western medicine, ischemic pain due to diminished blood flow can be very severe. There is symptomatic relief with pressure, a Yang form of "treatment" for Yin symptom. Qi deficiency symptoms include pallor and fatigue. Diet and lifestyle, especially those of the teenage girl, can aggravate symptoms. The weight-conscious young female sometimes ingests excessive salads which are energetically Cold to the system. Modern fashions often expose the umbilicus, CV-8, a major point for warming the Intestines and therefore predisposes the teenager to environmental Cold.

Abdominal Pain Associated with Dyspepsia

This is usually epigastric or upper abdominal pain that is temporally related to eating, with associated symptoms such as nausea, vomiting, heartburn, abdominal bloating, regurgitation of food, early satiety, excessive hiccups, and excessive belching. There may be altered bowel pattern such as diarrhea, constipation, or a sense of incomplete evacuation with bowel movements.

Chinese medicine explains these symptoms as primarily due to food retention, which can be caused by various energetic Stomach and Spleen imbalances, resulting in inefficient transformation and transportation of food. The diet, manner of eating, and the child's emotional state can precipitate this condition.

Diet

Excessive Cold foods would result in Coldness in the Spleen and Stomach, excess Hot/spicy and sugary/sweet foods would produce Stomach Heat and Spleen deficiency, excess dairy products and greasy/fried foods can lead to Phlegm and Dampness in the Stomach, and Spleen deficiency. Various chemicals such as drugs, artificial additives, or residual pesticides can all lead to various types of Stomach and Spleen dysfunction. For example, children are frequently given antibiotics, which are anti-inflammatory, i.e. anti-Heat, and therefore are Cold in nature and may result in excess Cold in the Stomach.

Manner of Eating

Children today tend to develop eating habits that predispose them to various Stomach and Spleen dysfunctions. Stomach Qi stagnation can result from eating too fast, eating too much, eating while studying or watching TV, studying immediately after eating, eating while emotionally upset, or constant nibbling. Stomach Qi deficiency can result from fasting, not eating breakfast, or eating irregularly. Stomach Yin deficiency results from eating late in the evening or night. Since Stomach and Spleen are couple organs, any disturbance in the Stomach would usually lead to Spleen deficiency and disruption of Spleen's function of transformation and transportation.

Emotional Association

Anxiety, resentment, frustration, and anger can all cause Liver Qi stagnation and Liver Yang rising, resulting in Spleen Qi deficiency due to Wood being the controlling element for Earth. The Five-Element Developmental Theory can further elucidate this condition as most of the children with RAP are in the Wood phase of development, when the Liver is most vulnerable, so that the child is prone to develop Liver Qi stagnation and Liver Yang rising.

Abdominal Pain Associated with an Altered Bowel Pattern

This pain has varied severity and typically is localized in the lower abdomen, and may be either relieved or exacerbated by bowel movement. Altered bowel pattern can be diarrhea, constipation, or sense of incomplete evacuation following bowel movement. Western medicine considers the colon as the major site of dysfunction.

Chinese medicine agrees that the pathology lies in the intestines, with the pathogenesis as Coldness in the intestines caused by ingestion of Cold foods or exposure to Cold. Girls' clothing often exposes the abdomen across the level of the umbilicus, so that ST-25, the Large Intestine Mu point, is also exposed to Cold, resulting in Cold contraction in the Large Intestine. The variation in bowel pattern can be explained by Spleen Qi and Yang deficiency causing diarrhea, and extreme Cold Intestines obstructing descending of Qi, causing constipation.

The familial predisposition that may occur in all three presentations corresponds to Kidney Qi and Jing deficiency in Chinese medicine. Stress and acute emotional trauma that precipitate symptoms in some children may also be due to acute Kidney Qi deficiency.

Evaluation

An evaluation from a Chinese medicine perspective necessitates taking a detailed history of dietary and eating habits, exposure to external Cold (including a girl's preference for stylish clothes), familial predispositions, stress, and emotional tendencies. Examination would focus on signs of Coldness, Yang deficiency, Spleen deficiency, and Kidney deficiency.

Treatment

All three presentations have excess Cold and Spleen deficiency with abdominal pain. Therefore, the general treatment for all three chronic, functional conditions would need to disperse both internal Cold and Coldness in the Spleen, tonify Spleen, and alleviate pain.

- Decrease or eliminate excess energetically Cold foods from the diet
- Diminish exposure to environmental Cold. Advise girls to wear clothing that covers CV-8
- KI-3, KI-7 to disperse Cold globally
- Warm the Middle Energizer with moxa of CV-8 or apply warmth to CV-8
- Disperse Spleen Cold with the four-point protocol:
    - Tonify SP-2, HT-8; sedate SP-9, KI-10
- Tonify Spleen with the four-point protocol (after dispersing Spleen Cold):
    - Tonify SP-2, HT-8; sedate SP-1, LR-1
    - ST-36, CV-12, PC-6 to regulate Middle Energizer and alleviate pain
- Auricular points: Shenmen, Point Zero, Stomach, Spleen, Kidney, Sanjiao.

Additional Treatment for Isolated Pain

- KI-3, CV-6 for general tonification of Qi
- SP-6, ST-36 to tonify Spleen and Stomach Qi.

Additional Treatment for Dyspepsia

- Eliminate or decrease the appropriate foods from the diet, e.g. excess sweets or dairy products
- Advise more regular eating habits
- For Stomach Qi stagnation:
    - CV-10 to promote descension of Stomach Qi
    - CV-6 to resolve food stagnation
- For Stomach Qi deficiency
    - ST-36 to tonify the Stomach and move Stomach Qi
    - CV-12 to tonify the Stomach and Middle Energizer
- For Liver emotional symptoms
    - LR-3, LR-13 to move Liver Qi; LR-3 to tonify Liver Yin and diminish Liver Yang
    - LR-14 to harmonize Liver and Stomach
    - Teach the child self-calming techniques
- Auricular points: add Liver.

Additional Treatment for Altered Bowel Pattern

- ST-25 moxa or apply heat to disperse Cold from the Intestines

- ST-37 the Lower He-Sea point of the Large Intestine to alleviate Large Intestine Cold, to regulate Stomach and Spleen
- CV-5 the Mu point of Sanjiao, to tonify and harmonize the Three Energizers
- Disperse Cold from the Large Intestine using the Five-Element four-point protocol:
  - Tonify LI-5, SI-5; sedate LI-2, BL-66
- Auricular points: add Large Intestine.

For Children with Familial Predisposition, or Pain Precipitated by Acute Stress/Trauma

- Tonify Kidney Yin and Kidney Qi with the Five-Element protocol:
  - Tonify KI-7, LU-8; sedate KI-3, SP-3
- Auricular points: add Kidney, Adrenals.

ACNE

Acne is the most common skin disorder affecting adolescents.[74,75] It is an expected physiologic phenomenon that occurs universally.[76,77] The incidence is approximately 80% worldwide[78,79] with higher prevalence in teenage boys, and peak age range of 14–17 years in girls and 16–19 years in boys.[77]

The disorder involves sebaceous follicles,[80] which have increasing sebum production as a normal maturation process in response to the increased activities of testicular, ovarian, and adrenal androgens.[77] Acne is a well known side-effect of systemic steroids. The Western diet does not appear to play significant role in the pathogenesis of acne.[77]

Although acne is self-limiting with age, treatment is necessary because the severe inflammation can result in permanent, disfiguring scars[78,79] that are socially disabling, and can have long-term psychological sequelae.[74–76,80]

Acne can be predominantly broadly classified into two types: obstructive as comedones, and inflammatory as pustules.[79–81] At this time, there is no cure for acne [1,2] but treatment with topical and oral medications, usually antibiotics, is directed toward controlling the progression of the process and preventing scarring.[74,75,80]

CHINESE MEDICINE

Acne in Chinese medicine is due to accumulation of Phlegm and Heat, which correlate well to the Western concept of obstructive and inflammatory types of comedones and pustules. The physiologic changes during puberty results in imbalances primarily in the Stomach and Lung channels, but may also involve Liver and Gallbladder channels.[82,83] The face is the most affected because many channels pass through the face and because it is the most exposed area of the body to Wind-Heat. Other common areas are the chest and upper back.[83] Since the skin corresponds to the Lung, excess Lung Heat can manifest as acne. Children in the Wood phase of development would be more prone to Liver and Gallbladder Heat, with distribution of acne lesions more prevalent along lateral aspects of the face and body.

Whereas diet does not appear to influence the pathophysiology or treatment in Western medicine, Chinese medicine posits that energetically Hot and Phlegm containing foods are significant in acne. One explanation for the efficacy of antibiotics from a TCM standpoint is that antibiotics are anti-inflammatory drugs and therefore are considered energetically Cold. Similar effects may be achieved by increasing Cold foods in the diet. Acupuncture treatment using body and auricular points seems to work synergistically in balancing the viscera and harmonizing Yin and Yang.[82]

Treatment

- Avoid Heat and Phlegm-producing foods in the diet
- Increase energetically Cold foods
- Use local points on the face and back, and connect with ion pumping cord to a distal point on the corresponding channel or to BL-60. For example, if acne lesions are on the forehead around Stomach points, use a local Stomach point on the face, and a distal Stomach point, e.g. ST-45 or use BL-60 as the distal point. Connect with ion pumping cord black on the Stomach face point and red on distal Stomach point or BL-60. If using magnets, place the bionorth (-) pole facing down on local point and the biosouth (+) pole facing down on the distal point, and connect with ion pumping cord as above
- ST-40, SP-6 to resolve Phlegm
- GV-14, LI-11 to clear Heat; which has been shown to be effective against acne pustules.[84]

For more chronic or severe acne, especially with pustules, use stronger treatment to clear Heat from the channels, such as the two-point or four-point protocols:

- Clear Heat from Lung channel: tonify LU-5, KI-10; sedate LU-10, HT-8 or use two points: tonify LU-5, sedate LU-10
- Clear Heat from Stomach channel: tonify ST-44, BL-66; sedate ST-41, SI-5, or use two points: tonify ST-44, sedate ST-41
- Clear Heat from Liver channel: tonify LR-8, KI-10; sedate LR-2, HT-8, or use two points: tonify LR-8; sedate LR-2
- Clear Heat from Gallbladder channel: tonify GB-43, BL-66; sedate GB-38, SI-5
- Auricular points: Shenmen, Point Zero, Master Skin point, Endocrine Hormone point, Lung points.[85]
- Kidney, Spleen, and Heart if there are pustules.[82]

ASTHMA

Asthma is the most common cause of chronic illness in childhood, with approximately 10% of children in the US carrying the diagnosis.[77,86] Significant numbers of school days are lost because of asthma. A wide variation of incidence is found in different countries, with the highest rates in the United Kingdom, Australia, and New Zealand, and the lowest in eastern Europe, China, and

India.[87,88] In recent years, prevalence of asthma is increasing worldwide, especially in children under 12 years of age.[89,90]

INCIDENCE OF YOUNG ASTHMATICS

Although asthma can have onset at any age, 80–90% of asthmatic children have their first symptoms before 4–5 years of age.[77] Children up to age 4 years have distinctive symptoms, and require special consideration.[91] They have increased health service utilization including a higher annual rate of hospitalization,[92] which has nearly doubled in the US from 1980 to 1992 for children 1 to 4 years of age. The same trend is observed by other nations worldwide.[93] Among American children aged 5 to 14 years, asthma death rates almost doubled from 1980 to 1995.[89,94] New Zealand and Canada have observed a similar increase in severity and mortality.[95,96]

PATHOPHYSIOLOGY

Asthma is a diffuse, reversible, obstructive lung disease with three major features: bronchial smooth-muscle spasm, edema and inflammation of the mucus membrane lining the airways, and intraluminal mucus plugs.[77,86] During the last two decades, chronic airway inflammation, rather than smooth-muscle contraction alone, has been recognized as playing the key role in the pathogenesis of asthma in adults.[97,98] Although this association is less well established in children, nonetheless, recent guidelines for managing asthma in the pediatric population have emphasized that treatment be directed toward the inflammatory aspects of the disease.[99–101] Chronic inflammation is due to the local production of inflammatory mediators and an increase in recruitment of inflammatory cells, predominantly eosinophils and mast cells. Studies in young adults suggest that the chronic inflammation may be responsible for long-term pulmonary changes including bronchial hyperresponsiveness, airway remodeling, and irreversible airflow obstruction.

Because of difficulties in conducting studies in infants and young children, information about them is incomplete.[102] Limited studies have detected increases in inflammatory cells and thickening of the lung basement membrane in infants and young children, and have found asthmatic children to have significantly lower lung function at 6 years of age compared to nonwheezers when both groups of children began with the same baseline at age 6 months. These data support the fact that asthma-like inflammation can be present at a very early age, and is associated with nonreversible impairment of lung function.[103]

The excessive inflammatory changes indicate that asthma is a disorder due to an "immunologic runaway response" that was poorly regulated so that instead of protecting the host, the hyperactive immune response destroyed normal structure. Increased concentrations of pro-inflammatory mediators, such as histamine and leukotrienes, are found in the airways, as well as in the blood and urine, of asthmatics[98] during an acute attack and after allergen and exercise challenge.[104] Cysteinyl leukotrienes are proinflammatory mediators that play an especially important role in the pathophysiology of asthma.[104] Lymphocytic and eosinophilic submucosal infiltrates appear to correlate with severity of disease.[97] In addition to inflammatory changes, epithelial destruction occurs at all levels of the tracheobronchial tree with exposure of the nerve endings, rendering the airways of the asthmatic patient hyperirritable.[105] The chronically inflamed and hyperirritable airways hinder mucociliary clearance, and become susceptible to acute obstruction by triggers such as allergens,[106] environmental irritants[107] including second-hand smoke,[108] exercise,[109] emotional stress,[110] and drugs. There is strong evidence that correlates asthma with respiratory syncytial virus infection; and children who enter day nursery before age 12 months and are exposed to viruses early in life thus build up immunity with decreased development of allergies.[111] In most children whose asthma is triggered mainly by respiratory infections at a younger age, asthma symptoms appear to remit by the adolescent years.[103] In older children and teenagers, emotions play a significant role both as the cause of symptoms and as the result of interplay of a chronic illness affecting the child's self-image and family dynamics.[77]

Diagnosis

The latest asthma management guidelines classify pediatric asthma into four groups of severity: mild intermittent, mild persistent, moderate persistent, and severe.[101] Mild intermittent asthma can be typified by exercise-induced asthma, a common pediatric condition.[101] Severe asthma, defined as increasing asthmatic attacks that respond poorly to conventional management, is becoming more prevalent in American children.[86] Status asthmaticus is the condition of a patient in progressive respiratory failure, in whom conventional forms of therapy have failed.[101] The exact definition differs between authors. For practical clinical purposes, any patient not responding to initial doses of bronchodilating agents should be considered to have status asthmaticus.[112]

Treatment

Avoiding allergens has been a successful management of asthma since the sixteenth century. It is a much more complex problem today, in view of the increasing amount of pollutants and chemicals in the environment that are potential allergens for children.[113] Parental education, especially in regards to smoking, can reduce hospital admissions.[114] Since infections that trigger asthma attacks are mostly viral,[115] antibiotics are not routinely indicated. Medication treatment consists primarily of bronchodilators and inhaled steroids, which are now justified as first-line therapy[116] both as long-term management[99] and for acute attacks.[117] Since growth suppression due to inhaled corticosteroids has been well documented,[118] it would be important to distinguish between infants with early-onset asthma from those with transient wheezing.[119] Recently, the FDA has also approved of leukotriene receptor antagonists for use in asthmatic children under 4 years of age.[120] These agents counteract the hyperimmune response so that there is diminished airway inflammation and decreased eosinophilia in the airway mucosa and peripheral blood.[104] Status asthmaticus requires aggressive treatments with multiple drugs. Efforts should be made to avoid mechanical ventilation as much as possible, since hyperinflation will worsen with positive-pressure ventilation.[86]

CHINESE MEDICINE

Current Acupuncture Data

Asthma epitomizes the Chinese medicine concept of "winter disease, summer cure." In China, many asthmatic children who were treated with herbal patches applied to acupoints during the summer had minimal or no symptoms during asthmatic seasons.[121,122] The few current studies and clinical reports on acupuncture treatment of children with asthma in general are favorable.[121,123,124] Empiric results using simple acupuncture regimes yielded good results in asthmatic children in Germany.[125] One study demonstrated that although acupuncture did not affect the basal bronchomotor tone; when administered 20 min before exercise, acupuncture was shown to be effective in attenuating exercise induced asthma,[126] which is common in children. One possible mechanism of acupuncture is in reducing the reflex component of bronchoconstriction, but not in influencing direct smooth muscle constriction caused by histamine.[127] For children who are fearful of or who cannot tolerate needles, non-needle treatments such as cupping and auricular press pellets[123] and massage of acupuncture points[124] have also been found to be effective.

Adult studies indicate that acupuncture was successful in treatment of allergic rhinitis accompanying allergic asthma and significantly affected serum IgE and lymphocyte count.[128] Even with treatment of just the master immunity point, Zusanli (ST-36) acupuncture was found to reduce the eosinophil count.[129] Two points on the Lung channel, LU-6 and LU-10, produced immediate effect in acute asthma attacks of the "Cold" type according to TCM diagnosis. Needle retention for 40 min produced long term benefits.[130] Combined electrical stimulation and topical herbal patches were synergistic, and more effective in both acute and maintenance situations.[121] When both auricular and body acupuncture points were used, steroid-dependent asthmatics were able to taper off of steroid doses.[123]

The most interesting future role for acupuncture in asthma lies in its potential both in stimulating an immune response and, more importantly, in regulating or modulating a hyperimmune response. At this time, there is ample biochemical support in the literature to indicate that acupuncture activates both the humoral and cellular immune system to protect the host.[131–136] Studies have also demonstrated that acupuncture can modulate the synthesis and release of pro-inflammatory mediators.[135,137,138] Current hypotheses suggest that this is most likely mediated through a common pathway connecting the immune system and the opioids,[139–141] which has been well known to be associated with analgesic effects of acupuncture.

Pathophysiology

Chinese medicine classifies pediatric asthma as acute Wind-Cold or Wind-Heat pathogenic invasion or as internal Kidney, Spleen or Liver imbalances. A careful history would decipher the etiology and facilitate a treatment plan.

History Taking in Asthma

Age of Onset

The onset of wheezing during the Water phase of development in infancy or early childhood is suggestive of weak Kidney constitution, which in general translates into more prolonged treatments. A child in the Wood phase of development tends to have Liver imbalance and emotional component to asthmatic episodes.

Dietary History

A detailed history must be taken that focuses on Phlegm-producing foods, sweets, and excess energetically Cold or Hot foods.

Family History

A strong family history of asthma would indicate hereditary—and therefore Kidney Yin/Essence predisposition.

History of Previous Other Illnesses

Other non-asthmatic illnesses can weaken the child; e.g., frequent episodes of viral gastroenteritis would result in lingering pathogenic influence and weakening of Spleen.

History of Emergency Visits and Hospitalizations for Asthma

Frequency and duration of emergency visits and hospitalizations are indications of severity of illness that may be more difficult to treat.

Precipitating Factors

Wind-Cold, Wind-Heat, external allergens, diet, and emotions are all precipitating factors for asthma.

Current and Previous Medication(s)

All medications being taken are important information, but especially steroids: dosage, frequency—since steroids interfere with acupuncture treatment.

Acute Episodes Due to External Pathogens

Wind-Cold Invasion

Wind-Cold invasion correlates to viral infection and airborne allergens, such as pollen, dust. The pathogen has passed through the Yang stages and has entered the Tai Yin stage so that the child is deficient with internal Cold. The Lung, being the organ that controls skin, is also susceptible to Wind invading the bronchi via the skin. Repeated exposures to Wind-Cold invasion can result in chronic lodging of Wind in the airways, making them more susceptible to future invasions. The Tai Yin stage of invasion also weakens the Spleen, which is already constitutionally deficient in children. A deficient Spleen cannot efficiently carry out transformation and transportation of fluids, resulting in increase of Damp and Phlegm that obstruct the channels and airways. When Lung Qi cannot descend, reversal of Qi flow or rebellious Qi ensues, causing symptoms of wheezing and cough with clear or white phlegm.

Both the Western lungs and the Chinese Lung actively participate in the immune protection of the host. The pathogen in the Tai Yin stage indicates that the Wei Qi was not strong enough to prevent the "burglar from entering the inner house." The presence of proinflammatory cells indicative of hyperimmune response even during an acute attack[104] suggests that the regulation of immune response is already affected. Both an ineffective immune response and an unmodulated immune response are biochemical correlates to Lung deficiency—a Lung unable to carry out its normal functions.

Treatment

During an acute attack:

- Dingchuan, special point for stopping wheeze
- BL-12, BL-13, PC-6, CV-17, LU-1[142]
- During the Wind-Cold illness, sequential treatments need to be instituted to shorten the course of illness:
  - First dispel Cold from the Lung, then tonify the Lung, and then tonify the immune system
- Tai Yin is the last stage when the pathogen, "the burglar," can be expelled. Tonification of the Lung or immune system without first dispelling Cold is equivalent to "locking the burglar inside the house." Since the Spleen is also directly or indirectly involved, similar treatment of the Spleen would be beneficial
- Dispel Cold: KI-3, KI-7
- Use the four-point protocol to dispel Cold:
  - Lung Cold: Tonify LU-10, HT-8; sedate LU-5, KI-10
  - Spleen Cold: Tonify SP-2, HT-8; sedate SP-9, KI-10
    (HT-8 and KI-10 are common points so that six points would disperse Cold from both Lung and Spleen)
- For infants and young children, only the Lung or Spleen points need to be stimulated
- Tonification: Use the four-point protocol for tonification:
  - Lung tonification: Tonify LU-10; sedate LU-5
  - Spleen tonification: Tonify SP-2; sedate SP-9
  - Use only Lung or Spleen points for infants and young children
- Tonify and modulate the immune system:
  - ST-36; back Shu points: BL-13, -18, -20, -21, -23
- Modify diet:
  - Decrease energetically Cold drinks and foods. Decrease sweet foods
  - Avoid Phlegm-producing foods: dairy products, sugar, honey, peanuts, almonds, or pork
  - Choose foods that tend to thin Phlegm: mushrooms, papaya, potatoes, pumpkin, radishes, strawberries, or string beans.

Wind-Heat Invasion

Wind-Heat invasion correlates to bacterial infection, which may be a secondary complication of viral infection, or may be a primary infection. Pulmonary symptoms indicates that the virulent pathogen has entered the Qi or even the Nutritive level. Spleen is similarly involved and becomes further weakened. Heat quickly combines with Phlegm, which now becomes thick and purulent. The invasion can quickly involve the larger airways and even lung tissue, causing bacterial bronchitis or pneumonia. Heat also quickly dries up Yin, causing great harm to the Lung which is vulnerable to Dryness. Lung functions are therefore much more compromised than in Wind-Cold invasion.

During an acute attack:

- Dingchuan, BL-12, BL-13, PC-6, CV-17, LU-1
- GV-14, LI-11 to disperse Heat

During the course of Wind-Heat illness, treatment needs to first dispel Heat from the Lung and Spleen, then vigorously tonify the Lung and Spleen with additional tonification of Lung and Spleen Yin; followed by tonification of the immune system.

Disperse Heat:

- GV-14, LI-11 to disperse Heat
- Use the four-point protocol to disperse Heat:
  - Lung Heat: Tonify LU-5, KI-10; sedate LU-10, HT-8
  - Spleen Heat: Tonify SP-9, KI-10; sedate SP-2, HT-8
  - (HT-8 and KI-10 are common points, so that six points would disperse Heat from both the Lung and Spleen in older children)
  - Use only the Lung and Spleen points for infants and young children
- Use the four-point protocols listed above to tonify Lung and Spleen
- Tonify Yin: KI-6 and SP-6
- Tonify and modulate the immune system
- Decrease energetically Hot drinks and foods. Decrease Phlegm-producing and sweet foods
- For thick and yellow "hot" Phlegm, white fungus is the most healing food. If it's not available, choose asparagus, apples, carrots, celery, pear, or mango; and avoid Hot foods such as garlic and ginger.

Chronic Asthma–Constitutional Weaknesses

Lung Deficiency/Kidney Deficiency

Children are constitutionally Lung deficient. The Lung is considered "immature" and vulnerable to Cold and Dryness. The increasing incidence of asthma in younger children can be explained by the Five-Element Theory of Development. Infants and younger children are in the Water phase of development, when the Kidney is vulnerable. The Kidney and Lung have a very close relationship. Kidney Jing or Essence correlates with Western concept of genetic predisposition. It is also closely related to the Corporeal Soul, which resides in the Lung and which provides physical sensations, such as breathing and itchiness. The Kidney Yang is the source of all the Yang in the body and is the root of the Defensive Wei Qi. The Kidney Yang enables the sorting out or filtering of clear fluid from dirty fluid that needs to be excreted. The clear fluid flows up the Bladder meridian, along the back and neck in the skin and muscles where it mingles with Defensive Qi. This becomes the first line of protection, the Tai Yang stage, against Wind-Cold invasion, or viral infection. In addition to diminished Wei Qi circulation and increased susceptibility to viral infection, there is also less clear fluid going up toward the Upper Energizer, making it more likely for the Western concept of formation of "mucus plugs" and diminished "mucociliary clearance." Lung deficiency results in inadequate descension and dispersion of Qi. The weak Kidney in turn cannot receive and anchor Qi, resulting in upward, "rebellious" Qi movement manifesting as cough and wheezing. With repeated occurrence, there is development of internal Cold which further contracts the channels, further diminishing circulation of Qi and fluid, making the child more easily susceptible to subsequent Wind-Cold attacks; to other external insults that are irritating to the airway, such as pollutants and smoke; and to ingestion of Cold foods. The Kidney and Lung relationship also explains prevalence of asthma during the autumn and winter seasons, because Lung is Metal, which corresponds to fall, and Kidney is Water, which corresponds to winter.[142]

Treatment

Acute attack: use the same protocol as for external Wind invasion.
Tonification between attacks as follows:

- Dispel Lung Cold
- Tonify Lung
- Tonify Kidney with the four-point protocol: tonify KI-7, LU-8; sedate KI-3, SP-3
- Decrease Cold foods
- Decrease spicy and salty foods that are harmful to the Lung and Kidney
- Minimize exposure to environmental allergens, e.g. smoke.

Spleen Deficiency

Children are also constitutionally Spleen deficient. The weak Spleen is further injured by modern diet that is high in Phlegm-producing foods—such as milk and dairy products—and artificially sweetened foods—such as cakes and cookies. Lung and Spleen have a close working relationship. Spleen extracts Food Qi and sends it upward to combine with air that Lung takes in through breathing to form Gathering Qi, the foundation for eventual formation of Nutritive Qi and Defensive Wei Qi. Spleen deficiency would therefore result in deficient Wei Qi.

Spleen deficiency impairs the transportation and transformation of fluids, resulting in formation of Damp and Phlegm, which accumulates in the Lungs and impedes Qi and fluid movements. Qi cannot descend in "clogged up" channels and fluid cannot move upward, and the child coughs and wheezes.

Treatment

Acute attack: use the same protocol as for external Wind invasion.
Tonification of Spleen between attacks as follows:

- ST-40 to transform Phlegm
- CV-8 moxa to warm the Middle Energizer
- Vigorous tonification of Lung and Spleen with tonification of the meridians, or two-point or four-point Five-Element tonification protocols
- Decrease spicy foods; Phlegm-producing foods, artificially sweetened foods
- For school-aged children, make sure they have a balance of studies, physical activities, and rest
- Auricular points: Shenmen, Point Zero, Spleen, Stomach, Lung, Asthma points.

Liver Yin Deficiency/Liver Yang Rising

In older children, emotions frequently precipitate an asthma attack. From the Five-Element developmental standpoint, these children are in the Wood phase of development when the Liver is most vulnerable. Children are constitutionally Liver Yin deficient, and at this Wood phase tend to easily become Yang excessed, manifest with Liver Yang rising symptoms such as motor symptoms of hyperactivity or emotional symptoms of being easily irritated, frustrated, angered and being very impatient. Liver Yang rising can dry up Lung Yin and quickly weaken the Lung.

Liver Qi can stagnate in the chest, obstruct the descension of Lung Qi and result in symptoms of shortness of breath, cough and wheezing. Since Wood/Liver has a destructive relationship with both Earth/Spleen and Metal/Lung in the Five-Element Cycle, an excess Liver can eventually weaken both the Spleen and the Lung, resulting in simultaneous deficiency of the two organs.

Treatment

Acute attack: use the same protocol as for external Wind invasion.

- Balance Liver:
  - LR-3 tonifies Liver Yin, subdues Liver Yang, moves Liver Qi
  - LR-13 moves Liver Qi
- Tonify Lung
- Tonify Spleen
- Decrease sour tasting foods, decrease fried foods, and medications
- Help the child explore factors that precipitate emotional stress and find ways to minimize them.
- Teach the child calming techniques such as Qigong or meditation
- Auricular points: Shenmen, Point Zero, Liver, Stress Control (Adrenal), Lung, Asthma points.

Maintenance Treatment for all Forms of Asthma

"Summer Cure"

A prophylaxis treatment described in the literature consists of massaging Bladder points for 3–5 min followed by application of an herbal mixture.[143] The TCM pediatric staff at the Xinhua hospital in Shanghai stimulates CV-22 and Bladder points.[122] Personally, I have had success in stimulating CV-22 and ST-36 and teaching parents to massage the Bladder meridian in the direction of flow during the summer when the asthma is in remission.

Tapering of Medications

It would be best for the acupuncturist to work with the physician in tapering medications, especially steroids, because of possible hypothalamo-pituitary-adrenal axis suppression with chronic steroid administration. Chinese medicine posits that steroids can cause Kidney deficiency.[38] Therefore, it would be reasonable to tonify the Kidney while the child is on steroids. The tapering of bronchodilators most likely would occur naturally, as the child would automatically require less medications with less wheezing (see Bibliography for further references on this topic).

ATTENTION DEFICIT HYPERACTIVITY DISORDER

Attention deficit hyperactivity disorder (ADHD) is the most common neurodevelopmental disorder of children.[144–146] The broad constellation of hyperactive, inattentive, and impulsive symptoms combined with the multiple comorbid conditions makes the definition of ADHD controversial,[147] and the diagnosis flawed.[148] The incidence in school-aged children ranges from 3 to 11%, averaging around 5%.[144,145–152] ADHD more commonly affects boys,[149] although it may be underidentified in girls.[150,153] It is a chronic, heterogeneous condition with academic, social, and emotional ramifications.[144,154] The disabling symptoms persist into adolescence in approximately 85% of children[155] and into adulthood in approximately 50% of cases[149,150,152,153,154,155] There is a developmental pattern[156] in the primary symptoms of the disorder: hyperactivity diminishes while attentional deficits persist or increases with age.[144] ADHD is also associated with numerous comorbid conditions.[153]

ETIOLOGY

The precise etiology is still not well understood,[148] but the complex debate of nature versus nurture continues to bring up multifactorial causes[147] and polarizing views.[158] There is general agreement that ADHD has a strong genetic predisposition.[145,152,153,157,159–162] The risk of developing ADHD in a first-degree relative is about five times higher than the general population.[153,156] Molecular genetic studies implicate at least three genes in ADHD: the D4 dopamine receptor gene, the dopamine transporter gene, and the D2 dopamine receptor gene.[156] Neurobiologic and neuroimaging studies suggest that both neuroanatomic and neurotransmitter defects contribute to ADHD symptomatology. Various dysfunctional central nervous system structures include prefrontal cortex,[163] frontal lobe,[156] corticostriatal pathway defect.[145,156,159,164,165] The neurobiologic abnormality involves dysregulation of neurotransmitters, especially dopamine and catecholamines.[166] Many ADHD experts posit that the central disability is impaired motor and behavioral inhibition, which leads to inability to manifest self-control, to acquire appropriate social skills, to organize time; all of which in turn lead to hyperactivity, learning disability, aggression, anxiety, and other primary and comorbid characteristics.[167-169] Currently, researchers are also studying the correlation between infant/child temperament, such as low frustration tolerance and low adaptability, with development of ADHD.[170]

Non-genetic "nurture" etiologies include prematurity, when hypoxia and ischemia can cause varying degrees of injury to a vulnerable central nervous system.[163,164] Various foods, including excess sugar, artificial colors, additives and preservatives, have been implicated to play a significant role in influencing the behavior and mood of children with ADHD.[145,171,172] Environmental chemicals, molds, and fungi, and neurodevelopmental toxins such as heavy metals and organohalide pollutants have all been found to correlate with ADHD symptoms.[145] Thyroid hypofunction[145] and abnormalities of fatty acid phospholipid metabolism[147] have also been implicated as potential causes of ADHD. On the other hand, there does not appear to be conclusive correlation of traumatic brain injury with development of ADHD.[173]

EVALUATION

Evaluation of the child with ADHD consists of a comprehensive medical and neurological examination, questionnaire from parents and teachers, and various rating scales and neurodevelopmental tests. Precise assessment is difficult because of a lack of specific biological or psychological test or marker for the disorder,[146,154,159,165,174] because of subjectivity in answers to questionnaires so that even father and mother can disagree on the child's level of hyperactivity or ability to concentrate; and because the DSM-IV diagnostic characteristics occur along a continuum that can be applicable to the normal population—for example, everyone can be impatient at times waiting in line—or can be associated with other neurodevelopmental and psychiatric disorders. The evaluation of the preschooler is even more difficult, as high activity level, impulsivity, and short attention span are—to a certain extent—age-appropriate characteristics of young children.[175] The 18 DSM-IV criteria are classified into three categories: inattention, hyperactivity, and impulsivity. Diagnosis is categorized as inattentive type, hyperactive type, or combined type that has both inattentive and hyperactive characteristics.

DSM-IV Diagnostic Criteria for ADHD[176]

- Either 1 or 2:
  - 1. Six (or more) of the following symptoms of inattention have persisted for at least 6 months to a degree that is maladaptive and inconsistent with developmental level:
  - Inattention
  - (a) often fails to give close attention to details or makes careless mistakes in schoolwork, work, or other activities

(b) often has difficulty sustaining attention in tasks or play activities

(c) often does not seem to listen when spoken to directly

(d) often does not follow through on instructions and fails to finish schoolwork, chores, or duties in the workplace (not due to oppositional behavior or failure to understand instructions)

(e) often has difficulty organizing tasks and activities

(f) often avoids, dislikes, or is reluctant to engage in tasks that require sustained effort (such as schoolwork or homework)

(g) often loses things necessary for tasks or activities (e.g. toys, school assignments, pencils, books, or tools)

(h) is often easily distracted by extraneous stimuli

(i) is often forgetful in daily activities

- 2. Six (or more) of the following symptoms of hyperactivity/impulsivity have persisted for at least 6 months to a degree that is maladaptive and inconsistent with developmental level:

  - Hyperactivity

  (a) often fidgets with hands or feet or squirms in seat

  (b) often leaves seat in classroom or in other situations in which remaining seated is expected

  (c) often runs about or climbs excessively in situations in which it is inappropriate (in adolescents or adults, may be limited to subjective feelings of restlessness)

  (d) often has difficulty playing or engaging in leisure activities quietly

  (e) is often "on the go" or often acts as if "driven by a motor"

  (f) often talks excessively

  - Impulsivity

  (g) often blurts out answers before questions have been completed

  (h) often has difficulty awaiting turn

  (i) often interrupts or intrudes on others (e.g. butts into conversations or games)

- Some hyperactive–impulsive or inattentive symptoms that caused impairment were present before age 7 years

- Some impairment from the symptoms is present in two or more settings (e.g. at school or work, and at home)

- There must be clear evidence of clinically significant impairment in social, academic, or occupational functioning

- The symptoms do not occur exclusively during the "course of a pervasive developmental disorder, schizophrenia," or one other psychotic disorder and are not better accounted for by another mental disorder (e.g. mood disorder, anxiety disorder, dissociative disorder, or a personality disorder).

In addition to the DSM-IV characteristics, this complex disorder also has numerous comorbid conditions: oppositional defiant disorder (ODD); conduct disorder (CD); antisocial personality disorder; tic disorder; depression, anxiety, and other mood disorders.[146,149,177–181] About 20 to 25% of children with ADHD have learning disability (LD).[177,182] The most common LD is reading disability or dyslexia;[183] but other difficulties include auditory processing disability,[184] communicative disorders,[185] motor and perceptual output problems,[186] executive dysfunction,[187] inability to understand causal relations,[182] difficulties in organizing, preparing, and inhibiting responses.[165] Some studies have demonstrated differences in baseline electroencephalogram (EEG) abnormalities in the parietal region for on-task conditions.[188] Currently, routine EEG is not recommended on children with ADHD. Academic problems lead to further behavioral problems, lack of peer acceptance, interpersonal difficulties,[165] low self-esteem,[144] and high level of alcohol and/or drug abuse.[149,189] The troublesome child with ADHD generates more complications, as families coping with these children tend to experience more stress and have more problems,[155] and the disruptive ADHD adolescent with chemical dependence is difficult to maintain in a treatment facility.[190] The child with ADHD tends to be more self-destructive and is more prone to injuries.[191]

TREATMENT

Because of the chronic, pervasive effects of the multiplicity of symptoms, ADHD management needs to be multifaceted and prolonged.[165] Medication continues to be the mainstay of treatment, with psychostimulants, especially methyphenidate (Ritalin), still being the most widely used drug.[144,146,153, 159,192,193] Although these drugs seem effective for improving attention and diminishing hyperactivity, their potential benefit on cognition and academic performance, on conduct and social behavior remain controversial.[144,194] The tricyclic antidepressants were added as an alternative medication in the 1970s,[195] with clonidine, buspirone (Buspar), and other antidepressants and neuroleptics added to the list in the 1980s.[196,197] These medications are currently recommended for stimulant nonresponders and children with more than one psychiatric disorder. Combined pharmacotherapy is sometimes prescribed for more complex cases of ADHD.[153]

Although it is generally agreed that drugs are beneficial on a short-term basis, there is a paucity of data on the long-term efficacy and safety of medications,[194,198] especially in children younger than 3 years of age.[175] Children with ADHD on medication should be monitored closely.[159,199] There is mounting controversy over the widespread use of Ritalin[145] because of concern of possible long-term side-effects that include poor weight gain and development of tic disorder, especially in children with a family history of Tourette syndrome. Pemoline, which is associated with possible increased risk of acute hepatic failure,[200] is no longer used. Clonidine is associated with many side-effects and has an increased risk for overdose.[201,202]

Besides pharmacotherapy, a multimodal approach using a combination of drugs and other methods such as cognitive behavioral therapy (CBT), psychotherapy, social skills training, and school interventions is frequently prescribed for ADHD. Cognitive-behavior therapies represent the most widely used alternative to pharmacotherapy. Previous studies showed disappointing results.[203–206] In 1992, the National Institutes of Mental Health began a 14-month, multisite clinical trial, the Multimodal Treatment of Attention Deficit Hyperactivity Disorder (MTA) study. The results indicated that high quality medication management (with careful titration and follow-up) and combination of medication and intensive behavioral therapy were substantially superior to behavioral therapy and community medication management. There is slight advantage of combination of medication and behavioral therapy over medication alone.[207] Psychotherapy can be an effective adjunct to medication,[144,154] but usually requires a long-term commitment to several years of treatment. Concerns about side-effects of medication, treatment acceptability, and compliance[208-210] are additional factors that complicate management of the child with ADHD. There is increasing interest in more natural, holistic integrative approaches to ADHD.[145]

CHINESE MEDICINE

There is minimal data on Chinese medicine treatment of ADHD. One clinical trial using a tonic herb demonstrated improvement of behavior and academic performance, and increased metabolism of dopamine and catecholamines.[211] Another trial using herbal preparation for balancing Liver and Spleen resulted in increase in intellectual function.[212] A thorough literature review of alternative treatments for ADHD identified 24 CAM therapies, and revealed that Chinese herbal treatment has promising pilot data. Simple sugar restriction seems ineffective.[213]

The author conducted a prospective, randomized, double-blind pilot study funded by the National Institutes of Health that integrated DSM-IV diagnostic criteria, conventional theories of frontal lobe dysfunction and neurotransmitter abnormalities with traditional Chinese theories of energetic imbalances. Laser acupuncture was used in the treatment of 7–9-year-old children newly diagnosed with ADHD. Preliminary data showed promise in reducing signs and symptoms of ADHD with improvement in behavior and cognitive function in children mild to moderately affected with ADHD.[214]

While Western medicine views ADHD as a complex neurodevelopmental disorder that encompasses all aspects of a child's life, Chinese medicine is equally concerned with the multifaceted condition that affects every major organ at all levels: energetic, physical, emotional, and even involves the spiritual level. The following exposition of the child with ADHD is based on the author's 20-year experience in working with children with ADHD, integrating Western information and incorporating the Five-Element Developmental Theory (Chapter 5) to help unravel the complicities that envelope the child with ADHD.

The strong genetic predisposition correlates to involvement of Kidney Essence and Kidney Qi. This is especially important in a young child in the Water phase of development, the preschooler. This child is naturally egotistical, curious, active and driven toward instant self-gratification. The child is pre-operational, manifests illogical and irrational thinking, as the child interprets the world according to his or her own experiences without regard for time or space. Activities and movements are not always purposeful, as they "run around" exploring this and that in the world. Growth and development are closely related to the maturation of the brain, the marrow in Chinese medicine. Kidney, the foundation of marrow, is the basis of all brain/marrow functions. This can be extrapolated to correlate familial predisposition to ADHD as transmitted through Kidney Essence, and neuroanatomic and neurotransmitter dysfunctions as Kidney Yang deficiency. The young Water child is also more susceptible to both explicit and implicit side-effects of medication. The physical side-effects listed for the ADHD medications do not disclose the potent energetic effects that usually injure Kidney Yang. Therefore, treatment of the preschool-aged child with ADHD is vigorous tonification of both the Kidney Yin and the Kidney Yang.

The Wood child is the operational school-aged child, who progresses from the unrealistic, Id-driven, one-dimensional thinking into the two-dimensional realm of cause and effect, right and wrong. Movements and activities become more purposeful as the child develops advanced motor coordination and social skills to participate in team sports. The Wood child is typically Liver Yang excessed as the young tree grows upward toward Heaven; the child learns to make decisions and take directions in his activities. The imbalanced Wood child would manifest motor "purposeless" hyperactivity and inability to understand right and wrong as the child becomes physically aggressive. A child acting without proper direction from the Liver, the Qi General, correlates to the Western terminology of having "impaired motor and behavioral inhibition." This child is particularly vulnerable to medication, which is metabolized in the Liver. Liver Yang leads to Spleen Yang deficiency through the destructive relationship of the Five-Element Cycle. Spleen is specifically involved with memory of facts and data, with concentration, therefore with academic learning. These influences are mediated through the Spleen Spirit, Yi. Spleen deficiency also explains the various sensitivities of the ADHD to foods, additives and preservatives. A deficient Spleen would in turn lead to deficient Lung because of the Earth–Metal nourishing relationship, and the child may have difficulty with organization and easily become sad and depressed. Lung deficiency would also predispose the child to become sensitive to chemicals and environmental toxins. Accompanying the Liver Yang excess is the constitutionally deficient Liver Yin— which is worse when accompanied by Kidney deficiency. Liver Yin houses the Ethereal Soul, the Hun, which spiritually connects human beings to each other. The child with ADHD has behavioral characteristics that alienate peer social interaction, which translates as a restless Ethereal Soul unable to settle down in a Liver Yin deficient environment. The Ethereal Soul is also intimately connected to the Mind, the Shen that is housed in the Heart. Inattentiveness and easy distractibility are manifestations of "brain" deficiency, but are Chinese medicine signs of disturbed Shen, a Mind that is not at peace. Therefore, the school-aged child with ADHD has multiple organ/system disturbance, manifesting primarily as Liver imbalance, but also encompass Kidney, Heart, Spleen, and Lung.

The teenager with ADHD is vastly different from the preschooler and the school-aged child with ADHD. As Western medicine points out, older children manifest less motor hyperactivity but are more troubled with inner restlessness. The excess movement of the Wood child gives way to a perturbed Shen in a fiery teenager, who is in the Freudian Genital phase of development with drastic hormonal and physical changes. Teenagers gradually discover their sexual identity, as they explore passionate relationships with the opposite sex and distance themselves from their parents. The adolescent Fire children are fearless and difficult to control. They experiment with drugs and alcohol and are rebellious in a treatment facility. Their excess Heart Fire or Yang is accompanied by Heart Yin deficiency secondary to Kidney and Liver Yin deficiencies. The Ethereal Soul and the Shen are restless, unable to find solace in deficient "houses." As Fire destroys Metal, depression and mood disorder can be more pronounced with Lung deficiency. The Spleen can have varying degrees of deficiency, depending on the extent of Liver–Heart imbalance of Yin and Yang. The teenager is also vulnerable to medications, because an excess bitter taste would further injure the Heart. Chinese medicine treatment would focus on the Heart, but also balance the Kidney, Liver, Spleen and Lung. Table 10.1 summarizes all the DSM-IV characteristics and their correlation to the Five-Element organs.

TABLE 10.1 *ADHD and the Five Elements*

DSM-IV characteristics	Wood/Liver	Fire/Heart	Earth/Spleen	Metal/Lung	Water/Kidney
Inattention					
Inattention to details, careless		X			X
Not sustaining attention		X	X		X
Not listening		X			X
Not understanding, not following through on instructions		X	X	X	X
Difficulty organizing tasks and activities					X
Avoids tasks requiring learning data					
Loses things necessary for tasks		X (memory)	X (memory)		X
Easily distracted					X
Forgetful		X (memory)	X (facts)		X (life events)
Hyperactivity					
Fidgety	X				
Restlessness	X				
Inappropriate behavior (inner restlessness, anxiety)	X (Ethereal Soul)				
Cannot stay quiet	X	X			
Large motor hyperactivity	X				
Talks excessively		X			
Impulsivity					
Blurts out answers—impatient	X	X			
Difficulty awaiting turn	X				
Interrupts or intrudes on others	X	X			
Associated affective characteristics					
Irritability, smoldering anger	X	X			
Explosive anger, temper outbursts	X	X			
Physical aggressiveness	X	X	X		
Sadness/depression	X	X	X	X	X
Worry/obsession			X		
Low frustration tolerance	X	X			
Low self-esteem		X	X		
Co-morbid conditions					
Learning disabilities	X	X			X
Oppositional/defiant disorder	X	X			X
Conduct disorder	X	X			X
Mood disorder		X			
Anxiety disorder	X				

Like its Western counterpart, acupuncture treatment of ADHD is also extremely complex. Management needs to take into account the age and stage of development of the child, the intensity and types of symptomatology, as well as dietary and environmental influences. Treatment has to be carefully planned so that all areas of deficiencies and excesses are treated, which must be done in increments as the child cannot possibly tolerate a massive, global treatment protocol. The regimen does not follow a fixed formula but must be flexible and devised individually, so that treatment is directed toward relief of the most immediate problem—such as disruptive hyperactive behavior or inattentiveness—with gradual overall balancing of all the Elements. A careful history about diet that includes excess types of foods, food additives, and medications or drugs and alcohol, would help steer treatment toward eliminating or tapering consumption. Lifestyle stresses, such as school pressures or dysfunctional family, would also be important information that provides a comprehensive understanding of the child.

General Treatment for all Phases of ADHD

- Sishencong—GV-20 with additional four surrounding points to potentiate effect
- A special point for the frontal lobe: 0.5 cm lateral to midpoint of forehead
- Yintang point for calming.

Preschooler—Water Child with ADHD

- Vigorously tonify Kidney Yin and Kidney Yang:
  - Individual Kidney points:
    - KI-3 tonifies both Yin and Yang
    - KI-6 tonifies Kidney Yin
    - KI-7 tonifies Kidney Yang
    - BL-52, Zhishi, "willpower room" to tonify the Kidney spirit, strengthen willpower
- Four-point protocol: tonify KI-7, LU-8; sedate KI-3, SP-3
- Eliminate salty "junk" foods, such as pretzels, chips, from diet. Decrease unnecessary intake of medications
- Begin tonification of Liver Yin: BL-18
  - LR-3 to subdue Liver Yang, nourish Liver Yin
- HT-7 to regulate the Heart
- BL-18 to tonify the Spleen.

School-Aged Wood Child with ADHD

The major focus is regulation of Liver and to calm the Hun and Mind:

- BL-18 to tonify Liver Yin
- BL-47 Hunmen , "Gate of the Ethereal Soul" to calm the Hun, improve relationship with others
- LR-3 to subdue Liver Yang, nourish Liver Yin
- LR-13 to regulate Liver Qi, to harmonize Liver and Spleen
- Diet should be a good balance of the five flavors:

- Decrease sour foods, such as pickles that are frequently put into hamburgers and sandwiches
- Minimize intake of medication
- Eliminate excess artificially sweetened foods
- Minimize salty foods
- Begin regulation of the Heart:
  - BL-15 to begin tonification of Heart Yin
  - HT-7 to regulate and tonify the Heart, calm Shen
  - CV-15 to regulate the Heart and calm the Shen
- Continue tonification of Kidney Yin: KI-3, KI-6
- Harmonize with the other organs:
  - BL-20 to tonify Spleen
  - BL-49 Yishe, "Thought shelter" to stimulate memory and concentration
- For children with affective component/depression:
  - LU-10, HT-7, LR-1 to harmonize Liver, Heart, and Lung
  - BL-42 Pohu, "Door of the Corporeal Soul" to sooth sadness, grief.

Teenage Fire Child with ADHD

The primary focus is to harmonize Heart Yin and Yang, and calm the Mind:

- HT-7, CV-15 to regulate the Heart, calm the Shen
- BL-44 Shentang, "Hall of the Shen/Mind" to strengthen and calm the Mind, stimulate clarity and intelligence
- Harmonize with the other organs:
  - BL-20 to tonify Spleen.
  - BL-49 Yishe, "Thought shelter" to stimulate memory and concentration
- Tonify Kidney Yin, regulate Liver, Spleen, and Lung as above (see Bibliography for further texts dealing with ADHD).

COLIC

Colic is a common condition of infants, affecting approximately one out of five infants, or more than 700 000 infants in the United States each year.[215] In spite of its prevalence, colic remains mysterious and puzzling to pediatric healthcare professionals.[216]

CONVENTIONAL MEDICINE AND COLIC

Review of pediatric medical literature indicates that infantile colic is difficult to define, both in terms of its etiology and symptomatology.[217]

Clinical Presentation

Colic usually begins between the second and sixth week of life and is rare after the fourth month of life.[218] The most common description of colic is intense, "paroxysmal" crying that is markedly different from normal fussing and crying. It can also occur as prolonged, unpredictable crying,[219] and the infant is restless and unconsolable.[220] The crying episode can last for minutes or even hours. Crying may occur any time of the day without obvious cause but is most common after the evening feeding.[218] The colicky episode is often accompanied by distension of the abdomen and cold feet. Often the baby seems to feel better after passing gas or a stool.

Etiology

Various etiologies of colic have been proposed that include variation in infant behavior and development, temperament, gastrointestinal and feeding abnormalities, and dysfunction in the mother–infant relationship.

Infant Behavior, Development, and Temperament

Early infancy is a developmental stage that represents a complex interaction between the baby and his environment. One conception of colic can be an expression of developmental stress,[221] possibly from unmet biological needs. A study on early infant behavior revealed that there was a progressive drop in colicky symptoms by the eighth week of life, so that it can be interpreted as a maturation process.[222] Some infants may have a temperamental predisposition to colic. A study of 40 infants and their mothers reveals that the irritable infants demonstrate an increase in the amount and intensity of crying, more disruption in sleep–wake states,[220] increased settled and awake periods.[222] Follow-up at 4 years of age revealed ex-colicky children displayed more negative emotions, more negative moods, and more reported stomachaches.[223]

Gastrointestinal

Colicky babies manifest various feeding difficulties and gastrointestinal variants. Hypermotility, an overagitated colon, may explain the symptoms.[77] One survey of 2773 infants revealed colicky babies tend to have slow or gluttonous feeding with various digestive symptoms.[224] Although no difference was found in the intestinal microflora between the colicky infants at the time of colic and the controls, a difference in bacterial cellular fatty-acid profiles at the age of 3 months was found to correlate with severe infantile colic.[225]

Colic has been attributed to feeding, both in the timing and the content. Early introduction of bottles may account for less effective suckling with more air swallowing that results in colic.[226] Cows' milk allergy has been repeatedly found in breast-fed babies with colic. When mothers were put on a diet free of cows' milk protein, colicky symptoms disappeared in many infants.[218,227–230]

Dysfunction in the Mother–Infant Relationship

The lack of synchrony in the mother–infant interaction has received a great deal of attention as the cause of colic. Studies are supportive of finding difficulty in mother–infant interaction.[220] Several possible factors contribute to the dysfunction: maternal perception of infant behavior; maternal age; inadequate parenting skills; mother's poor self-image. Colic may in fact begin during a woman's pregnancy or at birth.

A retrospective study of 25 4–8-month-old infants revealed mothers of infants with colic were more bothered by the infants' mood than mothers of infants without colic.[231] This was not attributed to the possible difficult temperament of the baby but to maternal perception. A prospective study of colicky infants with age-matched controls indicate that although there is no significant difference in temperament between the colicky and noncolicky babies, the mothers of colicky babies perceive them as more intense in their reactions, more distractible and negative.[232] Postpartum depression in the mother has also been found to correlate with development of colic in the babies.[233] A question survey of 76 747 infants in London revealed that the mother's young age, parity and socioeconomic status remain the most important risk factors for infantile colic.[234]

Parenting skills play a significant role in colic. In a survey of 2773 infants, the parents of colicky babies need more advice on diet and hygiene, and tend to give their babies more drugs.[224] Some parents who put forth a great deal of effort to console crying babies may actually be stimulating them excessively, resulting in the characteristic behavior of colic.[235] The mothers' own feelings of inadequacy may also play a role in colic. Compared to mothers with normal infants, mothers of colicky infants feel less competent as mothers and tend to have more separation anxiety.[236] Unable to calm her infant's distress, a mother may experience doubts as to her own mothering ability,[237] or even feel rejected.[238] This may be associated with abuse or thoughts of abuse, as 70% of mothers revealed explicit aggressive thoughts and fantasies and 26% admitted thoughts of infanticide during their babies' colic episodes.[239]

Colic may begin in the womb and at birth. A study from Finland looked at associations between characteristics of families during pregnancy and development of colic. Results indicate that when women experience emotional stress, physical symptoms, dissatisfaction with the sexual relationship during pregnancy, and negative experiences during childbirth, there was increased incidence of colic in the baies.[240]

It is, however, comforting to know that although colic causes added anxiety and conflict to a family, one study revealed that 3 years after the colicky period, families with moderate and severe colicky infants did not differ significantly from control families with respect to psychological family characteristics.[241]

Management

Treatment is advisable not so much because of the condition itself, but more because of the negative effect it can have on the parent–infant relationship. Since the precise etiology is not understood, the therapeutic goal of Western medicine is not aimed at "curing" colic, but at containment of the crying.[215] Removal of cows' milk protein from the mother's diet, changing the formula, and prescribing antispasmodic medications are the mainstays of conventional treatment and are sometimes helpful.[218] Parents may be referred for therapy to learn parenting and coping skills.

CHINESE MEDICINE AND COLIC

Currently, there is no data on acupuncture treatment of infantile colic. The TCM explanation of colic is a digestive problem due to inherent weak Spleen. Food accumulation and Qi stagnation result in abdominal distension, gaseousness, transformation into Heat, causing colicky symptoms. Since the infant is in the Water phase of development, the Kidney is vulnerable and fear is the underlying emotion that motivates many behaviors. These explanations correlate well with the proposed Western etiologies.

Gastrointestinal Symptoms

Spleen is the digestive Yin organ that is responsible for formation of Nutritive Qi, and for transformation and transportation of food, Qi and fluid.

Milk Allergy

Cows' milk causes Phlegm accumulation, and further weakens the Spleen.

Dysfunctional Relationship with the Mother

Chinese medicine posits that maternal physical and emotional health during pregnancy influences the physical and emotional health of the fetus. If mother experiences stress and worry during pregnancy, the fetus may be predisposed to developing various weaknesses, including Spleen deficiency. Western medicine has become concerned that colic may in fact begin during pregnancy. The mother's own weaknesses after pregnancy—Spleen, Kidney, Liver—predispose her to emotional states of excess worry, fear, anger, which can manifest as various maternal issues, such as poor self-image, and a more disturbed perception of the baby. The mother's mental state would in turn affect the mental state of the baby, who becomes more irritable.

Infant Temperament and Development

The infant is in the Water phase of development, when the Kidney that influences the marrow, the Western brain, is the dominant and the most vulnerable organ. The emotion associated with the Kidney is fear. The various irritating behaviors of the baby—increase in intensity and amount of crying, disruption in sleep–wake states—which Western medicine explains as based on unmet biologic needs, may be explained as motivated by fear, such as the instinctual fear of abandonment, especially when the mother is aloof due to depression or feelings of inadequacy.

Types of Colic

Colic can be classified in Chinese medicine as of two basic types:[242–245]

- *Excess colic*—signs of Heat and excess due to Spleen Yin deficiency: red face, warm extremities, intense crying, abdominal distention, agitation.
- *Deficient colic*—signs of Spleen Qi deficiency and Kidney deficiency: pale face, cold extremities, abdominal distension, cry prolonged but not intense, possible loose stools.

Management

The management is the same for both types of colic, and needs to be directed at both the infant and the mother.

Infant

- *Avoid overfeeding the baby*—excess milk or formula result in food and Qi accumulation in the Stomach and the Intestines. There is more tendency for parents to overfeed a bottle-fed baby, as parents usually want to "finish the bottle" even when the baby is full versus more natural, self-limiting with breast feeding.
- *Tonify abdominal Qi*: daily abdominal massage: clockwise in the direction of the Large Intestine flow: up the right side (ascending colon), across the top (traverse colon), down the left side (descending colon), and back across the bottom to the right side again.
- *Keep CV-8 warm*: babies should wear clothes that do not expose the umbilicus.
- *Tonify Spleen*: the mother can be taught to massage SP-6, ST-36. Although the infant's bony structures are not well formed, the mother can massage in the general area.
- *Tonify the Kidney*: massage KI-3.
- *Calm the baby*: Massage Yintang to calm the baby.
- *For infants with signs of Heat*: massage LI-11.

Mother

- *Diet*: breast-feeding mothers need to avoid Phlegm- and gas-producing foods: milk, milk products, cabbage, broccoli, cauliflower, brussel sprouts, tomatoes, citrus, garlic, onions, chocolate, coffee, beans, rhubarb, peaches, melons. Also avoid excess energetically Hot or Cold foods.
- *Treat mother's deficiencies*: find underlying weakness/deficiency in the mother, and treat the mother with acupuncture, herbs, and diet.
- *Calm the mother*: teach the mother to massage her own Yintang point, and calming exercises, such as simple breathing or Qigong exercises that take only a few seconds or 1–2 minutes, which she can practice throughout the day for calming effects.

CONJUNCTIVITIS

Conjunctivitis is very common in childhood. It can be caused by a wide range of both infectious and noninfectious agents. The infections are usually viral and bacterial; and noninfectious causes are due to a variety of allergens, irritants, and toxins. The cardinal sign is redness in the eyes, accompanied by different types of discharges and possibly other symptoms.

INFECTIOUS CONJUNCTIVITIS

Viral conjunctivitis is generally characterized by a watery discharge,[77] and may be associated with systemic viral infections, such as upper respiratory tract infection. *Bacterial conjunctivitis* is characterized by purulent discharge, often accompanied by edema or swelling of the eyes and some discomfort, but usually does not have any vision change or ocular pain. Sometimes children would give a history of morning crusting and difficulty opening the eyelids.[246] The majority of cases in children are caused by *Streptococcus pneumoniae* and *Haemophilus influenzae*,[246] less commonly by staphylococci.[77] Although conjunctival smears and culture are helpful in differentiating specific types,[77,247] they are rarely done in a pediatric outpatient clinic. The standard treatment is with broad-spectrum antibiotic eye drops and local measures, such as warm compresses. Complications of infectious conjunctivitis such as keratitis or abscess formation, should be referred for ophthalmologic evaluation and treatment.[247]

The newborn is given silver nitrate instillation immediately after birth to prevent gonorrheal conjunctivitis. Inclusion blenorrhea, a common form of ophthalmia neonatorum, is caused by *Chlamydia*. The infection is contracted from the maternal genital tract during birth. The incubation period is usually one or more weeks. The newborn develops an acute purulent conjunctivitis, but the discharge and scrapings are negative for bacteria and positive for the diagnostic intracytoplasmic inclusion bodies.[77]

NONINFECTIOUS CONJUNCTIVITIS

Allergic conjunctivitis is the most common noninfectious conjunctivitis in children. It presents with red, itchy eyes with profuse watery discharge and conjunctival edema. Children often rub the eyes, which aggravates the condition. History can often reveal the source of the allergen, onset of symptoms associated with being around cats or with seasonal pollen allergens. Treatment consists of avoiding the offending allergen, if possible. Using saline eyedrops is simple and nontoxic, and it is effective in up to 30–35% of cases.[248] Local treatment with cold compresses and topical antihistamine eye drops would resolve the majority of cases. Corticosteroid eye drops are rarely indicated and should be used only with the close supervision of an ophthalmologist.[247] Allergic conjunctivitis frequently accompanies allergic rhinitis in children[249] and would respond to oral antihistamines.

Chemical conjunctivitis is caused by an irritant to the conjunctivae. Silver nitrate can cause a chemical conjunctivitis in the newborn. Other common offenders are smoke, smog, industrial pollutants, and household cleaning substance sprays.

CHINESE MEDICINE

Chinese medicine correlates both viral and allergic conjunctivitis to Wind-Cold invasion and bacterial conjunctivitis to Wind-Heat invasion. There is no current study on acupuncture treatment of conjunctivitis in children. A report from Russia indicates that acupuncture increased 100 times the resistance to allergens and significantly reduced the content of IgE,[250] the immunoglobulin that increases with allergic reactions. A clinical report from China used acupuncture and bloodletting to treat acute, fulminant red eyes in adults.[251]

Treatment

Traditional treatment consists of expelling Wind invasions when there are systemic symptoms, and treating local and distal points for conjunctival symptoms of the eyes. For Wind-Cold and Wind-Heat treatments use the general protocols given in Chapter 7.

Local Treatment of Eyes

- Apply saline eye drops
- Local points: since it is difficult to insert needles or even apply noninvasive modalities such as electrical stimulation or magnets to points near or around the eyes in children, the best way to treat local points for conjunctivitis is with acupressure:
  - Massage BL-1, BL-2, GB-1, ST-1
- Distal points: GB-42, GB-43[39,243,244,252,253]
- In children with recurrent Wind invasions, tonify them with the immune tonification protocol.

CONSTIPATION

Constipation in children is defined by The Constipation Subcommittee of the Clinical Guidelines Committee of the North American Society for Pediatric Gastroenterology and Nutrition as a delay or difficulty in defecation, present for 2 or more weeks. It is a common pediatric problem encountered by both primary and specialty medical providers.[254] Constipation should refer to the character of the stool rather than to the frequency and to associated symptoms, such as abdominal discomfort, since constipation may represent the regular passage of firm or hard stools.[255]

Infants and toddlers often manifest hard and painful bowel movements by screaming and stool-holding maneuvers.[256] Because constipation is a common occurrence in childhood, it is easy for pediatricians to underestimate the pathology, and delay referral to the specialist.[257] The exact pathophysiology of constipation in children is not known[258] but the list of differential diagnoses for constipation is a long one: functional constipation; improper diet, such as excessive intake of cows' milk, lack of fiber; drug-induced, such as antihistamines that are commonly used by children; association with many gastrointestinal and anatomic disorders, secondary to endocrine disorder, such as hypothyroidism[259] metabolic disorder, such as renal tubular acidosis,[260] and neurologic disorders.[255,256,261]

Diagnosis is further complicated by familial, cultural, and social factors and normal childhood development. Psychogenic factors, such as various methods involved in toilet training, diet, and misuse or abuse of laxatives and enemas may influence the advent of constipation. Natural childhood motor and social development can also contribute to constipation: as the toddler becomes more ambulatory, he is distracted by many new and exciting activities so that he would pass just enough stool to relieve the pressure while continuing to play, and gradually he develops the capacity to ignore the rectal fullness. In the older child, school, games, social events, and the hurried pace of life may all interfere with any pattern of regularity. Many teenage girls, e.g., may become constipated because of reluctance to use toilet facilities other than at home.[255]

Diagnostic evaluation ranges from a simple history and physical examination,[255] to using sophisticated technical instrumentation such as anorectal manometry.[257] There is no single treatment protocol for constipation, and many children do not respond to multiple therapeutic trials and continue to have chronic problems.[258] Most treatment consists of fecal disimpaction, laxatives to prevent future impaction, promotion of regular bowel habits and retraining the child in toilet habits. New treatments consist of various prokinetic agents.[258] Behavioral and psychological interventions are not recommended for routine management[262] but would be beneficial in functional constipation. Parents should be reassured that although this disorder is not life-threatening, several months to years of supportive intervention may be required for effective treatment.[256,263] Young infants with constipation or older children with longstanding stool impaction should be referred to a specialist for further diagnostic and therapeutic management.[264]

HIRSCHSPRUNG'S DISEASE

Hirschsprung's disease, or aganglionic megacolon, is a congenital cause of severe constipation that occurs in approximately 1 in every 5000 live births. It is associated with a genetic defect on chromosome 10.[265] Intestinal motility is disrupted due to complete absence of enteric ganglia in an involved segment of the colon, resulting in constipation. Two-thirds of cases are identified by 3 months of age; a very small percentage are diagnosed beyond 5 years of age. The first sign frequently appears in the newborn infant, usually of average weight, who will fail to pass meconium; this is rapidly followed by reluctance to eat, bilious vomiting, and abdominal distention. Treatment is surgical resection of the involved colonic segment.[255,256] Although surgery provides near-normal gastrointestinal function for the majority of children, long-term follow-up shows significant residual problems with soiling in 12.6% of the patients.[266]

ENCOPRESIS

Encopresis is the constant or intermittent involuntary seepage of feces with a huge mass of feces in the rectal ampulla and sigmoid colon. It is common in children[265] especially in a young child under age 4.[261] It is known as psychogenic constipation, because it usually begins during toilet training, when the child needs to transform the natural, involuntary act of defecation into a voluntary process associated with parental approval and social taboos. This occurs during the preconcrete period of cognitive development when perception of reality can be easily distorted. The inability to completely hold back may reflect coercive attitudes toward rectal continence, or an inability to meet the high expection of a perfect daily performance.[255] Management in these cases must begin with educating parents that leaking of liquid stool onto underwear is completely involuntary, so the child should never be scolded or embarrassed.[267]

CHINESE MEDICINE

Currently there has only been one study from Israel on acupuncture treatment of chronic constipation in children. Ten acupuncture sessions increased the frequency of bowel movements.[268] Acupuncture has also been found to be effective in the treatment of postoperative rehabilitation in children who underwent surgery for Hirschsprung's disease. It may be recommended as a mode of treatment for postoperative complications.[269]

Physiology/pathophysiology

The physiologic process of bowel movement in Chinese medicine involves sufficient Qi in multiple organs and an adequate supply of Fluids, a Yin constituent. Digestion of Fluids begins in the Stomach, where Fluid is propelled downward. The Intestines rely on the Spleen to transform and transport fluids. The Liver directs smooth flow of Qi in the organs, including the Intestines. The Kidney is very important in being the foundation of Yin and Yang of all the organs, and therefore influences the Fluids and Yang Qi in the Lower Energizer; and in controlling both the urethra and the anus, therefore influences defecation.

Chinese medicine posits several factors that can interfere with normal physiologic function and produce constipation, and may offer explanations for pathophysiology that is puzzling to Western medicine.

Diet

The major causes of constipation relate to improper food intake. Whereas Western medicine concentrates on fiber, Chinese medicine focuses on excess Phlegm-producing foods, energetically Hot and Cold foods in children's diet of today. Constipation associated with cows' milk is due to excess Phlegm production. Energetically Cold foods and ice-cold drinks diminish Spleen's function of transportation which in turn results in colonic inability to move the stool downward. Energetically Hot foods dry up the fluids in the Stomach and in the Intestines so that stools become dry and hard, difficult to propel through the Intestines.

Excess Internal Cold

Excess internal Cold occurs frequently in children, secondary to recurrent invasions by Cold pathogens, from consuming excess energetically Cold foods or drinks, from medications that deplete Qi and Yang, and from any chronic conditions. Excess exposure to Cold such as repeatedly wearing clothing that exposes the umbilicus can also result in internal Cold. Cold causes contractions and slows down Qi and Fluid movement. Excess Cold in the Stomach would result in less Fluid being moved downward into the Intestines. Excess Cold in the Intestines slows down the normal peristalsis movement of the Intestines.

Stress

Today's children, along with their parents, live a lifestyle that is filled with stress. Worry, frustration, and anger can all cause Qi stagnation, specifically in the Liver and again the Spleen. This type of constipation is usually accompanied by abdominal distension and sometimes also pain.

Excess Mental Activity

Since Spleen is responsible for processing data, studying too much can deplete Spleen Qi, again causing constipation similar to Cold foods. Studying long hours without adequate rest would also deplete Kidney Yin and Yang. Kidney Yin depletion would lead to overall Yin or fluid deficiency, resulting in dry stools. Kidney Yang depletion would lead to Coldness in the Lower Energizer, in the Intestines, and result in slower peristalsis and constipation.

Excess Physical Activity

Children today are encouraged to excel in sports. Many families begin to enroll their children at a very young age in team sports, such as soccer. Some families and children become obsessed with competitive sports, especially in high school years, and the excess physical activity can often deplete Qi, especially Spleen Qi which governs muscles, leading to Spleen Qi deficiency constipation.

Lack of Physical Activity

The opposite of the competitive athlete is the "couch potato" child, as the incidence of obesity is increasing in childhood. Since an appropriate amount of exercise stimulates all metabolic activities, including peristalsis of the Large Intestine, lack of exercise would slow down movement of stool down the Large Intestine.

Repeated Illness-related Fevers

Infants and young children are more susceptible to developing infections or Wind invasions, and tend to run very high fevers with even mild illnesses. Repeat occurrences of fever results in interior Heat and dries up fluids, which can manifest as constipation. Frequent recurrences would result in a chronic state of Yin deficiency and constipation that is difficult to treat unless the Yin deficiency is corrected.

Medications

Pediatricians have routinely administered antibiotics for numerous common bacterial conditions in childhood, such as ear infection and streptococcal pharyngitis. While antibiotics are indicated for bacterial infections, they are frequently administered indiscriminately for viral illnesses, Wind-Cold invasions, such as URI.

Since antibiotics are anti-inflammatory, they are generally Cold in nature. Because they are chemicals, they exert much more potent Cold effects than energetically Cold foods. On an acute basis, the Coldness produces Spleen Qi deficient, Cold diarrhea, a common side-effect at the time when the child is taking antibiotics. The long-term, cumulative effect of multiple administrations of antibiotics is Coldness in the Lower Energizer, which would result in constipation. Children take antihistamines even more frequently than antibiotics, since they are available over the counter. Parents routinely give children antihistamines for URI symptoms and often concomitantly with antibiotics for an ear infection. Western literature lists antihistamine as a potential cause of constipation without an explanation for its pathophysiology. Chinese medicine can explain the role of antihistamine as a drying agent that depletes the child's Yin, resulting in constipation.

Constitutional Weaknesses

Children are constitutionally Spleen deficient. Some children also have a familial or pre-Heaven Jing predisposition for Spleen deficiency, which correlates to the Western diagnosis of anatomic anomalies.

Evaluation of the Constipated Child

Take a Detailed History

Note the age of onset, diet, previous illnesses, number and height of fever, mental and physical activities, emotional stress, medications—especially frequency of antibiotics and antihistamines; any associated symptoms such as abdominal distention or pain. It would be helpful to have a Western evaluation to rule out possible anatomic abnormalities, such as Hirschsprung's disease.

Determine any Possible Constitutional Weakness

Take a detailed family history of gastrointestinal disorders and constipation, physical and emotional health and well-being of the parents at conception, and mother's health during pregnancy—specifically if there were dietary factors or emotional stress such as excess worry that could have contributed to Spleen deficiency in the parents, and transmitted to the child in pre-Heaven Qi and Essence. A family history of Kidney deficiencies would predispose the child to Kidney Yin and Kidney Yang deficiencies.

Use the Developmental Theory to Help Determine the Origin

For children under age 6, consider Kidney deficiency as a contributing factor to constipation. For children over age 6, consider Liver Qi stagnation as a component of constipation.

Determine the Type of Constipation

- Constipation with excess Cold: facial pallor, general feeling of coldness, cold hands and feet, abdominal pain that improves with pressure

- Constipation with excess Heat: dry, hard, infrequent stools; thirst; dry mouth; red face; sometimes abdominal pain that worsens with pressure
- Constipation with Qi stagnation: firm stools every 3–4 days, abdominal distension with belching.

Diagnosis

There are three major diagnostic categories for childhood constipation, and many children may have a combination of two or all three types:

- Spleen Qi deficiency
- Liver Qi stagnation
- Yin deficiency.

Spleen Qi Deficiency

The constitutional Spleen deficiency in children may be aggravated by living in a Damp environment, consumption of excess Phlegm-producing or sweet foods; and familial predisposition. Internal Cold, excess mental activity, excess physical activities without adequate rest, and repeated illnesses can all contribute to further Spleen Qi deficiency. The Spleen is unable to properly transform and transport fluids, resulting in dryness in the Large Intestine and constipation. This type of constipation can explain the majority of Western diagnoses: functional constipation, improper diet, drug induced (causing internal Cold), and constipation secondary to chronic illnesses. Encopresis may be the concomitant occurrence of Spleen deficient constipation and Spleen Cold diarrhea, when loose stools seep around impacted dry stools. There may be other accompanying signs of Spleen deficiency, such as facial pallor, fatigue, abdominal distension, and muscle weakness.

Treatment

Expel Stool

The first goal is to propel the stool through the colon. Anatomically, the large intestine begins on the right with the ascending colon, then goes across the upper abdomen in the transverse colon, and down on the left side as the descending colon to the rectum. Teach the mother to massage the child's abdomen in a clockwise direction (with the child as the clock) begin at the child's right lower abdomen, massage upward to below the ribs, then across the top of the abdomen to the child's left, then down the left side. Massage 50 times at least once a day.

Modify Diet

Decrease or eliminate Phlegm-producing foods, artificially sweet foods, greasy/fried foods, and excess energetically Cold or Hot foods.

Modify Lifestyle

These children should have a balance of rest, study, and physical activities.

Acupuncture Treatment

- Tonify the Spleen
  - ST-36
  - SP-3, SP-6, BL-20
- Or use the four-point protocol:
  - Tonify SP-2, HT-8; sedate SP-1, LR-1
- ST-40 to expel Damp
- If there are signs of Coldness, expel Cold from the Spleen:
  - Tonify SP-2; sedate SP-9
- Or use the four-point protocol:
  - Tonify SP-2, HT-8; sedate SP-9, KI-10
- Moxa CV-8 to warm the Middle Energizer
- Avoid exposing the umbilicus (CV-8) to Cold
- Tonify the Kidney in children under age 6 in the Water phase of Development: KI-3, KI-6, KI-7, BL-23.

Liver Qi Stagnation

Dampness from Spleen deficiency can obstruct the flow of Qi and prevent the Liver from properly directing Qi circulation, resulting in Qi stagnation. There is usually fullness in the epigastrium accompanied by hypochondriac pain. Chronic intake of excess sour foods, greasy and fried foods, and medications (which are metabolized in the liver), as well as a stressful lifestyle, contribute to the development of Qi stagnation. Emotions associated with Liver imbalance, such as anger, anxiety, frustration, can precipitate an acute episode of pain in a constipated child. The pain is relieved with passage of stool. The school-aged child in the Wood phase of development is especially prone to constipation due to Liver Qi stagnation. This type of constipation often carries the Western diagnoses of functional or psychogenic constipation, and the child and family are often referred to a therapist.

Treatment

Abdominal massage is used as in Spleen Qi deficiency to expel stool. Modify the diet to decrease or eliminate excess sour foods, greasy and fried foods, and over-the-counter medications. Modify lifestyle to decrease stress, such as achieving a more balanced schedule with study, activities, and rest. Teach the child self-calming techniques.

- LR-13, LR-14 to promote the smooth flow of Liver Qi and relieve Qi stagnation
- ST-40 to expel Damp
- Tonify the Spleen
  - ST-36
  - SP-3, SP-6, BL-20

- Or use the four-point protocol:
  - Tonify SP-2, HT-8; sedate SP-1, LR-1.

Yin Deficiency

Children are constitutionally Yin deficient. Repeated Heat invasion illnesses with inadequate dispersion of Heat, chronic consumption of excess energetically Hot foods and over-the-counter antihistamines can consume and dry up Yin, causing further Yin deficiency. Accumulation of Dampness due to Spleen deficiency can transform into Heat. Yin deficiency can manifest as dryness in various organs, such as dry mouth, dry skin, and scanty urine. Yin deficiency in the intestines results in constipation. There may be accompanying Heat signs, such as low-grade temperature, and red rashes.

Treatment

- Abdominal massage to expel constipated stool
- Eliminate or decrease energetically Hot foods
- KI-3, KI-6, SP-6 to globally tonify Yin
- LI-11 to disperse Heat
- LI-2 tonifies Large Intestine Yin
- Use the two-point or four-point protocol to disperse Heat from the Large Intestine:
- Tonify LI-2; sedate LI-5
- Tonify LI-2, BL-66; sedate LI-5, SI-5
- Tonify the Spleen
  - ST-36
  - SP-3, SP-6, BL-20
- Or Use the four-point protocol:
  - Tonify SP-2, HT-8; sedate SP-1, LR-1.[38,39,77,242–245,252,270–274] (See Bibliography for further reading on this topic.)

DIAPER RASH

Diaper rash can occur at any time before the child is toilet trained. It usually peaks between 7 and 12 months of age.[275] Diaper rash not only causes discomfort to babies, but is also distressing to mothers and caregivers, who often feel guilty and ill-prepared for this problem.[275] The rash is caused by contact and irritation of a wet diaper and monilial overgrowth, usually appearing as red patches with "satellite" lesions. Excoriated skin can lead to secondary bacterial infection or impetigo. Both diarrhea and oral antibiotics predispose the infant to develop diaper rash. Diarrhea increases wetness, creating a favorable environment for yeast; while antibiotics alter normal bacterial flora, allowing yeast overgrowth.

The most effective prevention and treatment is keeping the diaper area clean and dry.[275,276] During the last decade, a number of technological innovations in disposable diaper designs and materials—such as using more absorbent material to keep the diaper area dry—have reduced incidence and severity of diaper rash.[277] Topical antimonilial ointments such as nystatin are usually prescribed. Although topical corticosteroids are in general contraindicated,[278] they are often used for their anti-inflammatory effects. Secondary bacterial impetiginous lesions are treated with antibiotic creams. Education of and support for the caregivers are also necessary components of diaper care.[279]

CHINESE MEDICINE

Diaper rash, like eczema, represents generalized accumulation of internal Damp Heat in the skin. There is no data at this time on acupuncture or herbal treatment of diaper rash. Traditional Chinese medicine recommendations would be to disperse Heat and Dampness.

- Keep the diaper area dry
- ST-40 disperses generalized Dampness
- LI-11 disperses Heat
- LR-8 Water point of the Liver channel, to sedate Heat in the Blood, and also Heat to the genital area
- KI-6 tonifies Yin
- Decrease energetically Hot or Phlegm-producing foods in the child's diet
- In children with recurrent diaper rash, overall tonification of the Spleen can decrease internal Dampness, and minimize recurrence
  - Single point: SP-3 or SP-6
  - Four-point protocol: tonify SP-2, HT-8; sedate SP-1, LR-1.[38,242,244,273,274]

DIARRHEA

Diarrhea is a significant cause of pediatric morbidity and mortality in both developed and under-developed countries,[255,280] and continues to pose diagnostic and therapeutic problems.[281] Diarrhea is defined as an alternation in normal bowel movement characterized by an increase in the water content (decrease in consistency), in volume, and increase in frequency to more than three stools per day. Acute diarrhea is an episode of diarrhea of less than or equal to 14 days in duration. The majority of pediatric acute diarrhea is "infectious diarrhea," an episode due to an infectious etiology. Persistent diarrhea is diarrhea of more than 14 days duration, whereas chronic diarrhea lasts more than 30 days.[282]

ACUTE INFECTIOUS DIARRHEA

Infectious diarrheal diseases are the second leading cause of morbidity and mortality worldwide.[282] Each year more than 4 million infants and young children die of acute infectious diarrhea.[255] Children under age 3 years have an average of approximately 2.5 episodes of gastroenteritis per year in the United States.[280,282] Internationally, the average is approximately 3.3 episodes annually.[255] As many as 30% of pediatric hospital admissions are for diarrhea, which accounts for more than 1/3 of all deaths in children younger than 5 years of age.[255] Infants under 3 months of age have the highest risk for hospitalization and mortality.[283] It is estimated that diarrheal diseases account for 10% of preventable infant deaths.[255] Preschoolers placed in child-care centers are at increased risk for diarrhea because of greater potential for person-to-person transmission.[284]

The infectious pathogens that cause acute diarrheal episodes in children include viruses, bacteria, and parasites.[285] Transmission is most likely via the fecal–oral route, from ingesting contaminated food or water,[286] or in infants and toddlers, by mouthing contaminated toys. The nature of food-borne diseases is changing as more mass-produced, minimally processed, and widely distributed foods result in nationwide and international outbreaks of diarrheal disease instead of just a few individuals who shared a meal.[282] The majority of cases are due to viral infections. Rotavirus is the most prevalent,[23] and human astrovirus (HAstV) is a significant cause of diarrheal outbreaks.[286] Frequently, children are co-infected by several viruses.[286] Viral diarrhea tends to involve the small bowel, producing large, watery, but relatively infrequent stools.[287] These illnesses usually have short, self-limiting courses,[285] typically lasting between 3 and 7 days.[23] However, they can be devastating to children with compromised immune systems or structural abnormalities of the gastrointestinal tract.[282]

The most common bacterial agents are enteropathogenic *E. coli*, *Shigella* and *Salmonella*, and *Campylobacter*.[23,287] These are much more virulent pathogens that usually cause mucosal injury in the small and large intestines, producing frequent, often bloody stools containing leukocytes.[287] *E. coli* has become an important public health problem in recent years, causing more than 20 000 cases of infection and up to 250 deaths per year in the United States.[288] Transmission of infection is most commonly linked to consumption of contaminated meat, water, unpasteurized milk, leafy lettuce, alfalfa sprouts and goats' milk,[288,289] and by exposure to contaminated water in recreational swimming sites.[289] The different strains of enteropathogenic *E. coli* produce an inflammatory diarrhea by attaching to the intestinal mucosa and releasing toxins that injure cells and cause hemorrhage and necrosis.[290] The acute diarrhea, accompanied by abdominal cramping, progresses to bloody stools, and often leads to serious complications such as hemolytic–uremic syndrome and thrombotic thrombocytopenic purpura.[288,289] *Shigella* and *Salmonella* cause similar inflammatory injury that results in bloody stools and fecal leukocytes.[23] The most common parasitic infection is *Giardia lamblia* which often causes secretory diarrhea without blood[23] and often leads to chronic diarrhea.[291]

Diagnosis and treatment are still inconsistent. Because most acute diarrhea is self-limiting, physicians often do not obtain stool cultures or examination for ova and parasites since the results are not available sometimes for several days. Stool culture can identify different types of bacteria, but detection of specific enteropathogenic strains of *E. coli* requires specific serotyping that is not performed in routine stool cultures.[288] It is expensive, time-consuming, and often not sufficiently specific or sensitive so that it is not recommended for routine diagnosis.[290]

The primary treatment focus is on correction of dehydration, which is the most important cause of morbidity and mortality in acute diarrhea.[292] Oral rehydration treatment (ORT) with solutions containing appropriate concentrations of electrolytes and carbohydrates is recommended by the World Health Organization (WHO)[293] and has significantly reduced mortality.[283,287,293–295] The rationale for ORT is that the intestinal sodium transport is enhanced by glucose and this mechanism remains intact despite entertoxin injury to the small intestine epithelium.[293] Following rehydration, early refeeding with lactose-free[287] or normal, age-appropriate diet[285] is important for reducing diarrheal duration, severity, and nutritional impact.[293] Supplementation with specific dietary ingredients that are lost in diarrhea, such as vitamin A, zinc, and folate, is also recommended.[293]

Since the majority of acute infectious diarrheas are viral, they do not need antimicrobial therapy. The rotavirus vaccine was put on the market in the United States in October 1998. This vaccine, as a natural infection, decreases the risk of acute rotavirus diarrhea by 50% and the risk of severe diarrhea with dehydration by more than 70%.[294,295] Breast feeding is one of the most important preventive measures.[296,297] Continuation of breast feeding has also been found to control acute diarrheal episodes.[293] Improving hygiene such as handwashing is also important, especially in daycare centers.

Treatment with antimicrobial therapy must be instituted carefully only upon specific identification of the pathogen and of drug sensitivity. There is increasing frequency of antibiotic resistance so that commonly used antibiotics are ineffective in acute diarrhea.[282,294–297] Treatment of salmonellosis with antibiotics can prolong the carrier state and lead to a higher clinical relapse rate.[282] Injudicious antimicrobial therapy can also lead to susceptibility to other infections, enhance colonization of resistant organisms,[282,298] and disrupt the normal intestinal flora, the body's natural defense against infection.[299]

PERSISTENT DIARRHEA

After acute gastroenteritis, delayed recovery and protracted diarrhea may occur, leading to postenteritis enteropathy. The diarrhea persists for more than 14 days, with continual small-intestinal mucosal damage.[255,300] It occurs most frequently in very young infants, especially those living in poor, crowded conditions,[255] in bottle-fed malnourished infants, and after rotavirus infection.[301]

In Denmark the incidence was estimated to be approximately 3 per 1000 pediatric hospital admissions for gastroenteritis.[255] Clinically, the infant is listless, irritable, often has a "worried look," and begins to show weight loss and wasting with persistent diarrhea. If the watery stool is profuse, the abdomen may become distended and tympanitic.[255] The precise pathogenesis for ongoing diarrhea following a bout of infectious gastroenteritis remains undetermined, but is most likely multifactorial: (1) persistence of the intestinal pathogen; (2) malnutrition from the acute episode exerts an adverse effect on the repair of the intestinal mucosa and on the recovery of normal motility; (3) dysmotility engenders bacterial contamination and overgrowth;[302] (4) young age with immature immune response to antigenic stimuli.[255] Secondary lactose[302] and sucrose malabsorption and small bowel bacterial overgrowth have been detected.[302] The finding of lymphocytic infiltration of the intestinal mucosa suggests a cell-mediated immune response to environmental antigens, such as dietary, microbial, or both.[303]

Whereas the major complication due to acute diarrhea is dehydration, persistent diarrhea even at 2 to 3 weeks' duration can result in malnutrition[255] and failure to thrive.[291,304,305] Despite intensive field-based and laboratory studies over three decades, many questions remain unanswered about prevention and the best approaches to management.[255] Children with secondary lactose intolerance would have more watery diarrhea, accompanied by bloating, flatulence, and crampy abdominal pain after ingestion of lactose.[23] A general elimination diet with lactose-free protein hydrolysate formula may be life-saving in some infants.[301]

CHRONIC DIARRHEA

Chronic diarrhea, defined as diarrhea lasting more than 30 days,[282] seems to be increasing globally in the pediatric population.[306] A long list of differentials includes congenital anatomic abnormalities, such as short bowel syndrome; enteric infections, extraintestinal infection, such as urinary tract infection; acquired sugar and protein intolerance, inflammatory bowel disease, immune defects, inborn errors of metabolism, and endocrinopathies.[255,307] Malnutrition due to chronic diarrhea affects hundreds of millions of young children and annually causes more than 3 million deaths in children aged under 5 years of age.[255] There is still no universal approach to diagnosis and treatment.[308] Infections remain the most common cause of chronic diarrhea in children of all ages,[307] with an expanding number of potential viral, bacterial, and parasitic pathogens.[309] Just as in acute diarrhea, identification of the specific pathogen and drug sensitivity is important for management of infectious chronic diarrhea. *Giardia* is a frequent parasite in children and medication treatment appears beneficial.[310]

Treatment of noninfectious conditions, such as inflammatory bowel disease, needs to be directed toward the primary disorder. In all cases of chronic diarrhea, malnutrition needs to be treated vigorously in order to prevent growth failure and mortality. Elimination diets generally only provide transitory, symptomatic relief.[311] Besides monitoring fluid and caloric intake, micronutrients such as zinc[312] and vitamins need to be supplemented.[306]

Newer treatment and prevention modalities, including probiotics and vaccinations, are assuming increasingly more important roles in management of chronic diarrhea.[309] Chronic diarrhea without malnutrition is toddler's diarrhea, or chronic nonspecific diarrhea (CNSD). It is the most frequent cause of chronic diarrhea in children between 6 months and 3 years of age.[255,313] The typical clinical presentation is a young child who was a colicky baby and gradually begins to have three to six loose stools per day. Most of the stools are passed early during the waking hours and contain undigested foods and mucus.[314] The child is otherwise active and healthy looking, with normal growth.[315] Stress and infection can precipitate bouts of diarrhea, which is made worse by a low-residue, low fat and high carbohydrate diet.[255]

The precise etiology is still undetermined. There is often a strong family history of functional bowel disorders[255,313] so that it may be an early manifestation of irritable bowel syndrome.[255] From an infectious standpoint, there is the possibility of bacterial invasion of the small intestine by the upper respiratory tract microflora.[255] Current evidence also suggests that CNSD is primarily a gut motility disorder, modulated by dietary factors.[255,316] Diminished upper small intestinal motility[304] may be a physiologic, developmental phenomenon.[317] Some children demonstrate intestinal mucosal injury[318] with villous atrophy.[291] The mechanisms that lead to mucosal injury are elusive.[306] Dietary factors include low dietary fat, high carbohydrate and high fluid consumption, especially apple juice.[319] The over-consumption of apple juice has received the most attention as the causative agent. Previously, children were given orange juice to prevent scurvy. In recent years, apple juice has become the juice of choice for the under-5 age group.[320] In many children with CNSD, apple juice makes up 25–60% of daily dietary intake.[321] Apple juice is high in sorbitol and has a high fructose to glucose ratio,[322] and therefore contributes to a carbohydrate imbalance. In addition, compared to the freshly pressed and unprocessed ("cloudy") apple juice, enzymatically processed ("clear") apple juice significantly promotes diarrhea. This suggests that the increased amount of nonabsorbable monosaccharides and oligosaccharides as a result of the enzymatic processing of apple pulp is an important etiological factor in apple juice induced CNSD.[319]

Normally, 95–98% of the intestinal fluid is reabsorbed. Disordered intestinal motility combined with excessive fluid and carbohydrate intake contribute to development of diarrhea.[255] Other proposed theories of pathogenesis include food allergy and intolerance,[314,323] behavioral problems,[323] hypogammaglobulinemia,[324] congenital sucrase–isomaltase deficiency[303] and iatrogenic causes of excess oral replacement therapy and elimination diet.[325] CNSD seems to be self-limiting, resolving spontaneously in a mean time of 1.7 years.[325] However, symptoms may resurface later in childhood,[255] such as in teenagers who have diarrhea while on a fruit and juice diet.[322]

Treatment generally consists of normalization of the child's diet, especially with regard to fat, fiber, fluids, and fruit juices[255,316] and alleviating parental anxiety. Unchilled beverages taken with meals seem to be beneficial.[313]

CHINESE MEDICINE

A few studies have demonstrated the efficacy of acupuncture in children with diarrhea. The treatment protocols in point selections generally depend on TCM diagnoses, with the majority of points on Stomach and Spleen channels, such as SP-3, SP-4, SP-6, ST-25, and ST-36.[326–330] Shallow needling that is more easily tolerated by children has been found to be effective.[331] In addition, acupuncture can induce favorable anatomic and biochemical changes in improving intestinal peristaltic function and in enhancing both humoral and cellular immunity.[331]

Acupuncture can be helpful in both the diagnosis and management of acute and chronic diarrhea. Chinese medicine explains acute diarrhea as external Cold and Damp Heat pathogenic invasions, which correlate to viral and bacterial infections. Chronic diarrhea is primarily due to internal imbalances of Spleen and Stomach deficiency and Kidney Yang deficiency. Improper diet can cause both acute and chronic diarrhea. Besides acupuncture treatment, acupressure and massage can be instructed to parents for home treatment programs to help alleviate symptoms and shorten the course of diarrhea. Chinese food recommendations can add another perspective to the dietary management of diarrhea.

Acute Diarrhea

Acute diarrhea is best managed with an integrative approach. It is important to obtain the appropriate laboratory studies: stool cultures for bacteria and examinations for ova and parasites—especially in bloody diarrhea or in watery stools of more than 7 days' duration. Antibiotic sensitivity should be determined in order to avoid giving medications indiscriminately. Fluid management with ORT should be part of the immediate treatment regimen. Acupuncture can be used to alleviate pain, to shorten the course by expelling the pathogens, and to strengthen the child's immune system.

External Cold Pathogenic Invasion

The Stomach and Intestines are prone to Cold invasion, which correlates to viral infection. In this instance, the Cold pathogen enters the Tai Yang or the Yang Ming level. Whereas the Wind-Cold pathogen that affects the respiratory tract enters the Tai Yang Bladder channel to affect the upper part of the body, the diarrhea Cold pathogen enters via the fecal–oral route, i.e. through the gastrointestinal tract and enters the Tai Yang Small Intestine level where sorting of clear from turbid fluid and absorption of fluid takes place. Stools become watery. The Shao Yang level is the Triple Energizer, whose overall function is regulation of body fluids. It is also the parasympathetic nervous system and influences intestinal motility. The next Yang level is the Yang Ming level, the Stomach and Large Intestine. Cold impairs the Yang function of the Stomach, which in turn affects the Yin couplet organ, the Spleen, which influences fluid absorption in the Large Intestine. The "rotting and ripening of food," the transportation and transformation of food and fluid are all affected, resulting in frequent watery stools, often containing undigested food particles. When the Cold pathogen enters the Tai Yin level, it directly injures the Spleen and the diarrhea at this point progresses to a more prolonged course, becoming chronic.

Treatment

All stages:

- Prevent dehydration with ORT
- Avoid raw and Cold foods, avoid Phlegm-producing foods that injure the Spleen
- Moxa CV-8 to expel Cold from the Middle Energizer and the Intestines
- KI-7 to expel Cold
- In the initial few days
  - ST-39 the Lower He-Sea point of the Small Intestine, to regulate Small Intestine and stop diarrhea
- Use the four-point Five-Element protocol for expelling Cold from the Tai Yang Small Intestine:
  - Tonify SI-5, TE-6; sedate SI-2, BL-66
- ST-25 to stop diarrhea
- CV-12, CV-6 to tonify the Middle and Lower Energizers
- CV-10 to stimulate the descent of Stomach Qi
- Begin tonification of the Spleen as preventive measure
- Tonify the immune system
- If diarrhea is more than 4–5 days use the four-point Five-Element protocol for expelling Cold from the Stomach and Large Intestine:
  - Stomach: tonify ST-41, SI-5; sedate ST-44, BL-66
  - Large Intestine: tonify LI-5, SI-5; sedate LI-2, BL-66

- In young children use only the two meridian points:
  - Stomach: tonify ST-41; sedate ST-44
  - Large Intestine: tonify LI-5; sedate LI-2
- Tonify Spleen: two points or four points
- Continue ST-25, CV-12, CV-6, CV-10, and warm CV-8
- ST-37 Lower He-Sea point of the Large Intestine to regulate Large Intestine and stop diarrhea
- If diarrhea is more than 1 week duration vigorously tonify Spleen and expel Cold from the Intestines
  - ST-37, ST-39 to regulate the Intestines
- After diarrhea has resolved, vigorously strengthen the immune system
- Home treatment: abdominal massage: with warm palms, parents can massage the child's abdomen in a counterclockwise direction around the umbilicus 50 to 100 times
- Warming CV-8.

Cold can be dispelled by applying warmth to CV-8. Parents can activate their Luogong point, HT-8, by vigorously rubbing their palms together, and placing the warm palm on the child's umbilicus. A warming herb, such as a slice of heat ginger, can be applied to CV-8. The ginger should be slightly heated so that it does not burn the skin.

- Tui Na: these are best done for children under age 3 years:
1. With thumb extended, massage along radial surface toward wrist
2. Counterclockwise massage of Qiji and Guiwei: Qiji means "the seven knots or divisions" and Guiwei means "the tail of the turtle"—this is the lower vertebral column from L4 to the coccyx. Massage in a circular motion. This cleanses the body by making the elimination process work better, therefore gets rid of waste products and toxins from the system.[332]

External Damp Heat Pathogenic Invasions

The external Heat pathogen correlates to bacterial infections. It is much more virulent than the Cold pathogen and quickly passes through the Tai Yang Small Intestine and enters the Yang Ming organs, Stomach and Large Intestine. Since Heat usually rises, the presence of Dampness would "drag" the Heat downward into the Lower Energizer. External Dampness enters the body by penetrating channels of the legs and flows up to the Spleen where it obstructs its function of transformation and transportation. The child could also have internal Dampness from eating greasy and Phlegm-producing foods, and from existing Spleen deficiency. Damp Heat in the Intestines is injurious to the intestinal wall and blood vessels, interfering with fluid absorption, resulting in diarrhea with mucus and blood. The child may manifest the "four bigs" of Yang Ming Heat: big fever, big thirst, big sweating, and big pulse. Fluid and Yin deficiency can occur quickly, so that there is greater risk for dehydration.

Diagnosis should be verified with stool culture and sensitivity. Treatment with acupuncture can be given concomitantly with medication, when it is indicated. The rapid progression of dehydration may necessitate intravenous fluid treatment, especially in infants and young children, as the Heat symptoms would result in red tongue and throat and the child would often refuse to drink.

Treatment

All levels:

- Prevent dehydration as soon as possible with ORT
- Avoid energetically Hot foods, avoid Phlegm-producing foods
- BL-25 to clear Heat from the Intestines
- BL-22, SP-9, SP-6 to resolve Dampness in the Lower Energizer
- GV-14 to treat fever
- LI-11 to resolve Heat
- ST-40 to resolve Damp
- BL-20 to tonify Spleen, resolve Dampness
- In initial Tai Yang stage, may be the first 1–2 days
  - ST-25 to stop diarrhea
  - CV-12, CV-6 to tonify the Middle and Lower Energizers
  - CV-10 to stimulate the descending of Stomach Qi
- Begin tonification of the Spleen as preventive measure
- Tonify the immune system
- ST-39 to regulate the Small Intestine
- Disperse Heat from the Small Intestine: tonify SI-2, BL-66; sedate SI-5, TE-6
- In small children, use the two Small Intestine points: tonify SI-2; sedate SI-5
- In Yang Ming stage, may begin within the first 24 hours, or after 2–3 days:
- Disperse Heat from the Stomach and Large Intestine:
  - Stomach: tonify ST-44, BL-66; sedate ST-41, SI-5
  - Large Intestine: tonify LI-2, BL-66; sedate LI-5, SI-5
- In small children, use only the channel points:
  - Stomach: tonify ST-44; sedate ST-41
  - Large Intestine: tonify LI-2; sedate LI-5
- Tonify Spleen: two-point or four-point protocol
- ST-39 to regulate the Large Intestine
- After diarrhea has resolved, vigorously strengthen the immune system
- Home treatment: abdominal massage and Tui Na as in Cold diarrhea, but do not apply warmth to CV-8.

Chronic Diarrhea

Spleen Deficiency

The Spleen is the most important organ in diarrhea. Spleen Qi usually ascends, carrying out the transforming function as digestion and reabsorption of fluid and nutrients and transportation of Qi to the body. In Spleen deficiency, the direction of Spleen Qi reverses and Qi descends. Food and fluid are not digested or reabsorbed properly, resulting in diarrhea. The child's constitutional Spleen deficiency can be aggravated by a diet containing excess Cold foods, sweets, greasy and Phlegm-producing foods; by exposure to Cold and Damp, such as living in a Damp environment; by chronic illness; by irregular eating habits. In older children in the Wood phase of development, excess mental work, stress, or excess emotions—such as anger, worry, frustration—can further weaken the Spleen with Wood invading Earth. Spleen Qi deficiency can explain postenteritis enteropathy that is puzzling to Western medicine. The external Cold invasion, the acute viral infection, has resolved. From a Chinese medicine standpoint, the acute illness has weakened the Spleen, resulting in lingering diarrheal symptoms. All the clinical signs and symptoms—listlessness, irritability, abdominal distension, carbohydrate intolerance, and even the "worried look" on the infant's face—point to Spleen Qi deficiency.

Spleen impairment can also explain CNSD of infancy and in early childhood. These children may appear "normal and healthy" to the Western physician, but may manifest subtle Spleen deficiency signs such as sallow complexion, slight abdominal distension after eating. The Spleen becomes weaker by an infection or a high carbohydrate diet, and diarrhea ensues. It is also interesting to note that apples are considered as energetically Cold foods and therefore injurious to the Stomach and Spleen. Since the Spleen is responsible for reabsorption and movement of fluid, excess juice or fluid intake would overwhelm the Spleen and cause diarrhea. These principles easily explain the association between excess apple juice and CNSD.

Treatment

- Vigorously tonify Spleen with the Five-Element four-point protocol:
  - Tonify SP-2, HT-8; sedate SP-1, LR-1
- Add BL-20, BL-21, SP-6, ST-36, CV-12 to tonify Stomach and Spleen
- Moxa CV-8
- ST-25, ST-37 to stop chronic diarrhea
- Avoid Cold, greasy, Phlegm-producing foods such as dairy products
- Avoid excess apple juice
- Modify the child's lifestyle: decrease school workload or extracurricular activities to allow more rest; decrease any stress that can precipitate worry and frustration
- Treat ear points: Shenmen, Point Zero, Stomach, Spleen, Small Intestine, Large Intestine
- Teach parents the same home treatment regimen as for acute Cold diarrhea.

Kidney Yang Deficiency

Early morning diarrhea with abdominal pain, and borborygmi during the bowel movement with a feeling of cold indicates Kidney Yang deficiency. Excess Cold and Spleen deficiency can lead to Kidney Yang deficiency. Coldness counteracts the warmth from the "Fire" of Kidney Yang. Spleen deficiency accumulates Dampness, which obstructs the movement of fluids, leading to Kidney Yang deficiency. Since the Kidney Yang is the basis of all Yang, Kidney deficiency would in turn cause further Spleen deficiency, and a vicious cycle ensues. Since Kidney corresponds with fear, a careful history can elicit if the child is fearful of something, e.g., failure in academic or athletic performance, or domestic violence.

Treatment

- Tonify Kidney Yang: KI-3, KI-7, CV-4, CV-6, BL-23
- Overall tonification of Kidney with Five-Element four-point protocol:

- Tonify KI-7, LU-8; sedate KI-3, SP-3 (obviously, cannot treat KI-3, KI-7 for tonification of Kidney Yang at the same time as the four-point Kidney tonification protocol)
- Tonify Spleen: tonify SP-2, HT-8; sedate SP-1, LR-11
- ST-25, ST-37 to stop chronic diarrhea
- Avoid Cold, raw foods; avoid greasy, Phlegm-producing foods such as dairy products
- Modify the child's lifestyle to minimize fear, e.g., taking a less rigorous class to allow more chances of success; family or individual counseling for any emotional situations or problems based on fear
- Treat ear points: Shenmen, Point Zero, Kidney, Spleen, Stomach, Small Intestine, Large Intestine
- Teach parents the home treatment regimen.

Improper Diet

Children's diet today often consists of an excess of unhealthy foods that are artificially sweetened, greasy, Phlegm-producing, salty, or energetically too Hot or too Cold for the child's constitution. Spleen deficiency is the most common end-result. Kidney deficiency and Liver Qi stagnation also occur frequently. The internal imbalances can predispose the child to acute episodes of diarrhea. For example, a child with Spleen deficiency develops acute abdominal pain and loose stools after attending a birthday party where cakes and cookies were served in abundance. The child may have other symptoms to indicate deficiency, such as abdominal distension with Spleen Qi deficiency. A progression of imbalances can lead to chronic diarrhea.

Treatment

- Eliminate excess inappropriate foods
- ST-21 to resolve retention of food
- ST-44 if retention of food is associated with Heat symptoms
- SP-4 to decrease abdominal distension
- CV-12, BL-20, BL-21, ST-36, SP-6 to tonify Stomach and Spleen
- ST-25, ST-37 to stop diarrhea
- Use the Five-Element four-point protocol to treat specific deficiencies:
  - Tonify Spleen
  - Tonify Kidney
- LR-3, LR-13 to move Liver Qi
- Treat ear points: Shenmen, Point Zero, Stomach, Spleen, Liver, Kidney (see Bibliography for further reading on this topic).

DROOLING (SIALORRHEA)

Drooling or sialorrhea occurs in normal infants until approximately 6 months of age, when muscular reflexes that initiate swallowing and lip closure are more developed. Later, the irritation of teething may lead to temporary drooling.[77] An estimated 10% of children with neurological impairment, such as cerebral palsy, have excessive drooling that interferes with everyday living.[333] Pathophysiology is primarily due to inefficient swallowing of saliva because of oromotor incoordination and not due to hypersalivation.[334,335]

Although it is not a serious health problem, drooling is difficult for parents and caregivers who need to constantly change bibs or clothing, and for children who may feel further social isolation with drooling added to their other handicaps.[336] Mild cases are usually not treated. More severe cases are managed by medications[337] and various surgical procedures such as submandibular duct relocation[335] and submandibular gland excision.[336,338]

CHINESE MEDICINE

There is little discussion of treatment of drooling in Chinese medicine. The best point appears to be the local point, ST-4,[39] which has recently been demonstrated to be effective in treating cerebral palsy children with the application of a biosouth (+) magnet facing downward on the point.[339]

- Treatment of excess Stomach water: sedate ST-44
- Tonification of Spleen can promote better movement and circulation of fluid:
  – Four-point protocol: tonify SP-2, HT-8; sedate SP-1, LR-1
  – Two points: tonify SP-2; sedate SP-1
- Or use meridian tonification: connect with ion pumping cord black on lower Spleen point, e.g. SP-3 or SP-6; red on SP-9. If using magnets, place bionorth (–) pole facing down on SP-3 or SP-6 and biosouth (+) pole facing down on SP-9 and connect with ion pumping cord as above
- Since the majority of drooling occurs in children with neurologic impairment, which correlates to Kidney deficiency, tonification of Kidney would help improve neurologic function: tonify KI-7, LU-8; sedate KI-3, SP-3
- Tongue acupuncture has been successful in treating severe drooling and may be tried by an experienced practitioner prior to considering invasive surgical procedures.[340]

ECZEMA

Atopic dermatitis (AD), or atopic eczema, is the most common chronic skin condition in children in the industrialized countries.[341] It affects between 5% and 20% of children from birth to 11 years at one time or other,[342] and accounts for 20% of all dermatological referrals. Recent data indicates that prevalence is increasing[342] and many cases persist into adulthood.[341]

The precise etiology and pathophysiology is still unknown.[341] Allergy, defined as an exaggerated response of the immune system to external substances, plays a role only in some but not all patients with eczema.[343] Various environmental allergens have been implicated, the most common are grass, tree pollens, the house dust mite, products from pets and other animals, agents encountered in industry, wasp and bee venom, drugs, and certain foods.[342,343] Food intolerance is a better term than food allergy, since many individuals with eczema do not demonstrate an alteration in the immune system with food challenges.[343]

Recent research has demonstrated that maternal atopy during pregnancy may have an important effect on the developing immune response of the fetus and may predispose the child to developing allergies. Maternal IgE, IgG and amniotic fluid cytokines, combined with the presence of allergen in the fetomaternal environment are all possible factors that influence infant responses to common environmental antigens. Immune modulation at this stage of development may, in the future, be a way forward in the prevention of allergy.[344]

The Canadian Cochrane Database examined preventive studies that prescribed an antigen avoidance diet to high risk mothers during pregnancy and lactation. A high risk woman is one with the atopic disease, and a high risk fetus or infant is one with eczema in the mother, father, or a sibling. Current data seems to suggest that when lactating mothers with high risk infants were given the diet, there is decreased incidence of eczema during the child's first 12–18 months of life,[345] whereas a small clinical trial of prescribing the diet to lactating mothers of infants who already have atopic eczema did not significantly affect the severity of the baby's eczema.[345] When a high risk mother was placed on the restrictive diet during pregnancy, there was no reduction in the incidence of giving birth to an atopic child, while such a diet may have had an adverse effect on maternal and/or fetal nutrition.[345]

Eczema has a wide spectrum of clinical presentation, ranging from a few patches of dry, pruritic, thickened skin to fulminant, severe, generalized dermatitis that fluctuates between acute flare-up of red, itchy skin with periods of relative quiescence.[341]

TREATMENT

Although eczema is not life-threatening, the discomfort from the symptoms, the unsightly rash, and chronicity of the condition are distressing to both the child and the parents.[341] The excoriated skin from scratching is susceptible to developing secondary bacterial infection as purulent, weepy impetiginous lesions. Treatment is therefore challenging and complicated, and needs to address not only the physical symptoms, but also the psychosocial impact on the lives of the child and the caregivers. As a result, eczema engenders significant cost for the family and health care systems.[342,346] The physical manifestations are treated symptomatically, mostly by allergen avoidance and by application of topical steroid. Dermocorticosteroids are anti-inflammatory and reduce itching; they also have immunosuppressive actions.[347] A short course of oral steroids may be prescribed for severe, acute flare-ups. In a few selected cases, in which other methods have failed, immunotherapy with desensitisation or hyposensitisation is recommended.[343] Mild impetigo is usually treated with topical antibiotic ointment. The more severe cases are treated with oral antibiotics

CHINESE MEDICINE

Acupuncture has been found to be successful in treating both the pruritic symptoms[348] and the skin lesions in eczema.[348–351] The possible mechanisms include an anti-inflammatory mechanism in minimizing IgE and eosinophils.[351]

The pathophysiologies of eczema are manifold: an accumulation of Heat and Damp, combined with Blood and Yin deficiency.[350] Multiple organ and channel dysfunction can be involved: Lung, Spleen, Kidney, Liver. Lingering Heat and Damp from previous illnesses, and a diet rich in Damp and energetically Hot foods would predispose children to accumulate Heat and Damp in the skin and in the Blood. The skin in Chinese medicine is part of the Lung, which explains the frequent manifestation of eczema in asthmatics. Spleen deficiency can manifest as accumulation of Damp. A child may have a prenatal predisposition to Dampness and to eczema when there is a strong familial tendency toward Spleen deficiency; when parents engage in excess mental work, have excess worry, or have digestive weakness due to poor diet or alcohol abuse during conception; and when the mother has these experiences during pregnancy. Living in a Damp environment, such as in the basement, close to the ocean, in rainy weather, and eating Damp-producing foods–such as milk products, greasy, fried foods, peanuts, sweets and white sugar—and engaging in excess mental activities can subject the child to Spleen deficiency and to the development of eczema. Although Dampness usually affects the lower part of the body, it can easily enter the Middle Energizer, from there it rises upward to affect the Upper Energizer, the Lung and its corresponding organ, skin. The Lung houses the Corporeal Soul, which gives us the capacity for physical sensations. When the Lung is not in balance, the Corporeal Soul is responsible for the manifestation of excess physical sensations, such as itching in eczema. Kidney and Liver Yin deficiencies can predispose the child to Blood and Yin deficiencies and Heat accumulation that manifest as red and dry skin. Treatment for eczema is directed toward dispersing Heat and Damp in acute flare-ups and tonifying chronic deficiencies.

Acute Eczema

- ST-40 to disperse Damp and Heat
- SP-10, BL-17, LI-11 to remove Blood Heat
- Avoid energetically Hot foods and Phlegm-producing foods
- Minimize application of dermocorticosteroids. From a Chinese medicine standpoint, these ointments tend to keep Dampness and Heat in the skin, which may predispose the child to develop Damp and Heat conditions elsewhere
- Treat lesions according to specific location
  - Local points and Ah Shi points: e.g. BL-40 for popliteal fossa, GV-14, GB-20, BL-12 for head and neck
- Combine proximal and distal points of the corresponding channels to the area:
  - Head, neck, upper back: Governor Vessel, and Bladder channels
  - Face: Yang Ming Stomach channel
  - Upper extremities:
    - flexor surface – Lung, Heart, Pericardium
    - extensor surface – Small Intestine, Large Intestine, Triple Energizer
  - Lower extremities:
    - flexor surface – Kidney, Bladder, Liver
    - extensor surface – Stomach, Spleen, Gallbladder

TABLE 10.2	Treatment for eczema		
	Source	**He (Sea)**	**Back Shu**
Spleen	SP-3	SP-9	BL-20
Kidney	KI-3	KI-10	BL-23
Lung	LU-9	LU-5	BL-13
Liver	LR-3	LR-8	BL-18

Chronic Eczema

- BL-17 to tonify Blood
- ST-40 to disperse Damp and Heat
- SP-10, BL-17, LI-11 to remove Blood Heat
- Avoid energetically Hot foods and Phlegm-producing foods
- Tonify Spleen to minimize Dampness: tonify SP-2, HT-8; sedate SP-1, LR-1.

The recommended treatment for specific channel and organs: select the Yuan (source) point, He (Sea) point, and back Shu points of each organ[350] (Table 10.2).

Tonification of the Immune System

Since there are immune components to eczema, use the immune protocol to strengthen the child (see Bibliography for further reading on this topic).

ENURESIS

Nocturnal enuresis, or bed-wetting, is a complex disorder with poorly understood pathogenicity and pathophysiology. It affects children all over the world:[77,352–354] approximately 5–7 million children in the United States[355] and as many as 30% of school-age children in Italy.[353]

Enuresis is defined as inappropriate or involuntary voiding during the night at an age when urinary control should be achieved.[77] It is classified as primary nocturnal enuresis (PNE) when the child has never been dry at night, or secondary nocturnal enuresis (SNE) when wetting follows a dry period usually after an identifiable stress.[77]

The majority or up to 85% of PNE is monosymptomatic in that the enuresis is not accompanied by other voiding disorders or daytime incontinence.[77,352,356] Most children with primary monosymptomatic bedwetting have either a large night-time urine production and a normal bladder capacity, or a small bladder capacity with normal urine production.[357]

By age 8 years, 87–90% of children should have night-time dryness. Enuresis improves with maturity, with a natural, spontaneous remission rate of 15% per year of age.[77] It is possible that different factors may be predominant in different age groups.[358]

ETIOLOGY AND PATHOPHYSIOLOGY

Both the etiology and pathophysiology of enuresis are still not well understood. There appears to be a wide spectrum of possible pathogenic factors for enuresis: functional/psychological causes, delayed maturation of the central nervous system, genetic predisposition, and infrequently, organic/anatomic dysfunction.

Functional/Psychological

Many investigators consider PNE as a disorder with a strong functional component.[359–361] Psychological factors may affect as many as 95% of children with enuresis.[361] It is interesting to note that fear reactions have been reported to be significantly higher in enuretic children.[354,362] Enuresis has been linked to night terror, nightmares, and sleepwalking.[363,364] Most likely, this disorder is a highly complex interaction between somatic and psychiatric factors.[360]

CNS

Nocturnal enuresis may be due to a maturational lag in the development of the central nervous system.[77] A popular theory posits that there is low nocturnal vasopressin secretion resulting in high nocturnal urine output, which explains why enuretics respond to DDAVP, an exogenous vasopressin. However, there may be a more complex, dual CNS developmental delay in both the afferent and efferent limbs: the central nervous system fails to recognize and respond to bladder fullness or contraction during sleep, and also fails to suppress the micturition reflex arc during sleep.[365] The pathology does not appear to relate to sleep physiology, since the sleep cycle appears normal and enuretic episodes have been found to occur in every sleep stage.[360] There may in fact be a close correlation between biological and psychological factors, in that extreme CNS disorganization may result in psychological symptoms.[366]

Genetic Predisposition

PNE has a strong hereditary component.[353,358,366] Many families seem to manifest an autosomal dominant mode of inheritance.[360] At this time, molecular genetics have identified numerous loci on more than 10 chromosomes.[360,367]

Organic/Anatomic Dysfunction

Organic factors are uncommon causes of PNE.[77] Anatomic anomalies include epispadias, ectopic ureter, spinal cord lesion, or urethral obstruction.[368] It can also be a feature of many conditions, including renal,[369] neurological and organic disease states.[370]

SECONDARY ENURESIS

SNE accounts for about one quarter of patients with bed-wetting.[371] There is significant association of psychiatric problems with SNE,[360,371] both causally and reactively following the enuresis.[360] The organic conditions that feature primary enuresis can also be the cause of secondary enuresis.[370] Enuresis has also been associated with behavioral disorders, such as ADHD.[372–375] SNE has also been reported with trauma such as car and motor cycle accidents, which may be due to psychological trauma or organic head trauma.[376] SNE has been reported to be associated with upper airway obstruction, which is difficult to explain in the Western paradigm.[377]

Treatment

Although the condition is considered benign and mostly self-limiting, treatment is warranted because of adverse personal, family, and psychosocial effects of the disorder.[355,358,378] Nocturnal enuresis delays early autonomy and socialisation due to decrease in self-esteem and self-confidence[356] and fear of detection by peers.[378] The child may be at increased risk for emotional or even physical abuse from family members.[378]

The conventional treatment modalities are still controversial. Since the vast majority of PNE resolves spontaneously with time, treatment should carry minimal or no risk. The moisture alarm is both safe and inexpensive and should be the treatment of choice in most cases[358] but is the least often prescribed.[366] Medical treatment should be placed in a biopsychosocial framework, with medication prescribed in conjunction with psychosocial interventions.[361,379]

CHINESE MEDICINE

Current Acupuncture Data

The current literature is supportive of acupuncture as a possible treatment modality for the enuretic child.[380] Worldwide reports give validation to acupuncture efficacy in the treatment of enuresis.[352,381–391] The reported success rate is as high as 98.2%.[392]

Acupuncture has been found to be successful both in decreasing occurrence of enuresis during treatment and in exerting a persistent, long-term effect after treatment.[352,385,386] Parents also report a decrease in sleep arousal threshold.[386] The therapeutic efficacy improves with combined treatment of DDAVP and acupuncture.[387] Although the precise mechanism of acupuncture is still unknown, a multidisciplinary approach that included acupuncture demonstrated on EEG that treatment normalized activities of the cerebral cortex,[389] and an Italian study and a Russian report showed that acupuncture treatment was effective in suppressing uninhibited bladder contractions and decreased bladder instability.[390,391] For those children who are fearful of invasive acupuncture, simple acumassage has also been demonstrated to be beneficial to the enuretic child.[393]

Etiology and Pathophysiology

Although it is not possible to precisely correlate the Western diagnosis of enuresis with TCM impressions, PNE can be explained in the acupuncture paradigm as Kidney Yang and Kidney Essence deficiency, and SNE as Spleen and Lung Qi deficiency, and Yin Deficiency.

Kidney Yang and Kidney Essence Deficiency—PNE

Kidney Yang and Essence encompass wide spheres of vital human functions, among them including Kidney Yang's influence in retention of urine in the bladder; and in production of marrow, the brain; Kidney Esssence correlates to heredity and developmental influences.

Kidney Yang enables the Bladder to hold and store urine and warms the Lower Energizer. Constitutional Kidney Yang deficiency results in a cold Lower Energizer, so that Bladder cannot regulate and store water well. This inability to hold urine is worst at night when Kidney Yang is at the lowest level during the Yin part of the diurnal cycle. A characteristic of Kidney Yang deficiency enuresis is the release of large amounts of usually clear urine during sleep. The child and the sheets are soaked and the child may wake up from the sensation of wetness. Along with nocturnal enuresis there may be other signs and symptoms of Kidney Yang deficiency: low pitched voice, facial pallor, cold extremities. Fearfulness and insecurity, the emotions that correspond with the Kidney, are frequently associated with enuretic children. In these children, the tongue may be pale, and the pulse slow, weak, and deep.

Kidney Yang deficiency results in insufficient production of marrow, the brain in Chinese medicine, which correlates well to the various postulates of CNS immaturity in Western medicine.

Part of Kidney Essence is pre-Heaven or ancestral, which represents hereditary influences on an energetic level that may translate in biochemical terms as chromosomal loci. Development and maturation of organs are also influenced by Kidney Essence, so that anatomic anomalies and organ dysfunctions may reflect Kidney Essence deficiency.

Developmentally, children are in the Water phase of development, so that Kidney and Bladder, the water organs, are most vulnerable.

Kidney Yang deficiency can also explain enuresis reported in Western literature that is associated with trauma or surgery: the "shock" to the system induces a transient Kidney Yang deficiency that manifests as enuresis.

Treatment

- Restrict fluid at and after dinner to decrease urine production
- Diet: avoid energetically Cold foods; avoid excess salt; increase Warming foods
- Keep warm, especially keep the abdomen warm, advise mothers not to dress young children with abdomen partially exposed
- KI-3 tonifies both Kidney Yin and Kidney Yang
- KI-6, CV-4, SP-6 tonifies Kidney Yin/Essence
- KI-7, BL-23 tonifies Kidney Yang

- Use the Five-Element four-point protocol to disperse Cold from the Kidney, and tonify both the Kidney Yin and Yang:
  - Disperse Kidney Cold: tonify KI-2, HT-8; sedate KI-10
  - Tonify Kidney: tonify KI-7, LU-8; sedate KI-3, SP-3
  - CV-6 to tonify Lower Energizer.

TCM and SNE

Spleen and Lung Qi Deficiency

In Chinese medicine, secondary enuresis that characteristically occurs after a period of dryness correlates to the presence of Spleen and Lung Qi deficiency. These deficiencies often occur due to poor recuperation after previous illnesses, due to the presence of other illnesses or stress that weaken the digestive and respiratory systems. The Spleen and Lung regulate the body's water and expel excess. Weak Spleen Qi cannot properly carry out the transformation and transportation of fluids. Whereas a healthy Spleen prefers dryness, a weak Spleen retains water. Weak Lung Qi cannot adequately carry out the functions of governing the Qi of the body and regulating body fluid in the Upper Energizer, which in turn interferes with proper water flow down to the Bladder. Nocturnal enuresis ensues. Therefore, TCM explains well the Lung and Kidney relationship that seems baffling to Western medicine.

Unlike PNE with Kidney Yang deficiency that typically manifests with copious urine, the enuresis associated with Spleen and Lung deficiency is due to inadequate regulation of fluid with inappropriate water retention, so that this type of bed-wetting characteristically would be of very small volume. Any illness or stress that diverts Qi away from the Lower Energizer would result in SNE: stress from school work, excess playing of computer games, emotional crises such as parental divorce or death of a close family member, could all divert Qi toward the Upper Energizer where it is needed the most. Possible associated symptoms may be facial pallor, poor appetite, lack of thirst, weak muscles, digestive and respiratory symptoms. The tongue is pale and the pulse is thin, deep and slow.

Treatment

- Avoid excessive sweet or spicy foods; also avoid Phlegm-producing, and Cold foods
- Change in lifestyle to provide plenty of rest and diversification of activities
- Calming exercises
- Tonify Spleen:
  - Two points: tonify SP-2; sedate SP-1
  - Four points: tonify SP-2, HT-8; sedate SP-1, LR-1
- Tonify Lung:
  - Two points: tonify LU-9; sedate LU-10
  - Four points: tonify LU-9, SP-3; sedate LU-10, HT-8
- Moxa CV-8 to tonify Middle Energizer
- CV-17 to tonify Upper Energizer.

Yin Deficiency Enuresis

Numerous conditions can lead to secondary Yin deficiency enuresis: all chronic illnesses can eventually lead to Yin deficiency; lingering pathogenic Heat that has not been appropriately expelled with Heat illnesses continue to exhaust Yin; excess consumption of energetically Hot foods, greasy and fried foods. Yin deficiency often manifests as Yang excess syndromes. The most common one in the enuretic child is Yang excess. This can be well explained by the Five-Element Developmental Theory: the child has strong Wood vulnerabilities either because of being in the Wood phase of development or because of having strong Wood tendencies in the Water phase. The heavy sleep that is characteristic of the child can be explained by Ethereal Soul, Hun. The Ethereal Soul resides in Liver Yin, which is constitutionally deficient in children. Hun leaves the body during sleep, and returns upon awakening. When there is Liver Yin deficiency, the Ethereal Soul would wander more at night, resulting in the child being difficult to awaken.

Treatment

- Avoid excessive intake of sour or bitter foods; avoid taking medication unnecessarily, especially over-the-counter pills
- Teach the child Qigong calming exercises; parents can massage Yintang point for calming
- KI-6, SP-6, CV-4 to tonify Yin
- BL-18 to tonify Liver Yin
- BL-47 Hunmen, "Gate of the Ethereal Soul" to calm the Hun
- LR-3 to subdue Liver Yang, and nourish Liver Yin
- LR-13 to regulate Liver Qi, to harmonize Liver and Spleen[38,39,242–245, 252,270,272,273,274]

FEVER

Human beings are homeothermic, which means that body temperature is normally maintained within a relatively narrow range, despite wide variations in energy intake and expenditure and environmental temperature.[394] The thermoregulatory center is located in the anterior hypothalamus.[395] Normal body temperature ranges from 36.1–37.8°C (97–100°F), rectal temperature is one degree higher and axillary temperature is one degree lower than body temperature measured by oral thermometer. Children tend to have higher body temperatures than adults, and may have a normal range to as high as 38.5°C (101°F).

The fever response can be mediated endogenously and exogenously: endogenous pyrogen is produced by immunologic cells, such as polymorphonuclear leukocytes and phagocytic cells; exogenous pyrogen, such as bacterial endotoxin, produces fever by acting on circulating leukocytes which, in turn, produce and release endogenous pyrogens.[394]

Each degree centigrade of fever increases the basal metabolic rate by 10 to 12% and increases basal cellular oxygen consumption by about 13%, with proportionate increase in carbon dioxide production, and requirements for fluid and calories. Elevated body temperature may engender beneficial effects, such as interfering with bacterial reproduction, and accelerating a variety of immunologic responses, such as phagocytosis, leukocyte migration, and lymphocyte transformation. On the other hand, very high fever can impair the immunologic response. The marked increase in insensible water loss requires large volumes of water intake. The increase in cellular energy expenditure requires significant amounts of nutrients. Both of these demands occur when the ill child has diminished oral intake, predisposing the child to dehydration and utilization of substrates contained within body tissues.[394] Fever can also precipitate febrile seizures in the susceptible child between 6 months to 5 or 6 years of age.[396] In children, infection is the most common cause of acute febrile episodes, and inflammatory diseases account for recurrent and persistent temperature elevation.[397]

TREATMENT

Western medicine directs specific treatment toward the disorder that caused the fever, such as antibiotics for an ear infection or an anti-inflammatory drug for IBD, chronic inflammatory bowel disease; and manages fever symptomatically with various cooling measures, extra fluids and antipyretics. Parents and caregivers often manifest "fever phobia"[398] and are quick to administer medications to control fever. Acetaminophen and ibuprofen are two of the most commonly used fever medications in children.[399,400] Aspirin usage is limited by adverse reactions, and the other nonsteroidal anti-inflammatory drugs have a limited role in pediatrics.[401] The dosage of medication should be carefully calculated according to both the age and weight of the child. However, children are frequently given improper doses, resulting in toxicity or inadequate symptomatic improvement.[400] Some studies have demonstrated that antipyretic therapy may actually prolong influenza A infection.[402] When febrile convulsion occurs, pediatricians in general reassure parents that they are benign, self-limiting, and that long-term prognosis in the vast majority of cases is good.[403] At this time, there are no modalities to increase the child's natural immunity to prevent further susceptibility to febrile illness. Temperature elevation due to hot weather is not considered pathological.

CHINESE MEDICINE

Chinese medicine defines fever as Heat accumulation due to external pathogenic invasion or to internal organ imbalances. Current data is in general positive for antipyretic effect of acupuncture. An animal study from Japan demonstrated that electroacupuncture stimulation to the point that corresponds to human LI-11 exerted an antipyretic effect.[404] Other major antifebrile points studied include GV-14 and ST-36.[405] Research also focuses on elucidation of the mechanisms of antipyretic effects and the potential interaction of acupuncture with drugs.[406] A review from Russia indicates that acupuncture exerts antipyretic effects by triggering adaptive mechanisms that are directed towards correction of disturbances in the homeostatic systems of the body.[407] One of these mechanisms may be related to the endogenous opioid system,[408] which has been demonstrated to be modulated by acupuncture in pain relief. Other possible antipyretic effects of acupuncture may be modulation of the hypothalamic thermoregulation.[405] One study from China suggests that acupuncture stimulation of LI-11 and LI-4 lowered body temperature through decreasing metabolic heat production and cutaneous vasodilatation.[409] An animal study from Russia indicates that when an antipyretic medication is used in combination with acupuncture, its effect is potentiated and lasts longer.[410]

Another important question is the effect of acupuncture on immune function in febrile illnesses. One study in China reports that when fever due to Wind-Cold invasion was treated with acupuncture on Dazhui (GV-14), Fengchi (GB-13), and Quchi (LI-11), in addition to a significant drop in axillary temperature, sometimes more than 1°C, respiratory rate, pulse, and blood pressure also decreased; symptoms were reduced; while the percentage of T-lymphocytes increased.[411] However, an animal study in China using acupuncture on points corresponding to human GV-14 and LI-11 revealed no change in Wind-Heat fever caused by bacterial endotoxins.[412] A clinical observation in China of pasting herbs on acupuncture points in 72 ill infants revealed an increase in humoral immune substances such as IgA, IgM, IgG. This is a better preventive—prophylaxis—for fever.[413] Acupressure can be considered as a potential modality for fever management at home.[414]

Chinese medicine posits that Heat accumulation in fever is due to either excess Heat or excess Yang with Yin deficiency. The Western medicine finding of children having a higher basal temperature and a tendency toward developing high fever can be easily explained by the TCM concept that children are constitutionally Yin deficient and have a relative abundance of Yang. They are also vulnerable to frequent febrile illnesses which further depletes Yin. The acute fevers are due to external pathogens. Wind-Cold invasion—viral infection—begins to manifest fever in the Shao Yang stage; whereas Wind-Heat invasion—bacterial infection—can manifest fever from the very beginning during the Wei Qi level. Heat due to hot weather is also considered an external pathogen because it can deplete Yin. Chronic Heat can be due to any disorder that causes Yin deficiency, to continuous consumption of Hot energy foods, to excess emotions that causes Qi stagnation, and may also be due to familial or constitutional predisposition to chronic conditions with underlying Heat disturbance, such as chronic inflammatory diseases.

Treatment

Chinese fever treatment parallels the Western system in symptomatic lowering of fever and expelling the pathogen. In addition, Chinese medicine would tonify Yin and the immune system.

- Lowering of fever due to any cause: GV-14, LI-11
- ST-36 can be used to lower fever and to increase immunity
- Conventional cooling measures such as tepid baths (children should take baths with lukewarm and not cold water, as the sudden chill would cause the child to shiver, which causes compensatory increases in metabolism and further elevation of temperature)
- Eliminate Hot energy foods; increase fluid intake
- Expel pathogen according to stage or level of invasion
- Five-Element four-point Heat treatment if specific organ is identified, e.g. Lung Heat for respiratory illness, Large Intestine Heat for bacterial diarrhea or inflammatory bowel disease
- Tonify Yin
- Tonify immune system.

HEADACHE

Headaches occur in about 40% of preschool children and up to 70% of school-age children.[415,416] The guidelines provided in the 55-page International Headache Society (IHS) handbook are widely used in classifying headaches in childhood and adolescence. There is, however, growing concern that the criteria need to be modified to increase sensitivity for pediatric headaches.[417–422] Childhood headaches can be broadly classified as acute or chronic. Acute headaches in children are mostly due to viral illnesses, sinusitis,[423] mild head trauma,[424] with a small percentage due to bacterial sepsis and meningitis, serious head trauma, or CNS abnormalities, such as brain tumor.[415] The majority of chronic headaches in school-aged children are idiopathic, which means that there is no specific etiology, and the pain is the main symptom and the primary disease entity itself. A small percentage of chronic headaches are secondary to a definite medical condition, such as hypoglycemia.[416] Idiopathic headaches in childhood fall into the migraine, migrainous disorder and tension-type categories.[418,425–427] Stress was the most frequently cited precipitating factor in all types of idiopathic headaches, while weather and environmental factors, and some foods also play a role.[428]

Diagnosis and differentiation can be difficult, especially in the very young.[429] Conventional medicine recommends systematic evaluations with careful history taking and neurological examination to identify the primary etiology,[418,430,431] and diagnostic testing based on individual findings and indications.[432]

Although very few studies have evaluated therapy of headache in young patients,[432] there is general agreement among medical practitioners that medications are first-line treatment for acute symptoms.[432,433] Appropriate medications are more limited in young children, with older children and adolescents having more options.[433] There is growing emphasis that nonpharmacologic modalities are becoming more important[432,433] so that modalities such as relaxation[434] and acupuncture[435] are being explored.

ACUPUNCTURE FOR HEADACHES

Because the etiology of headache can range from a benign, transient condition associated with a viral infection to serious, life-threatening brain tumor, it would be advisable to have an integrative approach in children. A proper neurologic evaluation can be helpful for ruling out significant pathology. In non-life-threatening headaches, TCM diagnoses and acupuncture treatment can be used either as a primary modality or as an adjunctive therapy to medication or can be incorporated in multidisciplinary approaches that may include relaxation training, change in lifestyle, and diet. Chinese medicine would be especially helpful in the management of "idiopathic" headaches that do not have an explanation in Western medicine but can be described as energetic disturbances from either internal or external causes. For those headaches that do have clear Western diagnoses, acupuncture can offer a complementary energetic perspective that can add another dimension to the diagnoses and treatment.

Although there are a number of studies on acupuncture treatment of headaches, there is a paucity of data in pediatrics. Many studies on adults are considered flawed scientifically. Nevertheless, available data do seem to support the value of acupuncture for treating headaches.[436] Reports of clinical improvement with acupuncture ranges from 20%[437] to approximately 67%[438] to as high as 95.6%.[439] A few studies report acupuncture as having no effect in prevention of tension-type headache[440] or making no difference in comparison with sham acupuncture treatment.[441]

Paralleling the paucity of research data is the lack of discussion of specific treatment protocols even in currently available pediatric acupuncture textbooks.[242,243] Both Western medicine and TCM have very complex classifications for headache. While some diagnoses can be correlated between two disciplines, such as migraine and headaches of acute viral infections, the majority of headaches are difficult to integrate because of very different TCM and Western approaches. This book proposes a classification that incorporates information from classical references, from adult acupuncture books, and from the author's own experience in integrating conventional and TCM pediatrics. This integrated approach broadly categorizes pediatric headaches as acute causes due to external pathogens and chronic, recurrent causes due to internal imbalances.

ACUTE/EXTERNAL CAUSES OF HEADACHES

Acute headaches are due to external pathogenic invasions and to acute head trauma.

- Wind-Cold—viral syndrome
- Wind-Heat—bacterial infection
- Wind-Damp
- Blood stasis—head trauma.

CHRONIC/INTERNAL CAUSES OF HEADACHES

The chronic headaches are associated with internal organ imbalance due to various causes: stress, emotional excesses, lifestyle aberrations, dietary imbalance, constitutional vulnerability. They are best classified according to location of headaches in relation to distribution of meridians.

- Tai Yang—occipital headache
- Shao Yang—lateral side of head and neck; migraines
- Yang Ming—forehead
- Shao Yin—inside the brain
- Tai Yin—heavy and tight sensation as if head is tightly wrapped with a band
- Jue Yin—vertex.

Variable location with history of head trauma.

ACUTE HEADACHES

The acute onset of headaches in children is usually due to external pathogens—Wind-Cold, Wind-Heat, Dampness—that obstruct Yang channels, resulting in

Qi and Blood stagnation that further block channels and collaterals. Blood stasis due to head trauma is also a common cause of acute headaches, especially in infants and young children.

Wind-Cold Invasion

Since Wind tends to affect the top of the body, headache is a frequent manifestation of both Wind-Cold and Wind-Heat conditions. Wind-Cold or viral infection headache usually affects the Tai Yang channels, the first stage in the six-stage Wind-Cold invasion discussed in Chapter 6. The Cold causes contraction of the channels and decreases defensive Wei Qi circulation, resulting in occipital headache or sense of stiffness in the back of the neck. The diagnosis is easily made, as the headache has an acute onset, and is usually accompanied by other signs and symptoms of Wind-Cold invasion. Further obstruction of Qi circulation in the muscles would lead to generalized myalgia. When Wind-Cold progresses to the Yang Ming stage, the headache becomes more severe and localized to the forehead.

Wind-Heat Headache

Since Heat also rises in the body, the combination of Wind and Heat causes a sharp, generalized headache. Just as in Wind-Cold invasion, the diagnosis here is easily made as other manifestations of Wind-Heat invasions are usually present. This correlates to bacterial infections, with the more severe forms being sepsis and meningitis.

Wind-Damp

Acute exposure to Dampness, such as walking barefoot in rainy weather causes Dampness to ascend the leg channels to the Middle Energizer then upward to the head. Dampness obstructs the orifices of the head and prevents clear Yang from reaching the head, so that this type of headache is characterized by a sensation of heaviness.

Blood Stasis—Head Trauma

Injuries are responsible for more deaths in the pediatric age group than all other causes combined,[442] and constitute the leading cause of death among US children over 1 year of age. Each year hundreds of thousands of children are seen in an emergency room for head injury. Fortunately, the majority of them are mild[443] which indicates a brief or no loss of consciousness, no abnormalities on radiographic examination, and no neurologic complications.[444] More severe injuries can result in skull fracture, epidural hematoma, subdural hematoma, cerebral contusion, and post-trauma seizures. Four-fifths of head traumas are due to accidents, with a mean age of 2.5 years, and the rest are from abuse, occurring primarily in infants, with a mean age of 0.7 years.[445] Skull fracture and intracranial injury are common among children younger than 2 years of age.[446] At this time, there are no formal criteria for obtaining laboratory studies or for admitting children with head trauma,[447] so that each institution has its own standards for evaluating pediatric head injury.

Chinese medicine considers a blow to the head as the cause of Blood stasis in the area of the trauma. This may result in localized or generalized headache. In mild cases, the headache resolves within a matter of hours or days. In more severe cases of head trauma, such as those associated with concussion, a brief loss of consciousness, or with epidural or subdural hematomas, children may not immediately complain of headache. Acute head trauma is best evaluated with the help of Western evaluation and technology. Head injury with abnormal neurological examination and positive laboratory substantiation, such as findings on skull X-ray, computerized tomography or magnetic resonance imaging scans of the head, usually indicates serious trauma and the child often needs to be hospitalized for close observation and for further interventions.

CHRONIC, RECURRENT HEADACHES DUE TO INTERNAL IMBALANCES

Chronic, recurrent headaches are due to impairment of Qi and Blood flow to the internal organ. The various causes include stress, emotional excesses, lifestyle aberrations, dietary imbalance, or constitutional vulnerability. Headache manifests along the path of the meridians to the head, so that the location of the headache would indicate pathogenic imbalance.

History

Six specific categories of information are important for assessing chronic headaches:

1. Location
2. Characteristics
   - Yang type: sharp, throbbing, presence of aura, relief with rest, aggravated by activity
   - Yin type: dull, achy, relief with activity
3. Relationship to food—types of food, manner of eating, e.g., spicy foods, caffeine; eating while working
4. Association with emotions that correspond to specific organs
5. Initial episode that precipitated the headache, such as exposure to Wind-Cold. Recurrence of headache is now associated with exposure to Cold along the Tai Yang channels
6. Evolution of headache—the relationship between the initial episode and current complaint is important to map out. For example, the first episode was precipitated by Wind-Cold invasion. The child now presents with Shao Yang type with exposure to Cold. The history reveals that the gradual evolution of symptoms along the Five-Element Cycle, and Shao Yang headache develops as a result of inadequate Water to nourish Liver Yin, resulting in Liver Yang excess headache. The treatment needs to address the root or the initiating factor as well as correct the current imbalances.

CHRONIC HEADACHES CLASSIFIED ACCORDING TO LOCATION

Tai Yang

A Tai Yang headache occurs along the Bladder Tai Yang channel. In acute instances, this is the result of Wind-Cold in the Tai Yang stage of invasion. Chronic, recurrent Tai Yang is compatible with the Western diagnosis of tension headache. However, taking a careful TCM history is very important in these cases. If Cold is not properly expelled from the Bladder channel during an acute invasion, Cold can chronically lodge in the Tai Yang channels, predisposing the child to Tai Yang headache each time the back of the neck is exposed to Cold. This headache occurs without the full development of Wind-Cold or viral illness. The child would also be vulnerable to developing tension headaches due to tightening of neck muscles that are already contracted by Cold.

Tension headaches occur in as many as one-third of childhood headaches,[448] and may present as sharp attacks that are sometimes difficult to distinguish from migraine without aura. Tai Yang headaches are usually less intense, do not have emotional components, and usually do not have gastrointestinal symptoms such as nausea, vomiting, or abdominal pain.

Shao Yang Headache/Migraine—Lateral Side of Head and Neck

Shao Yang headaches that occur on the lateral side of the head and neck correlate to the Western diagnosis of classic migraine, considered the most common headache in childhood.[418,425-427] Migraine affects as many as 5–10% of all children[449] and may represent as high as 54% of pediatric headaches.[448] The acute episodes can be triggered by numerous factors: emotional upset; stress—such as school pressure, lack of sleep; sensory stimulation—such as loud noise, bright light; and sympathetic stimulation—such as sports, physical exercise.[450] Headache is sometimes preceded by a visual or sensory aura. The characteristic attack consists of severe, throbbing or pulsating pain—usually unilateral but in children often bilateral—frequently accompanied by digestive symptoms (nausea, vomiting, abdominal pain) and sometimes hypersensitivity to light and sound.[450] The duration is 4–72 hours in adults, and 2–48 hours in children under age 15.[417]

Various hypotheses have been proposed for pathophysiology of migraine, but the precise mechanism is still poorly understood. The headache appears to involve both central and peripheral structures. There is vasodilatation and vasoconstriction of the neurovascular system,[417] possibly due to inflammation of cerebral arteries.[451,452] There may be altered neuronal excitability in the CNS.[453] Recent evidence suggests involvement of catecholamines,[454,455] serotonin,[456] and of some neuropeptides.[457,458] There is increasing focus on the role of dopamine, both in the prodromal symptoms (such as nausea, vomiting, drowsiness) and in the headache phase with pain perception and cerebral blood flow.[459,460] Migraine in children is often associated with abdominal pain[453] and cyclical vomiting.[461,462] A strong family history is supported by the finding of a dopamine receptor gene locus in migrainous patients with aura.[451,459]

Separation of migraine without aura from episodic tension-type headache may be difficult. The most important differential characteristics of migraine are the intensity of pain, association with emotions, aggravation by physical activity, and presence of nausea and vomiting.[425] Adolescents usually have migraine with aura and tension headaches, whereas younger children tend to present with migrainous-like headaches aggravated by physical activity, sometimes accompanied by photophobia.[419]

Much has been written about the "migraine personality," or the emotional make-up of the headache sufferers. These patients have a high prevalence of various neurotic and even psychotic symptoms:[463] excessive striving for tidiness and for perfection in performance,[464] exaggerated tendency in pain perception, in self-criticism;[465] and in symbiotic attachment to their own families.[464] They are at increased risk for comorbid affective and anxiety disorder: generalized anxiety disorder, panic disorder, obsessive–compulsive disorder; phobic disorder,[466] and depression.[464,466] Pediatric and adolescent patients have been found to be emotionally rigid with a tendency to repress anger and aggression.[467]

Migraine in children and adolescents is extremely disabling, causing loss of school days and extracurricular activities.[449,468] Rest and often sleep bring relief. Western treatment is mainly with medication, ranging from over-the-counter analgesics to specific oral and intramuscular injections of antimigraine medications for acute attacks and daily prophylactic pharmacotherapy. There is no wonder drug in sight. Effective treatments for both acute episodes and for prevention are therefore urgently needed.

In Chinese medicine, classic migraine is a Shao Yang headache because of the location along the distribution of the Gallbladder meridian on the temple or side of the head. The cause is usually due to the pathology in the couple Yin organ Liver: Liver Yang or Fire rising. Liver is one of two Yin channels (the other being the Heart channel) that flows directly to the head internally. (All the other Yin channels reach the head via divergent channels.) The typical Liver Yang rising headache is the classic migraine of intense, throbbing, pulsating pain, usually along one side, but may involve both sides of the head along the Gallbladder channel, to the temples, or behind the eyes. The visual aura described in Western medicine can be explained by Liver Yang excess blocking Qi flow to the eyes, the external orifices of Liver. Gastrointestinal disturbances, such as nausea and vomiting, are due to Liver Qi invading the Stomach and preventing Stomach Qi from its normal downward movement.

Various emotions that can trigger migraine attacks correspond to emotions that are directly associated with Liver as well as emotions associated with other organs and indirectly affect the Liver through the Five-Element Cycle. Liver Yang excess manifests as anxiety, anger, frustration, resentment. Kidney deficiency corresponds to fear, and in extreme cases depression, panic and paranoia. Spleen deficiency corresponds to worry and obsession. All chronic emotions eventually affect the Heart, which in turn can manifest as disturbance in self-perception and attachment. Various dietary indiscretions can also trigger migraines. Excessive sour foods can weaken the Liver: yogurt, grapefruit and its juice, sour apples, lemon, pickles, vinegar, spinach, rhubarb, gooseberries, redcurrants; excess Hot energy foods can cause Liver Fire: curries, spices, pepper (black, white, or red), red meat, alcohol. Caffeine in soft drinks and chocolate is a frequent cause of migraine in children.

Hereditary and constitutional vulnerability due to prenatal factors, such as stress, anger, excess alcohol or drug abuse of both parents at the time of conception or of the mother during pregnancy; weak pre-Heaven Essence and familial Liver imbalance can contribute to Liver Yin deficiency and Liver Yang excess in the child.

Liver Yang excess can also be due to imbalances in the other Elements, especially the Lung Qi. Excess worry weakens the Spleen and knots Qi, which can in turn affect Lung and Heart Qi. Spleen deficiency would lead to Lung deficiency, as there is insufficient Earth to nurture Metal. Lung deficiency would allow Liver Yang to rise, since there is insufficient Metal to control Wood. Reports on acupuncture treatment are usually favorable for adult migraines. The few studies that include children appear to show promise for acupuncture as a pediatric treatment modality. Several studies propose the possible biochemical effects of acupuncture on migraine as normalization of increased and slightly decreased levels of serotonin,[456] and in affecting serum catecholamine levels.[439,456] Needling LR-3 alone has been demonstrated to affect breakdown of catecholamine.[469] Increased activity of the opioid system has also been demonstrated.[470] An animal study posits that efficacy of SI-17 lies in its anti-inflammatory effects on blood vessels of the dura mater; it brings about inhabitation of the neurogenic inflammation on the affected side.[471] Acupuncture has been shown to be effective for both acute migraine attacks[472,473] and for prophylaxis.[473–476] When TCM principles are used to differentiate headaches, acupuncture can significantly improve symptoms and even cure migraines.[477] The long-term effect of reduction in frequency, duration, and intensity after treatment can persist for months and even many years,[478,479] or with up to 50% decrease in drug intake.[476] The effect of acupuncture was comparable to some of the potent antimigraine medications but does not cause any negative side-effects.[475] In a well-controlled randomized study of childhood migraine, acupuncture treatment significantly reduced both migraine frequency and intensity.[470]

A multidisciplinary approach that included acupuncture, dietary changes, medication, physical therapy, lifestyle adaptations, was effective in treating the majority of patients with various types of migraine-related dizziness and vertigo.[480] Age, sex, social status, and expectations of benefit did not show any relation to treatment efficacy, but those with fewer emotional issues reported a better response.[481]

Acupuncture has been demonstrated to be efficacious even for "German migraine." Germany is a unique country with reported 12%[482] to as many as 25% of the population afflicted with migraine.[482] The symptoms tend to be severe: sudden onset of usually unbearable headache that can last for up to 72 hours and can be accompanied by vegetative symptoms,[483] and can occur frequently. Patients often take numerous analgesics for symptomatic relief but suffer various side-effects. Acupuncture has been successful both for ameliorating acute symptoms and for prophylactic treatment.[482,483]

Yang Ming Headache—Frontal Headache

According to Western medicine, frontal headache is usually associated with sinusitis[484] and occurs in older children after the frontal sinuses are formed. In

Chinese medicine, headache located on the forehead generally indicates a Yang Ming Stomach imbalance, usually due to dietary indiscretions. Recurrent, sharp frontal headache can be caused by Stomach Heat, Stomach Qi obstruction, and food retention. When children consume too much red meat, spicy and fried foods, Stomach Heat accumulates and rises along the Stomach meridian to the forehead. Overeating weakens the Spleen and obstructs Stomach Qi; while eating too quickly or while studying may lead to food retention. Both of these can lead to sharp, frontal headache.

Migraine in children is frequently characteristically Yang Ming: frontal location accompanied by abdominal pain.[450] In recent years there is increasing advent of Yang Ming headache in children who spend long hours in front of a computer monitor. The eye strain and continuous electromagnetic stimulation to the Yintang point can lead to frontal headaches. A dull, achy frontal headache is caused by a deficiency of Stomach Yin, which occurs when children eat irregularly or eat very late at night.

Tai Yin Headache

This headache is characterized by a heavy and tight sensation as if the head is wrapped with a band. The pain is usually dull and achy, can be generalized or localized to the forehead. Western medicine reports that when patients regularly take analgesics, this type of headache occurs with drug withdrawal.[485] Chinese medicine attributes the cause of Tai Yin headache to Spleen deficiency with accumulation of Dampness in the head. There may be other Spleen deficiency signs, such as poor muscle tone, fatigue, and digestive problems.

A child may have a predisposition to Tai Yin headache when there is a strong familial tendency toward Spleen deficiency; when parents engage in excess mental work, have excess worry, or have digestive weakness due to poor diet or alcohol abuse during conception; and when the mother has these experiences during pregnancy. Factors that precipitate the headache consist of living in a Damp environment, eating excess Damp-producing foods, and engaging in excess mental activities. Living in a Damp environment, such as in the basement, close to the ocean, in rainy weather; and eating Damp-producing foods, such as milk products, greasy, fried foods, peanuts, sweets and white sugar can lead to Spleen deficiency. Although Dampness usually affects the lower part of the body, it can easily enter the Middle Energizer, from there it rises upward and obstructs the orifices that clear the head. Dampness then accumulates in the head, resulting in an achy, heavy sensation.

Tai Yin headache also occurs with excess mental activities. Today's children are faced with increasing pressures to perform academically while also participating in numerous extracurricular activities. From an early age, many children keep a busy schedule without getting adequate rest. Young students in middle school are often studying late into the night and are already beginning to worry about college competition, especially when they have parents with unrealistically high expectations. Excess mental activities, combined with worry and lack of sufficient sleep, can severely weaken the Spleen Qi.

Shao Yin—Headache "inside" the Brain

Children frequently describe the headache as just "pain inside the whole head." Western medicine does not have a diagnosis for this nonspecific type of pain, while Chinese medicine considers these as Shao Yin headaches due to Kidney and Heart deficiency. Characteristically, Shao Yin headache is a dull, achy pain in the whole head. It may also concentrate on the occiput, like tension headache. Since Kidney Essence nourishes the brain, a lack of nourishment in Kidney deficiency would manifest as dull, achy, generalized headache accompanied by a feeling of emptiness in the head. Other Kidney deficiency signs, such as enuresis, frequent urination, and lack of vitality, may accompany this type of headache.

Several factors can predispose a child to Shao Yin headache: (1) a strong familial tendency toward Kidney deficiency; (2) a father with history of promiscuity (Jing or Essence is lost through ejaculation) and a mother with polymenorrhea, history of miscarriages, or multiple pregnancies especially close together; (3) fear in either or both parents during conception; (4) studying long hours without adequate rest weakens Spleen Qi and in the long run, Kidney Yin; this is the most common cause of Yin deficiency in Western industrial societies and therefore also in children; (5) too much salty foods, such as tinned or processed foods often heavily salted; bacon, sausages, cereals, tinned soups, smoked fish, (pretzels, chips—both salty and greasy); (6) a chronic state of anxiety and fear can deplete the Kidney; (7) shock suspends Qi and can cause Kidney Qi and Jing deficiency.

Shao Yin headache can also be due to Heart deficiency, which can manifest as generalized dull, achy pain inside the head or localized on the forehead area. The child may have a bluish tinge on the forehead and chin, and may manifest other Heart deficiency symptoms, such as dream-disturbed sleep, nervousness, difficulty with concentration. The young child under age 3 may also wake up crying at night. Several factors can predispose the child to Heart deficiency: (1) A familial tendency toward Heart or Shen disorders; (2) any excess emotions that both parents felt during conception—since all emotions eventually affect the Heart—could result in Heart weakness in the child; (3) if the mother experiences physical Heart disorder or excess emotions during pregnancy, especially if there is any major physical or emotional experience that constitute a "shock" to the maternal system, can also cause Heart deficiency in the fetus; (4) excess worry can knot Heart Qi; (5) shock can also affect Heart Qi; (6) excess consumption of bitter foods or medications.

Jue Yin

The typical Jue Yin headache occurs at the vertex, the top of the head. This is most often due to metabolic imbalances, such as hypoglycemia, or when children adhere to a strict diet or are anorexic. The insufficient nourishment results in general deficiency of Qi and Blood that is felt as pain at the top of the head.

Variable Locations with History of Head Trauma

Chronic headaches can be due to severe accidents and falls causing Blood stasis in a particular area of the head. While some children may experience pain immediately following the trauma, many children may not complain of headache until years later. This is usually a localized headache that correlates with area of trauma. Sometimes, there may be a small purple spot near the tip of the tongue to indicate Blood stasis in the head. The injury creates a vulnerability for the particular channel or channels that circulate through the area of trauma, so that headache may be precipitated by physical or emotional factors specific for those meridians. For example, a child may fall on the side of the head and be mildly concussed. The child has transient headache immediately after the trauma. Many years later, the slightest anger or frustration would cause a sharp Shao Yang headache to occur.

Treatment

Treatment for headache can be general and specific.

General Treatment for all Types of Headaches

- GB-20 Fengchi is the most important point for headaches, and can be chosen as the first point for headaches of any type[486]
- GV-16 is a Window of Heaven point that is indicated for "hundred diseases of the head"
- LU-7 is a special point for any type of headache, stimulates clear Yang to ascend to the head[253]
- LI-4—a very strong dispersing point for headache, should be used with care in children who are deficient
- Ah Shi tender points are important in headaches[486]
- A combination of local and distal points are very effective in treatmet of headaches.[486–488]

Needle Treatment

- Simple needling: reducing method on the local points for sedation; tonification method for distal points
- Ion pumping cords: connect the black clamp on local point and red clamp on distal point.

Magnet Treatment

Place bionorth (–) pole facing down on local point, biosouth (+) pole facing down on distal point.

- Place black clamp on local point and connect with red clamp on distal point.

Acute/External Pathogens

For all external Wind pathogenic invasions, keep the child's occiput and back of the neck warm by wearing a scarf or a coat with a hood during cold and rainy weather. Treat the three major Wind "Feng" acupoints to expel Wind in the head: GV-16, GB-20, BL-12.

Wind-Cold

- Use the Five-Element protocol to dispel Cold from the Tai Yang Bladder channel:
  - Tonify BL-60, SI-5; sedate BL-66
- LU-7—helps to expel Wind-Cold from the head
- SI-17 a Window of Heaven point that is effective in expelling Wind from the head[489]
- BL-10 local point for Tai Yang channel Wind-Cold, combine with BL-60 as the distal point
- GV-14 to treat any fever
- Decrease cold drinks and energetically Cold foods; give the child warm drinks and energetically warm foods. Chicken soup is the universal "warming soup" for a cold.

Wind-Heat

- Use the Five-Element protocol to dispel Heat from the Tai Yang Bladder channel:
  - Tonify BL-66; sedate BL-60, SI-5
- GV-14, LI-11 to dispel Heat
- TE-5 expels Wind-Heat and relieves headache
- Decrease spicy or energetically Hot foods.

Wind-Damp

- ST-8 is the major local point combined with SP-3 or SP-6 as a distal point to eliminate Dampness from the head
- Dispel Wind-Damp acupoints: SP-9, ST-40
- Use the Five-Element four-point protocol to tonify Spleen:
  - BL-20 to tonify the Spleen: tonify SP-2, HT-8; sedate LR-1, SP-1
- CV-12 to tonify the Middle Energizer
- Yintang as local point if there is also forehead headache.

Blood Stasis

Acupuncture treatment should be instituted for head trauma headaches only if neurological examination and laboratory evaluations are negative for skull fracture or CNS bleed. These headaches can occur anywhere, depending on the site of trauma. Treatment can begin with Ah Shi tender points as local points, followed by a distal point along the channel that connects to the Ah Shi point. For example, if the tender point is on the forehead along Stomach line, treat the tender Ah Shi point, then choose a distal point on the Stomach channel; if the tender point is a Gallbladder point on the side of the head, treat the Ah Shi point as a local point, then treat a distal Gallbladder point.

- BL-17 the Hui-meeting point of Blood, invigorates Blood and dispels stasis
- SP-10 general treatment for Blood stasis
- Tai Yang acupoint for Blood stasis in the temple region
- TE-18 for Blood stasis in the occiput.

Chronic Recurrent Headaches

Tai Yang Headache Treatment

- Use the Five-Element protocol to dispel Cold from the Tai Yang Bladder channel:
  - Tonify BL-60, SI-5; sedate BL-66
- If recurrent episodes are associated with Cold exposure to the neck and occiput: keep the child's occiput and back of the neck warm by wearing a scarf or a coat with a hood during cold and rainy weather
- If recurrent episodes are associated with tension or stress teach the child deep breathing or Qigong exercises to relieve tension
- Modify lifestyle to reduce stress
- Use local points: BL-10, GV-16, GB-20 combine with BL-60 as a distal point.

Shao Yang—Migraine Headache Treatment

- Use the Five-Element four-point protocol to dispel Liver Heat:
  - Tonify LR-8, KI-10; sedate LR-2, HT-8
- GB-20 subdues Liver Wind and Liver Yang
- TE-5 moves Qi on the side of the head, subdues Liver Yang
- GB-41 can be combined with TE-5 to move Qi on the side, or with LR-3 to pacify Liver Fire[490]
- Tai Yang is a local, temporal point, also helps to subdue Liver Yang
- LR-3 is the main distal point to pacify Liver and subdue Yang rising
- LR-8 nourishes Liver Blood and/or Liver Yin
- LR-2 controls Liver Fire
- SP-6 as the meeting point of Liver, Kidney, and Spleen channels, it pacifies the Liver, nourishes Liver Blood, calms the Mind, promotes sleep, which is important in headache
- LU-7 tonifies the Lung, which controls Liver in the Five-Element Cycle therefore pacifies Liver Yang
- BL-18 back Shu point for Liver
- SI-17 as a local point; has been found in animal studies to have anti-inflammatory effect on the blood vessels of the brain on the affected side of migraine[471]
- Decrease sour and greasy foods in the diet
- Modify lifestyle to diminish stress
- Teach the child calming Qigong exercises.

Yang Ming/Frontal Headache

- Use the Five-Element four-point protocol to dispel Stomach Heat:
  - Tonify ST-44, BL-66; sedate ST-41, SI-5
- Local points: Yingtang, BL-2, ST-8, GV-23 combine with distal points along the Stomach, and Bladder meridians:
  - ST-34 the accumulation point of Stomach meridian, is effective as a distal point for pain relief
  - ST-40 the major point to clear Dampness
  - ST-44 main point to clear Stomach Heat
  - BL-60 distal Bladder point

    – CV-12 a strong point for Yang Ming headache for tonifying Stomach and Spleen[491]
- Decrease energetically Hot foods, greasy/fried foods in the diet.

Tai Yin Headache

- Use the Five-Element four-point protocol to tonify Spleen:
  – Tonify SP-2, HT-8; sedate SP-1, LR-1
- ST-40 major point for resolving Dampness
- ST-44 is an important distal point to pull Dampness downward
- SP-6 a good distal point to pull Dampness down, tonifies and regulates Spleen
- CV-12 tonifies Middle Energizer and resolves Dampness
- Modify the child's lifestyle, especially if there is excess mental activities, and insufficient rest
- Decrease Phlegm-producing and artificially sweetened foods in the diet.

Shao Yin Headache

Kidney deficiency:

- GV-20 and especially Sishencong are very beneficial for Kidney deficiency headaches[492] for nourishing the marrow, the brain
- Super Mingmen treatment: GV-4, BL-23, BL-52 as a strong Kidney tonification treatment
- KI-3 tonifies both Kidney Yin and Kidney Yang and Original Qi
- CV-4 tonifies Kidney Yin
- SP-6 tonifies Yin
- GB-19 is a special local point for Kidney deficiency as it attracts Kidney Essence up to the brain
- Use the Five-Element four-point protocol to tonify both Kidney Yin and Kidney Yang:
  – Tonify KI-7, LU-8; sedate KI-3, SP-3
- Decrease excess salt in diet.

Heart deficiency Shao Yin headache:

- HT-7 tonifies Heart Yin
- KI-3 tonifies all Yin
- PC-6 regulates functions of Heart
- Decrease bitter foods and medications
- BL-15 back Shu point for Heart.

Jue Yin

Metabolic disorders should be properly diagnosed and treated by Western evaluation with acupuncture instituted for pain relief: GV-20 as a local point combined with KI-1, BL-67, or LR-3 as distal points.

Blood Stasis

Acupuncture treatment for chronic, localized headache with history of head trauma should also only be instituted when neurological examination and laboratory evaluations are negative for the presence of CNS hematoma or abnormalities. The treatment can be the same as those for acute Blood stasis headache: combining local Ah Shi tender points with distal points along the same channel, and Blood moving and invigorating points: BL-17, SP-10. Local points such as Tai Yang for Blood stasis in the temple region, GV-20 or Sishencong for Blood stasis in the vertex (see Bibliography for further reading on this topic).

HICCUPS

Hiccups are due to brief, powerful involuntary spasms and contraction of the diaphragm and the auxiliary respiratory muscles during inspiration, followed by glottic closure. The movement of inspiratory air is rushed, producing a typical "hiccupping" sound.[493,494] Chronic hiccups is defined as recurrent episodes of hiccups or a duration exceeding 48 hours.[494] Hiccups is a physiologic gastrointestinal reflex that already exists *in utero*,[494] and appears to still occur frequently in young infants.[493] A possible etiology includes gastro-esophageal reflux,[494] or secondary to feeding gastrostomy,[495] tracheostomy,[494] and intubation.[493] While the physiologic effect from hiccups is generally considered negligible,[494] upper airway obstruction has been found in unintubated, young infants;[493] and respiratory alkalosis in tracheostomy[494] and gastrostomy[495] patients.

The majority of acute episodes of hiccups are self-limiting. Numerous remedies have been reported over the centuries, no single "cure" stands out as being the most effective.[496] Various home remedies include telling the child to hold his breath for as long as possible; or breathing in and out of a paper bag (a confined space)—both of which induce elevated levels of pCO_2 to stimulate respiration. Chronic and recurrent hiccups may be treated with medication, the most common being Baclofen.[494,495] More aggressive treatments in adults, such as the calcium channel blocker Nifedipine,[497] crushing of the phrenic nerve, or microvascular decompression of the vagus nerve[498] are not indicated in children.

CHINESE MEDICINE

Hiccups in Chinese medicine is due to rebellious Stomach Qi that disrupts the descent of Lung Qi during inspiration. Various causes that are applicable in children include improper eating and diet, such as eating too fast[499] or eating excessive Cold and raw foods,[499,500] Liver Qi stagnation, such as from emotional disturbances and prolonged illnesses that result in insufficient Qi in the Middle Energizer.[501] Body points[39,499–501] auriculopoints[502–504] and other microsystem points[505,506] have all been used for treatment of hiccups.

Treatment

Since children are not usually seen for acute episode of hiccups, acupressure of body points can be taught to the parents to administer during an attack. If the child is seen for recurrent or chronic hiccups, south pole, tonification magnets can be applied to the body points, and pellets can be applied to microsystem ear points.

- Main points: PC-6, CV-17, ST-36[39,500]
- "Hiccup relieving point" located at the middle of the posterior border of the sternocleidomastoid muscle, at the anatomic point where the phrenic nerve crosses the anterior scalenus muscle[499]
- Auxiliary points include: CV-14, LI-4[39] ST-25[501] Middle Sifeng, (extra point 29)[507] of the middle finger
- Auricular points: Shenmen, Point Zero, Stomach, Hiccups point[502–504]
- In rare, severe cases, needling of LI-18 (Futu) as a Yang Ming point[508] or electroacupuncture stimulation of the "hiccup relieving point", may be tried in children.[499]

IMMUNE SYSTEM

The human immune response is an extremely complex cascade of events that involves numerous different types of immune factors and biochemical mediators. The immune system can be broadly divided into humoral and cellular compartments. The humoral response refers to complement and immunoglobulin antibody-mediated B-cell system. The cellular response refers to delayed hypersensitivity mediated via T-cells, which consist of a wide variety of cells that include leukocytes, polymorphonuclear neutrophils (PMN), eosinophils, mast cells, macrophages, and natural killer cells. This classification is not precise, as there is a great deal of interaction and cross over of functions. Recent studies have focused in depth on the pro-inflammatory mediators, such as cytokines and leukotrienes. These mediators are a heterogeneous group of biochemical compounds produced by a gamut of cells that includes epithelial cells, fibroblasts, PMNs, and macrophages. They trigger or orchestrate an immune response by acting as signals between cells of the immune system, leading to inflammatory responses against pathogens. Neurotransmitters in the CNS and nutrition also actively participate in the immune response. While an immune reaction can be protective to the host, a hyperimmune response can be destructive by damaging normal structures so that regulatory process is necessary to prevent "immunologic runaway."[394]

Immune deficiency is associated with recurrent infections, malnutrition, trauma, and immaturity of the immune system. Children with recurrent infections often manifest immune insufficiency.[509,510] Abnormalities of the local defense mechanisms of the upper airways are very common.[511] Poor nutrition, especially a diet low in protein, can cause both humoral and cellular deficiencies. Iron, trace minerals and vitamin deficiencies can all affect the child's immune system.[512–518] Trauma can induce a potent inflammatory response.[519,520] Even hemorrhage alone may be a sufficient stimulus to activate the immune system.[519] Infants and young children have immature immune systems and are at greater risk for infections.[513,521] Neonates especially have very inadequate immune systems so that they are vulnerable to infections and often respond poorly to vaccines.[522–526]

While inadequate immune responses predispose children to illnesses and infections, current data also suggest that hyperactive immune or inflammatory responses are possibly due to poor regulatory control and result in destruction of normal tissues. Asthma, inflammatory bowel disease (IBD), juvenile rheumatoid arthritis (JRA), cardiovascular disease, diabetes and cancer are some of the chronic disorders attributed to uncontrolled hyperimmune response to an initial stimulus. There is evidence which suggests that juvenile rheumatoid arthritis is caused by T-cell infiltration of the synovial membrane.[527,528] Cardiovascular disease in children, such as rheumatic heart disease, are secondary immune response to infections.[529] The presence of pro-inflammatory mediators in diabetes suggests that a hyperinflammatory response to an infection causes pancreatic beta cell destruction.[530,531] Increased levels of mediators have also been found in cancer.[532] Recognition of the significance of pro-inflammatory mediators has generated fervent development of immune modulatory treatments. These treatments are costly and only a few are approved for usage in children. There is no medication that induces natural immune defense or regulation.

Western medicine also considers the skin, lungs, and liver to be immune organs. The skin is a protective organ. The lungs have important B-cell secretion of antibodies and T-cell mediated immune responses to foreign antigens.[533] The liver hepatocytes produce acute-phase proteins and complement in bacterial infections. Many cells participate in a T-cell immune response against bacterial infections and hematogenous tumor metastases.[534]

CHINESE MEDICINE

Chinese medicine traditionally incorporates strengthening of the immune system as part of the treatment of children. The immune system in TCM is Wei Qi, the Defensive Qi. Whereas the refined Nutritive Qi flows internally in the channels and Blood vessels, Wei Qi is the coarser form of Qi that flows exteriorly during the day and resides in the Liver at night. Wei Qi circulates outside the channels, in the skin and connective tissues, controls the opening and closing of the pores, and acts like a "shield" to protect the body against external pathogens. The Defensive Qi is intimately related to the Kidney, as it is influenced by Essence and transformed by Kidney Yang. It is nourished by the digestive organs, Stomach and Spleen, which supply the Food Qi. It is regulated by the Lung during the day. At night, it resides primarily in the Liver, which directs its flow to all the Yin organs.

When the body first contracts an infection, the external pathogen is in the superficial layers—the Wei Qi level of Wind-Heat invasion and Tai Yang level of Wind-Cold invasion. Treatment is directed toward expelling the pathogen and strengthening the body, i.e., chasing out the burglar and closing the windows and bolting the doors. At this time, there is ample biochemical support in the literature to indicate that acupuncture activates both the humoral and cellular immune systems to protect the host, as well as regulate a hyperinflammatory response.[531] Acupuncture treatment has been demonstrated to stimulate humoral immune factors.[535–538] Animal studies demonstrated that when acupuncture points that correspond to human CV-2 and HT-8 were stimulated, an active humoral response ensues.[539] Acupuncture also significantly enhanced T-cell population and activities in both clinical and animal studies.[536,540–544] There can be an increase in lymphocyte proliferation[544] in phagocytosis[545,546] or in enhanced killer cell cytotoxicity.[547] There may be a close relationship between the Stomach meridian and mast cell population, since stimulation of many Stomach points seem to result in an increase in mast cells.[548] An animal study using a point that corresponds to BL-23, the Kidney Shu point, increased T-cell activities.[541] Acupuncture can improve immune function in trauma-induced immunosuppression.[544,549] Noninvasive laser acupuncture, which is well tolerated by children, was demonstrated to positively affect both humoral and cellular immunity.[536,550] Acupuncture has also been shown to affect the nervous system arm of the immune response.[535] Animal studies have demonstrated increased immunity with stimulation of the catecholaminergic[538,540,551,552] and serotonergic neurons.[538] The immune response may also be mediated via the autonomic nervous system.[553] Acupuncture seems to stimulate the sympathetic nervous system,[554] resulting in activation of the release of helper T-cells from the bone marrow.[555] In fact, stimulation of the Kidney Shu point, BL-23, has been demonstrated to stimulate T-cells.[541]

While acupuncture stimulates the immune response as a protective mechanism, it also appears to exert a regulatory effect on hyperinflammation. Acupuncture seems to be able to modulate the synthesis and release of pro-inflammatory mediators.[540,556,557] Current hypotheses suggest that there is a common pathway connecting opioids and the immune system.[535,544,546,549,558] Acupuncture is well known for its efficacy in the treatment of pain. Acupuncture analgesia is mediated through the stimulation of large myelinated nerve fibers which conduct the impulse to the spinal cord and higher centers. Opioids such as endorphins are released to block the ascending pain signals. It is possible that along with the opioids, other neurotransmitters that modulate the inflammatory response, such as substance P and serotonin, are also released.[559]

Magnetic resonance imaging has demonstrated the coupling of pain and immune processes via the same afferent and efferent signals.[560] Acupuncture immunomodulation may also be mediated through the release of acetylcholine from the parasympathetic nerve endings.[561]

Animal studies have also demonstrated specific immune effects of acupuncture in various conditions. Acupuncture treatment minimizes the hyperinflammatory response in asthma,[562] stabilizes mast cells of gastric ulcer,[563] reduces anticollagen-specific antibody level,[564] enhances the cellular immune functions in cancer,[565–567] and diminishes inflammation in rheumatoid arthritis.[564]

The most frequently used overall immune point is Zusanli ST-36,[271,535,546,548,556,557,564,565,568,569] followed by Hegu LI-4. Other points include Lanweixue, Dazhui[568] Bladder Shu points,[271] and even local points for specific conditions, such as LI-20 for rhinitis.[569] Since the majority of pediatric illnesses are acute infections, the simple "immune tonification" protocol can be carried out along with expelling the pathogen while the invasion is still in the superficial stages or levels. In chronic illnesses, such as inflammatory bowel disease, the priority of treatment is to first balance the internal organs, and add immune tonification points as adjunctive therapy.

Simple, General Immune Tonification Protocol for Children

- ST-36
- LI-4 if used together with ST-36
- Shu points associated with Wei Qi production and movement:
  – BL-13 Lung Shu
  – BL-18 Liver Shu

- BL-20 Spleen Shu
- BL-21 Stomach Shu
- BL-23 Kidney Shu.

INFLAMMATORY BOWEL DISEASE

CHRONIC INFLAMMATORY BOWEL DISEASE

Chronic inflammatory bowel disease (IBD), comprised of ulcerative colitis and Crohn's disease, is now being recognized with increasing frequency in children of all ages,[570] and has become one of the most significant chronic diseases affecting children and adolescents.[571] IBD presents unique challenges for diagnosis and management because physically and psychosocially developing children often do not present with the classic symptoms.[572]

Ulcerative colitis (UC) and Crohn's disease (CD) are probably syndromes rather than single entities,[573] since they share many similarities in epidemiology, immunologic, clinical and therapeutic characteristics.[255]

Twenty-five to 30% of all patients with CD and 20% of those with UC present before age 20.[574] Four percent of pediatric IBD occurs before the age of 5 years, with a peak age of onset in the late adolescent years.[572] In North America, the incidence for 10- to 19-year-olds is approximately 2 per 100 000 for UC and 3.5 per 100 000 for CD.[575] The incidence of IBD is worldwide,[576] primarily occurring in industrialized countries with well-nourished populations.[255] The possible environmental risks include lack of breast feeding or early weaning, perinatal infections and "Western diet" with high fatty acid intake.[255] Although infectious gastroenteritis may be the triggering event,[572] there is no convincing or direct evidence that links an infectious agent with IBD.[255] There is strong evidence for genetic influence[577] and specific loci on chromosomes have been identified.[578,579] Currently, the dominant view of IBD pathophysiology is hyperactive immune response of the gastrointestinal mucosa to triggering factors present in the gut lumen, resulting in chronic inflammation and ensuing tissue injury.[255]

Colonic malignancy is a major complication of both UC and CD patients with pancolitis beginning in childhood.[580] The chronic, lifelong disease process also leads to significant psychosocial impact on the child and adolescent.[581]

Crohn's Disease

Crohn's disease has an equal incidence in boys and girls.[575] Thirty percent of children have a positive family history.[575] In addition to the environmental triggers for IBD, tobacco smoking seems to affect the familial type of CD.[582]

The enteric pathology in CD is transmural inflammation, which is characteristically asymmetric and segmental with skipped areas. Granulomas are pathognomonic for the disorder. Any segment of the bowel may be involved: aphthous ulcerations can occur in the mouth, esophagus, stomach or duodenum;[255] and perianal lesions including skin tags, fissures, fistulas and abscesses[583] can occur in 15% of pediatric patients with CD.[583] The majority of children (50–70%)

with CD have involvement in the terminal ileum, with more than half of these patients also having inflammation in variable segments of the colon, usually the ascending colon.[255,584] Ten to 20% of children have isolated colonic disease, and 10–15% have diffuse small bowel disease involving the more proximal ileum or jejunum.[570]

The clinical presentation of CD depends on the part of the gastrointestinal tract involved. The majority of the time, the child presents with small intestine symptoms, consisting of recurrent, poorly localized abdominal pain; chronic diarrhea; lassitude; late afternoon and evening low-grade fever, anorexia; and weight loss of several months' duration.[255,570] CD involving the colon may be clinically indistinguishable from UC, with symptoms of bloody, mucopurulent diarrhea, crampy abdominal pain, and urgency to defecate.[255]

Growth failure, seen in 30% of pediatric CD,[572] is a disconcerting problem in young children[585,586] and in the adolescent whose sexual development may be delayed.[572] Growth deceleration is usually insidious, and may precede the onset of intestinal symptoms by years,[587] thereby delaying diagnosis.[588] Inadequate nutrient intake, anorexia, malabsorption, increased losses, and increased metabolic demands all contribute to poor growth.[570]

The transmural inflammation leads to bacterial overgrowth and the formation of fistulas and strictures that can cause obstruction. The risk of adenocarcinoma of the colon for Crohn's colitis is 4 to 20 times that of the general population.[570] Perianal disease may precede the appearance of the intestinal manifestations of CD by years, and is seen most commonly in patients with colitis. When perianal disease does not respond to medical therapy, surgical management is necessary.

Ulcerative Colitis

UC is a diffuse, chronic inflammation restricted to the mucosal lining of the rectum and large intestine, and extends proximally in a symmetric, uninterrupted pattern to involve parts or all of the large intestine.[589] The rectum is involved in more than 95% of cases.[255] In addition to the environmental triggers for IBD, UC patients report a higher incidence of cows' milk allergy.[255]

The most common presenting symptoms are rectal bleeding, diarrhea, and abdominal pain. Children usually have more extensive disease at the time of diagnosis than adults.[589] Mild disease is seen in 50–60% of UC, characterized by increased mucosal blood flow with erythema and mucosal edema, which can lead to granularity and friability, resulting in spontaneous bleeding. The disease is usually confined to the distal colon, the child does not have any systemic signs and symptoms.

Thirty percent of pediatric patients present with moderate disease characterized by bloody diarrhea, cramps, urgency to defecate, and abdominal tenderness. Systemic signs, such as anorexia, low-grade fever, and mild anemia, may be present. Fifteen percent of pediatric UC patients have growth failure.

Severe colitis occurs in approximately 10% of patients, presenting with more than six bloody stools per day, abdominal tenderness, fever, anemia, leukocytosis, and hypoalbuminemia. In less than 5% of pediatric patients, UC may present with extraintestinal manifestations, such as arthropathy, skin manifestations, or liver disease.[255,590]

The major gastrointestinal complications of UC are massive bleeding, toxic megacolon, and carcinoma. Toxic megacolon is rare in young patients, but is a medical and surgical emergency because there is a high risk for colonic perforation, gram-negative sepsis, and massive hemorrhage.[591] Children who develop UC before 14 years of age have a cumulative colorectal cancer incidence rate of 5% at 20 years and 40% at 35 years.[592] Children who develop the disease between 15 and 39 years of age have a cumulative incidence rate of 5% at 20 years and 30% at 35 years. Therefore, it is estimated that there is an 8% risk of dying from colon cancer 10 to 25 years after diagnosis of colitis if the disease symptoms are not controlled.[593]

Extraintestinal Manifestations

Twenty-five to 35% of patients with CD or UC have at least one extraintestinal manifestation, which may be diagnosed before, concurrently with, or after the diagnosis of IBD is made.[594] Skin manifestations, aphthous ulcers in the mouth, ocular findings such as uveitis, arthritis (occurring in 7–25% of pediatric patients), hepatobiliary disease, urologic complications including renal stones (occurs in approximately 5% of children with IBD), and hydronephrosis have been reported.[570] Rarely, arthritis can be the first and sometimes only initial symptom for months to years in children with IBD.[572] CD also has characteristic erythema nodosum (raised, red, tender nodules that appear primarily on the anterior surfaces of the leg, and affects 3% of children).[595] It is estimated that 75% of patients with erythema nodosum ultimately develop arthritis.[596]

Diagnostic Evaluation

Physical examination and initial laboratory evaluations can all be nonspecific. Once infectious causes have been ruled out, it is best to refer the child to a pediatric gastroenterologist for further diagnostic evaluation, which would include flexible colonoscopy with colonic and terminal ileal biopsy specimens. The flexible, small-caliber endoscopes allow colonoscopic evaluation of pediatric patients of all ages, including infants,[597] by direct visualization and biopsy of the colon and terminal ileum. An upper gastrointestinal with small bowel follow-through X-ray contrast study is performed on younger children, whereas double-contrast radiography (enteroclysis) is the state-of-the-art technique for examining fine mucosal details to detect early ulceration in the small bowel in older children. When there is suspicion of abscesses and fistulas in CD, computerized tomography and ultrasonography are useful additional studies.[570] The pediatric CD activity index, which includes growth parameters, was developed in 1990 and validated at 12 pediatric gastrointestinal centers as a scoring system for diagnosing CD. At this time, a disease activity index is being developed for pediatric UC.[598]

Management

The general goals of treatment for children with IBD are to achieve control of the inflammatory process, to promote growth through adequate nutrition, and to permit the child to function as normally as possible, such as attending school or participating in sports.[570] Nutrition is a very important part of management since growth failure is a major concern.[572] Recommendations for nutritional therapy include an increase in energy and protein intake to 150% of recommended daily allowances for height and age. Some studies recommend nocturnal nasogastric infusion as supplements of daily intake. Nutritional support has been shown to be as effective as steroids in achieving remission of disease in children.[572,586,599]

Antibiotics may be helpful in CD. Omega-3-fatty acids has been shown to reduce relapse rates.[600] Various pharmacologic agents are being used in IBD. Recently, there is growing preference for immunosuppressive therapies[255,601–603] for controlling the hyperactive mucosal immune system. Steroids are used in acute flare-ups, but are usually not beneficial in maintaining long-term remission in CD.[604,605] Growth retardation can occur in children even with small doses of steroids and is not overcome by administration of growth hormone.[605] Other immunosuppressive drugs also have significant toxicities that include potential risks of infection and malignancy so that they should not be used indiscriminately,[606] especially in children. Refractory inflammatory bowel disease can be treated by surgery.[603] Various surgical, endorectal pull-through procedures have been used to treat UC. CD is often more difficult to manage because surgery does not cure the disease. It is considered only for uncontrollable bleeding, stenotic bowel, or fistulas unresponsive to medical therapy.[570,604]

CHINESE MEDICINE

Acupuncture Data

Approximately 51%[607] of IBD patients have resorted to complementary healing practices, including acupuncture.[608] Concern about side-effects of medications and lack of effectiveness of standard therapies were the most commonly cited reasons for seeking complementary medicine.[607]

There are very few studies on acupuncture treatment of IBD. Current literature strongly suggests that acupuncture modulates the immune system.[531] There is one animal study that used an herbal tablet to treat induced Spleen deficiency in guinea pigs, resulting in amelioration of symptoms and decrease in size of colonic ulcer and edema.[609] There are no human studies at this time that specifically examine mucosal biopsies with acupuncture treatment. However, since acupuncture has been demonstrated to be successful in modulating immune response[531] it would be reasonable to assume that acupuncture can have a beneficial effect on the hyperimmune inflammatory response of gastrointestinal mucosa in IBD.[610] Acupuncture treatment is based on TCM differentiation.

TCM Differentiation

There are several possible TCM diagnoses that correlate with the Western diagnosis of inflammatory bowel disease:

- Spleen deficiency
- Damp Heat in the Intestines
- Liver Qi stagnation
- Kidney deficiency.

Spleen Deficiency

Children are constitutionally Spleen deficient, which can be aggravated by: living in a Damp environment; by consuming excess sweets, greasy and fried foods, and Phlegm-producing foods; by hereditary Spleen deficiency; by chronic illnesses; and by irregular eating habits. In older children, excess mental work, stress, or excess Wood emotions—such as anger, worry, frustration—can further weaken the Spleen with Wood invading Earth. Spleen deficiency results in insufficient transformation and transportation of food and fluid, resulting in accumulation of Dampness and turbidity that can obstruct the circulation of Qi and Blood, leading to abdominal pain and diarrhea. There are usually other signs of Spleen deficiency, such as fatigue, pallor, and abdominal distension.

Treatment

- ST-40 to expel Damp
- SP-3, SP-6, BL-20 to tonify Spleen
- Vigorous tonification of the Spleen with the Five-Element four-point protocol:
  - Tonify SP-2, HT-8; sedate SP-1, LR-1
- CV-12 tonifies Middle Energizer
- Decrease intake of sweets, greasy/fried foods, and Phlegm-producing foods.

Damp Heat in the Intestines

Children can have lingering Heat when external Heat invasions are not adequately expelled. Chronic consumption of an excess amount of energetically Hot and spicy foods can also cause Heat accumulation. Physiologically, Heat usually rises. However, the presence of Dampness would "drag" the Heat downward into the Lower Energizer. External Dampness enters the body by penetrating channels of the legs and flows up to the Spleen where it obstructs its function of transformation and transportation. Internal Dampness can result from the Spleen deficiency factors listed above. Dampness and turbidity from Spleen deficiency can accumulate in the Intestines and also transform into Heat. Damp Heat in the Intestines is injurious to the intestinal wall and blood vessels, and interferes with fluid absorption. It prevents the Intestines from performing their functions of food and Qi conduction, resulting in abdominal pain and diarrhea. Damp Heat coagulates with Qi and Blood, causing Blood stasis that further obstructs Blood vessels and Qi channels. Bleeding occurs in the presence of Blood stasis because non-coagulated Blood cannot pass through the blood vessels and leaks out of the vessels. The Large Intestine is more affected because of its Yang Ming–Tai Yin relationship with Stomach and Spleen.

CD correlates to Damp Heat in the Small Intestine, and UC correlates to Damp Heat and Blood stasis in the Large Intestine, manifesting as bloody diarrhea and severe abdominal pain.

Treatment for Damp Heat in CD and UC

- Eliminate or decrease energetically Hot foods, greasy/fried foods; excessive sweets, and Phlegm-producing foods
- LI-11 to clear overall Heat
- TE-6 clears Heat from the Intestines and promotes bowel movements
- CV-10 resolves Dampness and stimulates descending of Qi in the Intestines
- Resolve Dampness:
  - ST-44 to resolve Dampness
  - SP-9 to resolve Damp Heat
- ST-25 to stop diarrhea
- CV-6 to tonify Lower Energizer
- Tonify Spleen.

One clinical report from China suggests that strong moxibustion at ST-25, CV-4, and BL-23 can theoretically improve microcirculation of the intestinal mucosa.[611] Another clinical report used moxa on ST-25 and CV-4 and demonstrated marked improvement.[612]

Additional Treatment for CD

Use the Five-Element four-point protocol for clearing Heat from the Small Intestine: tonify SI-2, BL-66; sedate SI-5, TE-6.

Additional Treatment for UC

- ST-25, BL-25 Large Intestine Mu-Shu points, stimulate Large Intestine Qi, alleviate diarrhea and pain
- ST-37 Lower Sea point for Large Intestine to stop diarrhea
- Also treat Blood stasis and bleeding:
  - SP-1 to stop acute bleeding
  - SP-10, BL-17 to remove Blood stasis
- Use the Five-Element four-point protocol for clearing Heat from the Large Intestine:
  - Tonify LI-2, BL-66; sedate LI-5, SI-5.

Liver Qi Stagnation

A child in the Wood phase of development is especially vulnerable to development of IBD due to Liver Qi stagnation. The Wood child is naturally Liver Yang excessed and constitutionally Liver Yin deficient. Emotional disturbances such as anger and frustration may block the Liver function of directing smooth flow of Qi. Since Liver is in a destructive cycle with the Spleen, Liver Yang excess or Liver Qi stagnation would lead to further deficiency of the constitutionally weak Spleen.

Treatment

- CV-12, PC-6 for feeling of stuffiness in the epigastrium[613]
- Explore issues that caused emotional disturbance; teach the child calming exercises; massage Yintang for calming effect

- Avoid excess sour foods and medications
- Resolve Liver Qi stagnation
  - LR-14 promotes smooth flow of Liver Qi
  - LR-13 harmonizes Liver and Spleen
  - LR-3 to tonify Liver Yin, move Liver Qi
- CV-6, GB-34 together to move Qi in the abdomen, and diminish abdominal pain
- Tonify the Spleen:
  - CV-12, ST-36, BL-20 to tonify the Spleen
- Use the four-point protocol: tonify SP-2, HT- 8; sedate SP-1, LR-1
  - Clear Heat from the Small Intestine or Large Intestine, depending on symptoms.

Kidney Deficiency

This correlates to the strong genetic predisposition in IBD. It is often associated with watery stools or diarrhea in the early morning, and is more serious and therefore more difficult to treat.[613]

Treatment

- GV-4, BL-23 to warm the Fire of Mingmen and invigorate Kidney Yang
- CV-6 to warm Lower Energizer to stop diarrhea
- KI-6, SP-6 to tonify Kidney Yin
- Strong moxibustion at ST-25, CV-4, BL-23
- Auricular points: Shenmen, Point Zero, Large Intestine, Small Intestine, Lower Rectum; add Spleen, Kidney accordingly[613] (see Bibliography).

OBESITY

Obesity in childhood and adolescence is increasing in the US and all over the world[614–616] in epidemic proportions with an upward trend of 0.2 kg increase in body weight/year at any given age.[619] It has become a major pediatric health issue.[620] Statistics of obesity in children range from 10%[621] to 20%[617] to 25%[622], and even at 30% the condition is still considered to be underdiagnosed and undertreated.[623] There is increased prevalence among some minority subgroups, such as African Americans.[617] Obesity is usually evident by age 5–6 years.[255]

Obesity in children is difficult to define, as it is influenced by age, by developmental stage, by physical fitness and individual variations in caloric needs. Skinfold thickness is difficult to apply to children.[624] In general, a body mass index (BMI; in kg/m^2) between the 85th and 95th percentiles indicates a risk of being overweight and a BMI greater than the 95th percentile indicates being overweight,[617] or children whose weight exceeds 120% of that expected for their height are considered overweight. Since obese children are at increased risk of becoming obese adults and of developing obesity-related complications later in life, it becomes of utmost importance for early identification and treatment.[615,617,618,625] The potential for persistence of obesity into adulthood increases with obesity at an early age or in adolescence, severity, and parental obesity.[626] The risk of adult obesity is greater if at least one parent is obese, especially when the child is obese before 10 years of age.[627]

ETIOLOGY

Endogenous obesity such as metabolic or hormonal disorders, or syndromes such as Prader–Willi, are uncommon in children.[255,623] A comprehensive history and examination can usually elicit any medical causes of obesity.[614] The majority of cases of obesity in children are exogenous, due to a disproportionate intake of calories to expenditure. Genetic factors influence the inheritance of obese phenotypes, the major affectors of body fat content, energy intake and expenditure, and responsiveness to dietary intervention.[618,624] Most likely obesity is a complex polygenic trait.[628]

The most important issue in exogenous obesity is the balance of energy intake with energy expenditure. The major determinants of energy expenditure are basal metabolism, metabolic response to food, physical activity and growth; these are age-related in children.[255] The traditional view that obesity occurs when intake exceeds expenditure or in individuals with lower metabolic rate are now controversial, especially with respect to the pediatric population. Studies have demonstrated that obese individuals can have comparable metabolism as nonobese individuals[621] and some obese people in fact can have higher metabolic rates.[628] Obese and nonobese individuals often have similar energy intakes and expenditures.[617,624] This implies that the difference between obesity and nonobesity can result from very small imbalances of energy intake and expenditure,[617,624] possibly due to very small differences in basal metabolic rate or the thermic effects of food[624]. In addition, children go through distinct developmental periods with different energy needs, such as early infancy and adolescence. Since there is inherent individual requirement for energy[255] and susceptibility to the balance in energy[617] and since changes in intake or expenditure in children may occur concomitantly with physiologic changes, such as hormonal levels in adolescence, weight gain especially during critical developmental periods is not always directly related to energy expenditure.[617]

The hypothalamus is the center for regulation of energy balance. It integrates neural, hormonal, and nutrient messages from the gut and circulation and sends signals to higher centers leading to feelings of hunger or satiety. The hypothalamus also controls energy expenditure via the autonomic nervous system and pituitary hormones. The hypothalamus nuclei contain over 40 neurotransmitters that affect food intake and thermogenesis. Those that stimulate appetite, such as opioids, and neuropeptide Y, suppress sympathetic nervous system activity and thus reduce energy expenditure, while the neurotransmitters that inhibit food intake, such as serotonin, dopamine, cholecystokinin, have the reverse effect of decreasing appetite and stimulating energy expenditure. There is evidence that hormones such as insulin and the concentrations of nutrients such as glucose and amino acids all play a role. Leptin is a recently discovered hormone, which is synthesized in fat and acts on the hypothalamus to suppress food intake and increase energy expenditure. Its concentration is high in nearly all obese people, and falls with weight loss, possibly suggesting some resistance to the central effects of leptin in obesity.[617]

Obesity in children is often associated with high intake of sweets and fattening foods, which is often under-reported by children.[621] This, coupled with an increasing sedentary lifestyle in children,[624] an increase in television viewing[629] and a decrease in regular physical activity[621] especially in prepubertal girls[617] result in development of obesity in the pediatric population.

COMPLICATIONS

Obese children are predisposed to developing physical and psychoemotional complications. The physical complications include hypertension,[630,631] and cardiovascular disease[623,632] as autopsy findings reveal progression of atherosclerotic plaques can begin in the very young,[617] and fatty liver, which can occur without correlation to severity of obesity.[255] One of the most dramatic and disturbing findings in the past decade is the tremendous increase in the incidence of type II diabetes in children and adolescents with obesity.[617,633,634] Other physical complications include orthopedic problems due to increased weight on the hips and knees,[623] and obstructive sleep apnea with symptoms of snoring and difficult breathing during sleep.[635]

Psychologically, the obese child carries emotional burdens[622] such as low self-esteem, resulting in less social interaction with peers and less participation in team sports.[255] The negative psychosocial effect can be long-term, as women who were overweight adolescents are less likely to marry, have lower paying jobs, and complete fewer years of school. Overweight men are also less likely to marry.[617]

TREATMENT

Childhood obesity is among the most difficult problems to treat. It is frequently ignored by the pediatrician or viewed as a form of social deviancy, and blame for treatment failure is placed on the patients or their families.[624] Management is often unsuccessful.[614] There is increasing trend to direct treatment at prevention and early identification, with dietary and lifestyle management. At well child examinations, pediatricians need to identify high risk infants and children and discuss preventive measures such as dietary changes, change in lifestyle and behavior modications.[615,623] In the future, new information from molecular biology—such as more research on the role of leptin in obesity—and molecular genetics may provide definitive early identification of individuals who are susceptible to developing obesity.[636]

Diet and exercise remain the cornerstones in the Western management of obesity.[628] A multidisciplinary team consisting of a pediatrician, a nutritionist, a psychotherapist and other ancillary personnel—the number increases with the level of academic involvement of the clinic—devise an appropriate treatment regimen. Weight management usually tries to set reasonable weight-loss goals[623,626] consisting of a combination of healthy diet and physical activities to change the sedentary lifestyle.[614,623] The theory is that a reduction of 500 kcal/day would result in the loss of 1 lb (500 g) of fat per week.[255]

The specialists recognize that family involvement is crucial in management of childhood obesity.[614,620,621,623,626,637] Children's food preferences and physical activity (or inactivity) are often influenced by parents.[621] Family readiness to change would also influence therapy.[626] Long-term success requires parental support to motivate the child in continuing the healthier lifestyle and eating habits.[621] Anorexic medications have significant side-effects such as heart disease, pulmonary hypertension, and are not approved by the US Food and Drug Administration for use in pediatric populations. Gastric bypass surgery for pre-morbid obese adults should at best be considered as experimental in children and adolescents.[626]

CHINESE MEDICINE

Current Acupuncture Data

There are a number of studies, mostly adult clinical trials, which have demonstrated efficacy of acupuncture in the treatment of obesity. Acupuncture offers a safe, simple, economical, and effective treatment that can be used in conjunction with conventional managements. Whereas Western medicine treats all children with obesity as having one pathology, Chinese medicine considers a variety of Qi imbalances as the cause of obesity, each requiring a specific treatment regimen. Through energetic balance of the internal viscera, acupuncture treatment has been successful in reducing weight, often with long-lasting effects.[638,639] In addition, acupuncture treatments have been shown to correlate with normalization of Western bioanatomic and biochemical parameters.

Acupuncture has demonstrated impressive effects on the hypothalamus and autonomic nervous system in weight control. Auriculoacupuncture alone has successfully treated obesity[640,641] and can reduce weight even in nonobese subjects.[642] One theory proposes that stimulating the auricular Stomach point blocks the afferent signal of the hypothalamus, and thereby suppresses hunger, resulting in less food intake.[638,639] A Japanese study indicates that auriculoacupuncture improves the hypofunction of the hypothalamus, inhibits weight increase and the deposition of lipid.[638,639] A clinical study that included 19-year-olds measured fasting blood-glucose, noradrenaline, dopamine, adrenalin and cortisol levels indicates that patients with simple obesity had hypofunctioning of the sympathetic–adrenal system and the hypothalamus–pituitary–adrenal system. Acupuncture treatment enhanced the functions of both the sympathetic–adrenal system and the hypothalamus–pituitary–adrenal systems and brought about weight loss.[643] The same investigator in China also demonstrated improved functions of the hypothalamus–hypophyseal–adrenal axis and the sympathetic–adrenomedullary systems.[638,639] In an animal study, electroacupuncture stimulation at ST-36 and ST-44 resulted in weight loss by stimulating the center of satiation in the hypothalamus.[644]

Western medicine also posits that the hypothalamus controls energy expenditure via the autonomic nervous system. Nogier in France noted that stimulating the Lung point on the ear (which has vagus nerve innervation) resulted in appetite and weight loss.[638,639] A Japanese study revealed simultaneous sympathetic hypofunction and parasympathetic hyperfunction in obese patients, and acupuncture balanced the autonomic nervous system by enhancing the function of the sympathetic nerve and inhibiting the hyperfunction of the parasympathetic nerve.[638,639]

Current data also reveals various effects acupuncture has on lipid and carbohydrate metabolism, on regulation of salt and fluids, and on endocrine functions. Acupuncture has been shown to regulate hyperlipidemia,[645] cholesterol and high density lipoprotein metabolism,[646] and increases cAMP, which can activate lipase and promote decomposition of lipid.[638,639] In a Russian study on 62 children, electroacupuncture decreased fatty tissue content, and normalized serum lipids.[647] Auricular and body points seem to work synergistically to reduce cholesterol and triglycerides with resultant weight loss.[648] Acupuncture treatment can also have a positive effect on carbohydrate metabolism, with a decrease in serum glucose and an increase in lactic dehydrogenase.[649] Acupuncture has been shown to decrease edema in obesity by regulating water and salt metabolism through lowering serum sodium and aldosterone levels.[650] Other studies have demonstrated that acupuncture can regulate endocrine and metabolic functions that are important for control of obesity. A Japanese study showed acupuncture increases basal metabolic rate[638,639] and a European study demonstrated increased levels of pituitary and thyroid hormones with acupuncture.[638,639]

Acupuncture has also been effective in preventing complications of obesity, by reducing the arteriosclerotic index, the indicator for development of cardiovascular disease,[651] and by lowering blood pressure.[652] Even when acupuncture fails to reduce weight, it can improve the psychological outlook of the obese patient.[653] An integrated approach with auricular acupuncture, diet control and aerobic exercise resulted in 86.7% success in weight reduction.[654]

Chinese Medicine Differentiation of Obesity

The majority of the studies use a TCM paradigm for differentiation of various syndromes as the cause of obesity. This is an important adjunct for Western medicine.

Many children with exogenous obesity do not have a wide discrepancy between intake and energy expenditure and do not respond to conventional dietary management. These children have different Qi imbalances in the viscera that are not manifested in conventional examinations or laboratory studies, and would respond well to acupuncture. The key to successful acupuncture treatment is in the correct differentiation of different types of obesity and in selection of specific points to regulate each imbalance. The Five-Element Developmental Theory can augment understanding of the dysfunctions that result in obesity in children.

The primary organs of dysfunction in obesity are Stomach, Spleen, and Liver and Kidney. Current acupuncture thinking posits three major obesity syndromes that are applicable in children:

- Spleen and Stomach Qi deficiency
- Liver Yang excess/Liver Qi stagnation
- Kidney Qi or Yin deficiency.[640,641,643, 648, 649]

Spleen and Stomach Qi Deficiency

This is the most common TCM syndrome for obesity in pediatrics. Children have constitutionally weak Spleen and are prone to developing Spleen and

Stomach deficiency, which can in turn lead to Dampness in the Middle Energizer. Children are also susceptible to Wind invasions and tend to accumulate Heat as each fever with Wind invasion would use up Yin. The end result is inefficient transformation of food into Qi and transportation of Qi throughout the body, and insufficient transformation of fluids would further increase accumulation of Heat. Food and fluid tend to be retained in the Stomach. These children gain weight easily. If there is more predominance of Stomach Heat, the children would have increased appetite. These are the ones who seem to "stuff their faces" when they are stressed. If there is more predominance of Spleen Qi deficiency, the appetite would be poor. In both cases, the children would not respond to a Western dietary regime for two reasons: (1) the foods that cause continuing imbalance are not high caloric foods but Heat foods and spices, such as ginger, or garlic, which do not have calories; (2) even small amounts of food of any type would still accumulate without being transformed or transported, resulting in weight gain. These overweight children tend to be sedentary, partly due to the weight gain, but partly also due to muscle weakness with Spleen deficiency and Dampness that make the legs feel heavy, so that they are easily fatigued with very little activity. The emotional manifestations tend to be excess worry, often about their weight which is made worse when they receive attention from peers, parents, and doctors. In extreme cases, the worry becomes an obsession about weight that can lead to depression and a referral to psychiatry. The complication of snoring and obstructive sleep apnea can be explained by an accumulation of Phlegm due to Spleen Qi deficiency. The treatments that are successful in the various studies have been dispersing Heat, resolving Dampness, and harmonizing the Middle Energizer. Acupuncture treatments of Spleen and Stomach have been shown to decrease weight by having a positive effect on carbohydrate metabolism with a decrease in serum glucose and an increase in lactic dehydrogenase[649] and by reducing cholesterol and triglyceride levels.[648]

Evaluation

History and physical examination would reveal signs of Spleen Qi deficiency in the presence of Heat and Dampness.

Treatment

- Disperse Heat
  - Eliminate Hot spices and foods from the diet, decrease Warm foods, increase Cooling foods
  - Use the Five-Element four-point system to disperse Heat from the Stomach: tonify ST-44, BL-66; sedate ST-41, SI-5
  - LI-11 to disperse Heat overall
- Resolve Dampness
- Eliminate or decrease artificially sweetened foods, specifically candies, cookies, cakes
- ST-40 to resolve Damp
- Tonify Spleen and Stomach, harmonize Middle Energizer
- Tonify Spleen with the four-point protocol: tonify SP-2, HT-8; sedate SP-1, LR-1

- Tonify Middle Energizer: CV-12
- Tonify Stomach: tonify ST-41, SI-5; sedate ST-43, GB-41
- Specific "big points" from the studies: ST-25, ST-36, ST-37, ST-40, ST-44, SP-6, SP-9
- Treat auriculopoints: Shenmen, Point Zero, Hunger, Mouth, Esophagus, Stomach, Spleen, Sanjiao, Endocrine
- Exercise.

There should be no increased physical activities at the beginning of treatment, as the child would become discouraged with an inability to perform. Exercise or increased physical activities can be added to the treatment regime once the child has shown some response to the treatment: such as less Heat and Dampness signs, less Spleen Qi deficiency, some weight loss. The activities need to be increased slowly as tolerated.

Liver Yang Excess/Liver Qi Stagnation

The majority of obese children are in the Wood phase of development when they have Liver vulnerability with a tendency toward Liver Qi stagnation and Liver Yang excess. The basis for this is Liver Yin deficiency. Since Liver has a destructive relationship with Spleen, Liver excess would result in Spleen deficiency and imbalances listed above. These children may respond to lower caloric diets, since greasy and fattening foods are injurious to Liver. Excess medications may also cause Liver imbalance. These children are sedentary because Liver Qi stagnation impairs the overall movement of Qi throughout the body, resulting in easy fatigability. The emotional manifestations from Liver Yang excess tend to be frustration, irritability, smoldering anger, and sometimes withdrawal and depression. These children are resistant to psychiatric intervention as it is very difficult for them to make any affective changes. The emotional manifestations of Liver Yin deficiency reveal a disturbance of the Ethereal Soul and therefore Shen: mental restlessness such as anxiety, fidgetiness that worsens later in the day, and insomnia. Successful managements in the studies have been to move Qi, subdue Liver Yang, tonify Liver Yin. Lipid metabolism was found to be abnormal in obese patients with Liver Yang excess syndrome, which can explain the Western complication of finding fatty livers that do not correlate with severity of obesity. Acupuncture brought about better lipid metabolism and also decreased blood pressure.[651]

Use the Five-Element Developmental Theory to assess the root of the child's obesity. If obesity began in infancy or early childhood, or if there is a strong family history of obesity, then the root of the Wood child's obesity is in the Water phase of development. There is Kidney Yin and Kidney Essence deficiency, to cause Liver Yin/Ethereal Soul deficiency. Kidney Yang is not deficient as there is Liver Yang excess.

Treatment

- Dietary management
  - Eliminate greasy and fattening foods, diminish sour foods
  - Decrease intake of medications, especially over-the-counter drugs which tend to be taken indiscriminately

- Treat Liver Yang excess
- LR-3, LR-13 to move Liver Qi
- Yintang for overall calming effect
- Diminish stress that precipitates frustration and anger
- Tonify Liver Yin
  - LR-3, LR-8 to tonify Liver Yin
- BL-47 Hunmen, Gate of Ethereal Soul, to settle the Ethereal Soul
- HT-7 to tonify Heart Yin, calm the Mind
- BL-44 Shentang, Hall of the Shen, to settle the Shen
- KI-6 nourishes Kidney Yin
- Auriculopoints: Shenmen, Point Zero, Liver, Heart, Spleen, Kidney
- Exercise.

The same principles on excercise should be followed with no increased physical activities at the beginning of treatment. Exercise or increased physical activities can be added to the treatment regime once the child has shown some response to the treatment, and activities increased slowly as tolerated.

Kidney Qi or Yin Deficiency

The Kidney deficiency type of obesity usually has early onset in infancy or early childhood before 6 years of age, and usually has a strong family history of obesity with one or both parents being overweight. It is normal for babies to be chubby with puffy face, hands and feet—the Water phenotype as they are in the Water phase of development. Older children may have a tendency to continue with the Water physique in being shorter, having a puffy appearance and edematous extremities. The Kidney in Chinese medicine is the basis for marrow, the brain. This correlates to the involvement of the hypothalamus and the autonomic nervous system in Western medicine. The Chinese Kidney corresponds to both the kidney and adrenals in Western medicine. Water imbalance is due to both kidney and adrenal dysfunction, which in turn affect the sympathetic system and the adrenal–pituitary–hypothalamic axis. Numerous acupuncture studies quoted in the last section demonstrate the effect on the hypothalamus, the autonomic nervous system, and the sympathetic–adrenal and hypothalamus–pituitary–adrenal systems.

Since Kidney Qi and Yin are the basis of the Qi and Yin of all the organs, there are usually other imbalances concomitantly. Kidney Yin has a more specific and direct effect on Heart and Liver because of the mother–child nurturing relationship with Liver and the Fire–Water destructive relationship with the Heart. The child in the Wood phase of development would be more likely to develop both Kidney and Liver Yin deficiencies, manifesting both physical signs of Kidney Yin and Liver Yin deficiency, as well as emotional signs of fear and frustration or anger, and Ethereal Soul and Mind disturbances listed above. When Kidney and Heart are not harmonized, there is usually Heart Fire flaring due to inability of Water to control Fire. The child would manifest more disturbances of Shen: an inability to concentrate or think clearly, restlessness, and agitation. This would be more likely in a child in the Fire phase of development, i.e. the teenager. These children are usually frustrating for a psychotherapist, since they may become passive and deliberately say nothing or look bored during therapy, manifesting more Water characteristics; or they may become "fiery" during the sessions and become verbally aggressive toward the therapist or toward family members for sending them there.

Kidney Yang deficiency has more specific effects on the Lung and Spleen because of the Lung–Kidney mother–child nurturing relationship and the Spleen–Kidney destructive relationship. An obese child with both Kidney and Spleen Yang deficiency would manifest physical signs and symptoms of both deficiencies—with more exaggerated Spleen Qi deficiency signs because of concomitant Kidney Yang deficiency. Puffy weight gain would continue in spite of very poor appetite. These children tend to dislike exercise as both Yang deficiencies make them become tired very easily, feel very heavy in the lower limbs that tend to be edematous, and to develop soreness in the knees and muscles with little movement. They may respond slightly to a diet eliminating candy. However, as a rule, these children are refractory to conventional treatments. Emotionally, these children may appear dull and lack willpower or motivation to "stick to a diet," or tend to give up easily with any project or school work. They are fearful and worried on the inside, but outwardly may appear apathetic: "I don't care if people call me fat." Their "I don't care" attitude presents a challenge to the psychotherapist. The Kidney and Lung deficiency combination would have manifestations of both Kidney Yang and Lung Qi deficiency. These children have a difficult time with exercise because they easily become short of breath and start coughing when they do anything physically strenuous. Hypertension and cardiovascular complications would be the most common in this group. Emotionally, these children are sad and fearful, a combination that makes them withdrawn and depressed. It usually takes many sessions before these children would look at the therapist in the eye and open up to talk about themselves. This group of children would include "normally obese" children who developed obesity at an early age, and "abnormally obese" children with congenital syndromes, such as Prader–Willi or Beckwith syndromes that have other anomalies, including renal and CNS (Kidney–marrow) abnormalities.

In view of the complex factors of weight gain due to Kidney deficiency—an early onset with positive family history, secondary involvement of other Yin organs—this type of obesity in children is the most difficult to manage. Treatment entails strengthening a genetic or constitutional predisposition (Kidney Essence deficiency) that may have been in the family for many generations, bringing about overall Yin and Yang balance, and correcting individual organ dysfunctions. Treatment of these children would definitely need involvement of the family, and it would in fact be wise to treat the parents and siblings, who most likely would share similar characteristics. The dietary management should be applicable for the whole family.

Evaluation

The early onset of obesity and positive family history would point toward Kidney deficiency diagnosis. Look for signs and symptoms of other organ involvement.

Treatment

Keep in mind that the Kidney deficiency is the root of the problem, and manifestations of other organs are the branches. The treatments would need to alternate between tonification of the Kidney Yin and Yang and treatment of the dysfunction of the secondary organ of involvement. However, since Kidney is the root of the imbalance, some Kidney points should always be incorporated into the treatment of the secondary organs.

- If possible, evaluate the family members to gain a better understanding of the child, or even incorporate the family members for treatment
- Diet—may be appropriate for the whole family
  - Eliminate any excess salt in foods: no extra added salt, no salty foods such as pretzels or chips
  - Presence of Liver Yin symptoms: eliminate or decrease sour foods; decrease medications
  - For Heart Fire symptoms: eliminate bitter foods in the diet; also be careful in taking medications which are usually bitter
  - For Spleen deficiency: eliminate artificially sweetened foods; some medications for children also contain artificial sweeteners
  - For Lung deficiency: eliminate spicy foods
- Tonify Kidney Yin and Kidney Qi
- If there is no Liver Yang excess, can overall tonify Kidney with the four-point protocol: tonify KI-7, LU-8; sedate KI-3, SP-3
- BL-52 to increase willpower; diminish fear
- In treating any secondary organ dysfunction, always include some Kidney points: KI-3, to tonify both Kidney Yin and Yang or KI-6 to tonify Kidney Yin, KI-7 to tonify Kidney Yang
- Treat the specific secondary organs:
  - Tonify Spleen with four-point protocol
  - Add ST-40 to disperse Damp
  - Tonify Lung with four-point protocol: tonify LU-9, SP-3; sedate LU-10, HT-8
  - Tonify Heart with four-point protocol: tonify HT-9, LR-1; sedate HT-3, KI-10
- BL-44 to settle Shen
- Balance Liver
- Treat emotional problems with the respective "Soul" points; modify lifestyle to minimize situations that precipitate frustration and anger, or fear, or sadness
- Acupuncture treatment can be provided concomitantly with individual or family therapy
- Auricular points: Shenmen, Point Zero, Kidney, Adrenals, Sanjiao, Hypothalamus, Pituitary
- Add specific organ points in the ear accordingly: Spleen, Liver, Lung, Heart.[655–658]

OTITIS MEDIA

Otitis media, infection of the middle ear, can occur in children as acute otitis media (AOM), and as two types of chronic otitis: chronic suppurative otitis media and chronic serous otitis media (CSOM).

ACUTE OTITIS MEDIA

AOM is one of the most common pediatric infectious conditions. It is most prevalent in young children of 8–24 months of age. Approximately two-thirds of all children will have had at least one episode of AOM before age 3 years, and half of them will have recurrences of chronic otitis media with effusion (OME) into early elementary school years.[659] By the time the child reaches adolescence, AOM occurs infrequently.[660] Nearly one-third of pediatric office visits are for treatment of AOM.[394] The majority of ear infections are caused by upper respiratory tract viruses and bacteria. The most common viral culprits are respiratory syncytial virus (RSV),[661] influenza virus,[662] and adenoviruses.[394] Viruses cause ear infection by direct invasion of the middle ear and disrupt eustachian tube function,[663] or by inducing inflammatory injury that facilitates attachment of bacteria to respiratory epithelial cells.[664,665]

Two-thirds of middle ear infections are due to bacteria.[394] The predominant organisms are pneumococci, *Haemophilus influenzae*, *Moraxella catarrhalis*,[666–669] and group B streptococci.[670] Bacterial pathogens adhere to mucous membranes and colonization ensues. The severity of infection or response to the invading bacteria depend on the health of the child's immune system.[668] The humoral system is especially significant in protecting the middle ear cavity from disease, and the nasopharyngeal lymphoid tissues are the first line of defense against bacterial colonization.[671] The sterility of the eustachian tube and tympanic cavity depends on mucociliary system and secretion of antimicrobial molecules, such as lysozyme, lactoferrin, and beta-defensins.[672] There is evidence that a number of children with recurrent episodes of AOM have minor immunologic defects.[671] Pneumococcus is by far the most virulent of AOM bacteria. It causes approximately 6 million cases of otitis media annually in the US.[673] Uncontrolled pneumococcal otitis can lead to meningitis.[674] Pneumolysin, the pneumococcal toxin, is especially injurious to cell walls and can induce severe tissue injury.[674] Other etiologic agents include *Mycoplasma* and *Chlamydia*.[394] Incidence of AOM is higher in winter and early spring.

The pathogenesis of otitis media is primarily mediated through eustachian tube dysfunction. The eustachian tube protects the middle ear from nasopharyngeal secretions, provides drainage into the nasopharynx of secretions produced within the middle ear, and permits equilibration of air pressure with atmospheric pressure in the middle ear. Infants and children are vulnerable to developing middle ear infection because: (1) their eustachian tubes are shorter and more horizontal so that drainage of middle ear is impaired; (2) they are prone to develop congestion from acute upper respiratory tract infection, from smoke or environmental allergens and pollutants.[668,675,676] The congestion generates a negative middle ear pressure, resulting in intermittent obstruction of the eustachian tube[676] that can lead to bacterial colonization.[394] Children have inadequate mucociliary function that is necessary for maintaining eustachian tube sterility.[677]

Clinically, the child with AOM presents with earache, and fever, usually accompanied by upper respiratory tract symptoms such as rhinorrhea. The tympanic membrane on otoscopic examination varies from hyperemic with preservation of landmarks, to a bright red, tense, bulging, distorted appearance. In the advanced stage of suppuration, the tympanic membrane ruptures with a gush of purulent, or bloody tinged fluid from the ear.[394] Since viral or bacterial otitis usually cannot be distinguished by otoscopic examination, AOM is usually treated empirically, using antibiotics such as amoxicillin that have a high concentration in the middle ear fluid.[678,679]

However, the widespread use of antibiotics has resulted in increasing resistance to the more common medications.[666,668] Currently, 10% of children with acute otitis media are recalcitrant to antibiotic therapy.[680] The prevalence of resistant organisms tends to increase in the winter months.[681] Economically, treatment failure due to drug resistance has been responsible for further escalating the billions of dollars spent treating acute otitis media.[682] In addition, antimicrobials suppress the normal flora, which is beneficial to the host because it has the capabilities to interfere with and therefore prevent pathogenic infections, and may enhance recovery from upper respiratory tract infections.[681] On the other hand, since the advent of antibiotics, complications such as mastoiditis and intracranial infections have significantly decreased.[77,394]

The current focus is on prevention. Breast feeding confers lifesaving protection against infectious illness, including otitis.[683,684] Pneumococcal conjugate vaccine (PCV), approved in 2000 for use in the US, covers the seven serotypes that account for about 80% of invasive infections in children younger than 6 years of age. This vaccine was demonstrated to have more than 90% efficacy,[673] and has resulted in a modest reduction of total episodes of AOM.[685] The goal of pneumococcal vaccine is to prevent symptomatic infections in the middle ear and to prevent colonization of pneumococci that can cause subsequent middle ear infections.[686] It may eliminate nasopharyngeal carriage of pneumococci.[687] However, since PCV only prevents disease due to the most common serotypes, there is concern that the nonvaccine serotypes will become more common, especially in children less than 2 years of age.[685] An effective RSV vaccine for the infant and young child could markedly decrease otitis media disease.[661] Intranasal spray of attenuated viruses is currently under investigation, in the hope that early antiviral therapy would reduce the risk of otitis media following respiratory tract infections.[662,665]

CHRONIC OTITIS MEDIA

Chronic otitis media is divided into two categories: chronic suppurative otitis media and chronic OME. Chronic suppurative otitis media is not temporally related to acute otitis, since the pathologic changes in the middle ear are different. The classic symptoms of established chronic suppurative otitis are otorrhea and deafness (some form of hearing loss).[394] Chronic suppurative otitis media can lead to the formation of cholesteatoma, a cyst that contains desquamated epithelial cells, that can cause local bone erosion and lead to retention of infected material.[394] Chronic OME is one of the most common diseases in childhood.[675] It is related to infection, eustachian tube obstruction, allergic or immunologic disorders, and enlarged adenoids.[394] The serous fluid in CSOM still contains bacteria, such as *H. influenzae* and pneumococci.[688] OME has been implicated to be an immune-mediated disease,[675] since immune complexes have been demonstrated in the middle ear effusion[689,690] and highly organized lymphatic tissue has been found in the middle ear mucosa.[691]

The rationale for treating OME is prevention of recurrence of AOM. Currently, a once daily antibiotic regimen is the recommended prophylaxis. The benefit is also weighed against the increasing risk of emergence of resistant bacteria.[684] When antibiotics fail to control recurrent otitis, a short trial of prednisone is sometimes prescribed.[680] Surgery is recommended when medical treatment fails,[680] especially when the child has hearing loss.[667] Tympanostomy tubes appear to be beneficial in OME, but is of less value in chronic suppurative otitis.[684] An increase in hearing loss has been reported with insertion of ventilation tubes.[692] Adenoidectomy is sometimes recommended,[664] especially after tympanostomy tube failure.[684]

CHINESE MEDICINE

There is a total lack of recent acupuncture data on treatment of otitis media in children. Only one clinical trial was reported, in 1985.[693] Traditional Chinese medicine diagnoses correlate well with Western categorizations of acute and chronic otitis media.

AOM—Wind-Cold and Wind-Heat Invasion, Dampness

AOM correlates to the Shao Yang stage of Wind-Cold invasion and to the Wei Qi level of Wind-Heat invasion. Dampness—the Western medicine congestion and fluid accumulation in the eustachian tube—predisposes the child to external invasions, and suppuration correlates to Chinese diagnosis of Damp Heat. An integrative approach would be beneficial, both with diagnosis using otoscopic examination, and with follow-up audiologic evaluations, such as tympanograms and other hearing tests. Acupuncture treatment can be given concomitantly with antibiotics, as Chinese medicine's goal in expelling the pathogens and tonifying the immune system complements the Western regimen.

Treatment

- Treat the local ear points: GB-2, SI-19, TE-21; parents can be taught to massage these points
- Can "pull down" the inflammation by using ion pumping cord connecting local and distal points: connect the black clamp to GB-2 local point and red clamp to BL-60; if using magnets, place the bionorth (–) downward on GB-2 and biosouth (+) downward on BL-60, connect with black clamp on GB-2 magnet and red clamp on BL-60
- Use the Shao Yang protocol (Chapter 7):
  - GB-16, GB-20 to dispel Wind
  - LI-4 + KI-7 to cause sweating
  - GV-14 if there is fever
- Prophylactically tonify the Stomach and Large Intestine to prevent further progression into the Yang Ming stage of mastoiditis
- If there is Cold, use the four-point protocol to dispel Cold from the Gallbladder channel: tonify GB-38, SI-5; sedate GB-43, BL-66
- In infants and young children, use two points: tonify GB-38; sedate GB-43

- If there is Heat, use the four-point protocol to disperse Heat from the Gallbladder channel: tonify GB-43, BL-66; sedate GB-38, SI-5
- In infants and young children, use two points: tonify GB-43; sedate GB-38
- If there is Damp, resolve Damp:
    - GB-34 transforms Shao Yang Damp
    - SP-9 clears Damp Heat
    - ST-40 to resolve Damp
- Tonify Spleen: SP-3, SP-6 or use four-point protocol
- After the ear infection has resolved, tonify the immune system.

Prophylactic Treatment

Since AOM is prevalent during winter and early spring, the TCM principle of "winter disease summer cure" would be prophylactically tonifying Wei Qi or the immune system, treating the local ear points, or tonifying the Shao Yang Gallbladder channel during the summer months.

- Tonify Gallbladder: tonify GB-43, BL-66; sedate GB-44, LI-1
- Tonify Kidney Yin
- Since the ears are the external orifice for Kidney, tonification of Kidney Yin during an acute invasion is comparable to prevention of suppurative complications
- KI-6 tonifies Kidney Yin.

Chronic OME

Spleen Qi Deficiency

The lingering effusion is indicative of Dampness due to Spleen deficiency. Children are constitutionally Spleen Qi deficient. They may become more Spleen deficient due to inheritance of weak pre-Heaven Spleen Qi, such as a strong family history of Spleen Qi deficiency, Spleen deficiency in both parents during conception, in mother during pregnancy; due to a diet with excessive sweets, dairy and greasy foods; due to chronic illnesses; or from living in a Damp environment. Spleen Qi deficiency results in Dampness accumulation. Chronic Dampness would in turn further injure the Spleen. Spleen corresponds with the emotions worry and obsession, and with excess mental activities. A careful history would uncover any situations that would predispose to worry, and academic overload or lack of rest due to school or extracurricular activities.

Treatment

- Treat the local ear points: GB-2, SI-19, TE-21 (Figure 10.1)
- Treat local–distal points as indicated for acute treatment
- Avoid artificially sweetened foods.
- Vigorously tonify Spleen with the four-point protocol
- Modify lifestyle to allow the child to feel less pressure from school work and other activities, to minimize worry.

FIGURE 10.1　*Points on the ear for the treatment of otitis media.*

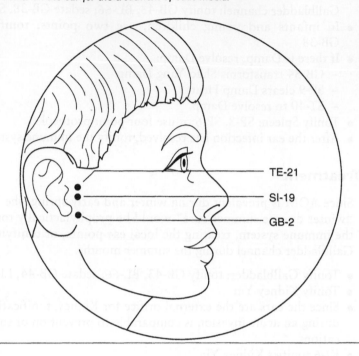

TE-21

SI-19

GB-2

Shao Yang Heat

This condition tends to affect children in the Wood phase of development when Gallbladder is vulnerable. Heat in the Gallbladder channel may be due to lingering pathogenic Heat from previous illnesses that was not completely expelled, or to consuming excess greasy food or medications that injure the Wood Element. While Liver is the "General" that directs Qi, Gallbladder has the important function of carrying out the decisions. This child, then, would have chronic otitis with other Heat symptoms and indecisiveness.

Treatment

- Treat local and distal points
- Avoid greasy or sour foods; minimize medications
- Clear Gallbladder Heat: four-point protocol: tonify GB-43, BL-66; sedate GB-38, SI-5
  - Two points: tonify GB-43; sedate GB-38.

Chronic Suppurative Otitis Media—Kidney Yin Deficiency/Spleen Damp

The hearing loss associated with chronic suppurative otitis media is indicative of injury to the Kidney Yin, and Kidney Essence, with persistence of Spleen Damp.

Treatment

- Treat local and distal points
- Avoid excess salty foods

- KI-6 tonifies Kidney Yin
- Tonify Spleen with the four-point protocol
- Transform Damp.

Prophylactic Treatment

During periods of remission, tonify the immune system.

PHARYNGITIS

Acute pharyngitis and tonsillitis are common in healthy children and adolescents. The tonsils and adenoids, located at the portal of entry of many airborne and alimentary antigens, prevent bacterial colonization and form antibodies. They influence both local and systemic immunity, and are often considered the first line of defense against respiratory infections.[694,695]

The majority of pharyngitis cases have a viral etiology—such as rhinovirus, adenovirus, Epstein–Barr virus (mononucleosis), influenza A and B.[696,697] Younger children have frequent episodes, while adolescents experience two to four nasopharyngeal infections annually.[698] Bacterial pharyngitis occurs when the pathogens adhere to and colonize in the mucous membranes. The extent of pathogenic injury varies according to the host immune system. In a healthy individual, there may only be mild edema and swelling.[699] The most important bacterial agent is group A beta-hemolytic streptococcus (GABHS). The incidence of GABHS in children ranges from as low as 5%[700] to 20%[701,702] to 35%.[703–706] Even during the peak streptococcal infection seasons, winter and early spring,[696] it occurs in less than 40% of pharyngitis cases.[707] GABHS is primarily a disorder of children between 5 years and 15 years of age.[696] The clinical presentation of GABHS consists of sudden onset of sore throat, fever, and pain on swallowing.[696,708] Headache, nausea, vomiting, and abdominal pain may also be present in children.[696,708] Physical examination reveals tonsillopharyngeal erythema with or without exudates, and tender anterior cervical adenopathy.[696,708] However, only about 15–30% of children present with classic clinical signs,[708,670] so that clinically viral pharyngitis and GABHS are often indistinguishable.[696] Infrequently, other infectious agents that produce sore throat include non-group A streptococci, *Haemophilus influenzae*, *Mycoplasma*, *Chlamydia*, *Neisseria*, and *Moraxella catarrhalis*. They can be distinguished from GABHS because they are usually accompanied by other concomitant clinical illness.[705,706, 709]

Because of the prevalence of viral pharyngitis and unreliable clinical findings, the Infectious Diseases Society of America[696] and the American Academy of Pediatrics Principles on Management of Common Office Infections[710] recommend throat culture and/or rapid group A streptococci antigen detection test (RADT) to precisely diagnose GABHS.[700,703–705,708] Their use has been shown to be cost-effective and to reduce antibiotic overprescribing substantially.[670] Newer immunoassays and nucleic acid techniques being developed will be more sensitive and specific.[711]

Viral pharyngitis is benign and self-limiting, needing only symptomatic care without antibiotics.[680,696,712] Penicillin has been the treatment of choice for group A streptococcal tonsillopharyngitis since the 1950s,[700,708] and is currently recommended as first-line therapy by the American Academy of Pediatrics and American Heart Association.[670]

A 10-day course of oral penicillin or an intramuscular injection of penicillin G benzathine are considered equivalent treatment. Erythromycin is used for patients who are allergic to penicillin.[696,705,708,712] Early antibiotic therapy reduces the duration of pharyngitis, and minimizes formation of peritonsillar retropharyngeal and parapharyngeal abscesses.[664,676,698,708] The primary objective for antibiotic therapy of GABHS infection, however, is the prevention of rheumatic fever.[670] The incidence of rheumatic fever has declined in industrialized countries since the 1950s and now has an annual incidence of around 0.5 cases per 100 000 children of school age. In developing countries it remains an endemic disease with annual incidences ranging from 100 to 200 per 100 000 school-aged children and is a major cause of cardiovascular mortality. The risk of developing rheumatic fever following untreated tonsillopharyngitis is 1%.[701,702] The current understanding is that there is a genetically determined predisposition[713] that results in the host's autoimmune response to GABHS.[701,702] In France and most of Europe there is tacit agreement that all cases of pharyngitis and tonsillitis should be treated with antibiotics without identification of the causal agent.[701,702]

Empiric and widespread over-treatment of pharyngitis with antibiotics has resulted in emergence of bacterial resistance.[699,705,670,709] Up to 35% of children may experience recurrence,[676,699,704,670] which is more prevalent in children younger than 8 years of age.[706] The high failure rate after penicillin treatment[706] prompts some to recommend against using penicillin as the solo drug of choice.[714]

Explanations for recurrence include poor compliance with taking medication,[715] co-colonization by other organisms, and reacquisition from a family member or peer.[705,690] Currently, routine laboratory evaluation or treatment of close household contacts are not recommended.[696] Compliance can be improved with shorter-course nonpenicillin antibiotics, which tend to be broader spectrum and are often more expensive,[716] although they may have less gastrointestinal side-effects.[717] There is also concern that antibiotics can also suppress natural immune responses by eradication of normal pharyngeal flora that act as natural host defenses[705] in interfering with pathogenic activities and prevent infection.[676] Evidence is mounting that antibiotics may have little impact on the duration of sore throat symptoms, regardless of etiology. Complications of sore throat are now so rare that an adverse drug reaction from antibiotic therapy is more likely.[718] Tonsillectomy and adenoidectomy for recurrent pharyngitis remains controversial.[694,719]

CHINESE MEDICINE

At this time, there is very little data on acupuncture treatment of pharyngitis. Chinese medicine diagnoses can correlate to both Western categories of acute and recurrent pharyngitis. The best approach would be to integrate the Western diagnosis and treatment with Chinese medicine: examination of the throat and palpating for cervical adenopathy is much easier than Chinese pulse taking and tongue diagnosis in children. Laboratory confirmation for GABHS is important.

Acute Pharyngitis

Wind-Cold Invasion

This correlates to viral pharyngitis with negative laboratory findings for GABHS. The "mild sore throat" throat indicates that the invasion is beginning to enter the Yang Ming stage involving the Stomach organ and meridian.

- Extra fluids to prevent dehydration
- GV-16, GB-20 to expel Wind
- LU-7, LI-4, BL-12 to expel Cold
- Add CV-22, KI-27 as specific points for throat treatment
- Dazhui point, GV-14, can be used to treat pain[720] or for any fever
- Tonify the immune system after infection has resolved.

Wind-Heat Invasion

This correlates to bacterial pharyngitis, including GABHS. The Wind-Heat invasion or bacterial infection is much more virulent than the Wind-Cold invasion, and enters quickly into the Qi level that correlates in this case to deep penetrating of the Yang Ming organs and meridians. Acupuncture treatment can be given concomitantly with antibiotics.

- Extra fluids to prevent dehydration
- GV-16, GB-20 to expel Wind
- Add CV-22, KI-27 as specific points for throat treatment
- Dazhui point, GV-14, can be used to treat pain[720] and for fever
- Use either two points or the four-point protocol to disperse Yang Ming Stomach Heat:
  - Tonify ST-44; sedate ST-41
  - Tonify ST-44, BL-66; sedate ST-41, SI-5
- Gastrointestinal side-effects of antibiotics can be minimized with tonification of Spleen.

Stomach Heat

In addition to Wind invasions that cause Yang Ming Heat, Chinese medicine also posits that the sensation of soreness in the throat can be due to Stomach Heat derived from excess consumption of energetically Hot foods, sweet foods, or greasy and fried foods. Since Western medicine does not recognize the relationship between sore throat and foods, the negative culture in this case would be diagnosed as viral pharyngitis. One distinguishing feature is that these children often complain of abdominal pain that may be temporally related to eating.

- Eliminate excess Heat foods, sweets, greasy and fried foods
- Clear Stomach Heat with the Five-Element four-point protocol: tonify ST-44, BL-66; sedate ST-41, SI-5
- SP-6, CV-12 to tonify Stomach Yin.

Chronic, Recurrent Pharyngitis

Yin Deficiency

Two conditions can predispose to chronic pharyngitis with Yin deficiency: pathogenic Heat lingers and accumulates when Heat is not adequately expelled in acute invasions, and continual consumption of excess Heat foods. Both of these can cause chronic state of Heat that exhausts Yin. Since Kidney Yin is the foundation of all the Yin, tonification of KI-6 has been found to be important for treating recurrent sore throat.[721]

Treatment

- Eliminate excess Heat foods, sweets, greasy and fried foods
- Use the four-point protocol to clear Stomach Heat
- KI-6 to tonify Kidney Yin
- SP-6, CV-12 to tonify Stomach Yin
- Immune protocol to increase immunity.

Home Treatment

Parents can be taught to do acupressure on CV-22, KI-27 for acute symptoms and SP-6, KI-6 for tonification of Spleen and Kidney Yin in chronic, recurrent pharyngitis. Although the current Western approach is to not treat close family contacts with medication, acupressure can be used as a preventive measure since it does not encompass antibiotic concerns of potential side-effects and overuse (see Bibliography for further reading on this topic).

SEIZURE (EPILEPSY)

Epilepsy, or seizure disorder, is considered primarily a pediatric disease as over two-thirds of all seizures begin in childhood. It is an important disorder since it can significantly affect not only the health but also the quality of life of the child and the family.[722] A study from the UK estimates that approximately 0.7–0.8% of school-aged children have active epilepsy.[723] Childhood seizure represents a broad and complex range of disorders which vary from benign to severely disabling diseases.[724] The spectrum of causes encompasses genetic predisposition, birth and perinatal complications, congenital anomalies, metabolic disorders, infections, head trauma, and brain tumor. A significant number of seizures are considered idiopathic—without known cause.[415] Various non-neurologic disorders, such as breath-holding spells, can mimic seizures.[725] Seizures in children are frequently misdiagnosed and inappropriately managed.[726] Epileptic children have a higher incidence of psychiatric disorders.[722]

By definition, an epileptic seizure is a paroxysmal disturbance of consciousness, motor function, sensation, perception, behavior or emotion resulting from a cortical neuronal discharge. The symptoms can occur singly or in any combination.[723] The immature and developing brain of children, especially infants, has a lower seizure threshold and therefore is vulnerable toward developing epilepsy.[727]

Neuronal hyperexcitability is the common pathophysiology in the various epileptic syndromes.[728] Neurochemical mechanisms include neurotransmitters gamma-aminobutyric acid (GABA) and catecholamines and opioid peptides.[728]

The International Classification of Seizure Disorders broadly categorizes seizures into generalized, partial (focal, local), and unclassified seizures. Each class has a long list of differentials that have complex dimensions.[415] This section focuses on the major seizures of childhood and correlates them with TCM diagnoses: generalized seizures: grand mal, febrile, and absence seizures; and partial, focal seizures.

GENERALIZED SEIZURES

The generalized seizures have clinical presentations that indicate involvement of both cerebral hemispheres. Consciousness may be impaired, and may in fact be the initial manifestation and motor manifestations are bilateral. The electroencephalogram (EEG) reflects widespread neuronal discharges in both hemispheres.[415]

Grand Mal Seizures

Grand mal seizures are the most common type of convulsive disorders in children.[729] The seizures are characterized by generalized tonic–clonic movements that reflect involvement of both hemispheres. There is usually impairment of consciousness, as well as a postictal period of drowsiness or confusion. The EEG reveals higher amplitude of waves during the tonic phase, and slower waves during the clonic phase.[415]

There are numerous causes for grand mal seizures. Convulsions are often associated with CNS infections, such as viral encephalitis or bacterial meningitis. Generalized seizure may be the first presentation of bacterial sepsis and meningitis in infants and young children. Mechanisms of seizure production in infection include venous thrombosis, cerebritis, abscess formation, and subdural effusions. In neonates and infants, grand mal seizures may be due to congenital anomalies, prenatal and perinatal complications, or metabolic dysfunctions. The majority of primary grand mal seizures in older children are idiopathic, often with a strong genetic predisposition.[729] Vascular lesions, and even brain tumors, usually present with focal seizures. Head trauma seizures tend to be focal when the onset is within 24 hours, and generalized when the onset is delayed, usually within 3 years after the injury.[415]

Diagnosis is made by neurological evaluation, examination of cerebral spinal fluid, and brain imaging studies. Treatment with long-term anticonvulsants is important, because hypoxemia during an acute episode of seizures can have serious central nervous system sequelae. Overall, epileptic children have diminished mental processing abilities, poorer concentration, and are less alert than age-matched controls.[730] Because seizure medications have significant side-effects, physicians are often confronted with the difficult decision of maintaining a child on long-term treatment versus discontinuation of drugs and risk the relapse of seizures.[731] Medically intractable, disabling seizures may be treated with surgery.[724,732,733]

Infantile Spasm

Infantile spasm is one of the most severe forms of epilepsy of the infant. It has distinct recognizable seizure types—spasms or epileptic spasms—associated with definitive electrographic features and hypsarrhythmia. The seizure is generally resistant to treatment, with adrenocorticotrophic hormone still being the drug of choice.[734] More effective newer drugs are associated with more adverse side-effects[735] and have contributed to therapeutic confusion.[726] The neurologic and cognitive prognosis is poor.

Benign Epilepsy of Childhood

This form of partial or generalized seizure is associated with a genetic predisposition and maturational process. Some cases have transient worsening, including cognitive troubles.[736]

Febrile Convulsions

Febrile seizures are the most common seizure disorder in childhood, occurring in 2–5% of children.[737] Most often febrile seizures are generalized tonic–clonic convulsions. They usually occur hours after onset of a febrile illness, are usually self-limiting and brief, lasting only a few seconds to a few minutes. They occur in children between 3 months and 5 years of age, with predominant presentation between 18 and 22 months.[738] There is no precise temperature elevation for seizure to occur, since the temperature threshold varies from one child to another, and varies even within the same child during different illnesses.[738]

Although children with pre-existing neurologic or developmental abnormalities may be more vulnerable to febrile seizures, they usually occur in normal children and are considered benign.[724] The recurrence rate is 30–40%.[739] There is specific genetic defect associated with a child's vulnerability to febrile seizures.[728] About 10% of parents of children with febrile seizures have had seizures themselves, chiefly the febrile type. Maternal illness and smoking during pregnancy also contribute to increased risk.[415] Treatment of most simple febrile seizures consists of fever control and counseling parents,[740] who understandably become very upset on seeing their young child convulse. The American Academy of Pediatrics determined that simple febrile convulsions are not associated with long-term adverse effects, and the risk of developing epilepsy is extremely low. Furthermore, even in those children who do become epileptic, there is no evidence that recurrent simple febrile seizures produce structural CNS damage. Therefore, long-term treatment of simple febrile convulsions is not recommended, since the potential toxicities associated with antiepileptic therapy outweigh the relatively minor risks associated with simple febrile seizures.[737] In these cases, EEG changes tend to resolve even within hours or days after the acute episode, and is of limited diagnostic and prognostic value.[415] Neuroimaging is not recommended.[738] Antipyretic treatment does not reduce the recurrence rate.[739] Intermittent diazepam prophylaxis at times of fever may or may not reduce the recurrence rate significantly. There is no data to suggest that it improves the long-term outcome, as compared with short-term seizure control, in terms of IQ, cognition, academic progress, motor control, and subsequent epilepsy.[739]

Absence Seizures

Absence, or petit mal epilepsy, remains one of the most enigmatic of neurological disorders. There is no widely accepted theory of its etiology.[741] In a typical simple absence attack, the child abruptly loses consciousness and ceases ongoing activity without even change in posture. The child's eyes stare vacantly straight ahead or may roll upward. There is no movement except possibly some subtle fluttering of the eyelids and twitching of the perioral muscles. The episode lasts for a brief moment, usually a few seconds, and the child suddenly resumes previous activity as if nothing had happened. There is no postictal confusion or drowsiness. Dozens to hundreds of seizures may occur in a single day. Intellectual and school performance may deteriorate because of the frequent interruptions of concentration. The child may be labeled as a daydreamer, lazy or dull. These attacks tend to abate by adolescence[724] although many children continue to suffer absence seizures well into adulthood.[741] EEG exhibits a typical pattern of bilaterally synchronous, frontally predominant 3-Hz spike-and-slow-wave activity. These are thought to be abnormal oscillations between the thalamus and cerebral cortex.[742] There is overwhelming evidence of genetic predisposition in absence seizures.[741] Research has demonstrated neurochemical basis involving GABA, catecholamines, and "endogenous" epileptogens[741] that activate burst firing of thalamic neurons, initiating an absence seizure.[743] These seizures are usually managed with medication.[724]

PARTIAL, FOCAL SEIZURES

Partial, focal seizures have clinical and EEG changes that indicate initial activation of neurons limited to part of one cerebral hemisphere. The seizures may or may not have impaired consciousness, and often progress to generalized motor convulsions.[415] Some may become generalized so quickly that the initial focal nature of the seizures is masked. Others become generalized after an appreciable time has elapsed. EEG tracing may indicate initial activation of neurons limited to a localized area in one cerebral hemisphere.[415] The mechanisms that initiate, promulgate, and terminate seizures remain unknown.

In children, approximately 30–50% of focal seizure have no known etiologic cause. There appears to be a genetic factor that determines whether a focal lesion becomes epileptogenic. Cerebral damage during or near the time of birth may result in seizures in early infancy or later in childhood. CNS tumor is rare in children. Head trauma is the most common cause of focal seizures. Closed head injuries, which constitutes most of pediatric injuries, are associated with only 5% incidence of epilepsy. The best results (of head trauma) were associated with normal computerized tomography scans.[744] Linear or depressed skull fractures have approximately 50% incidence of post-traumatic seizures. Fifty percent of seizures have their onset within 24 hours of injury, and tend to be focal in nature. Seizures occurring within 3 years of injury are more frequently generalized tonic–clonic grand mal seizures.[744] The pathogenesis of seizure due to head injury may be extravasation of blood which stimulates epileptogenic processes. Management may require neurosurgical evacuation of subdural hematomas, followed by long-term anticonvulsant medications.

CHINESE MEDICINE

The first description of grand mal seizures appeared in Emperor's Classic of Internal Medicine *Huang Di Nei Ching* (770–221 BC).[745] Pediatric textbooks have indicated successful treatment with acupuncture. Current acupuncture data has demonstrated varying degrees of success in treatment of adult epilepsy—mostly the chronic, medically intractable seizures,[746–750] which may not be applicable in pediatrics. Scalp acupuncture has been shown to improve cerebral blood flow in children, which would increase the delivery of oxygen and nutrients to the cortical tissues. This can theoretically be beneficial in childhood epilepsy.[751] An animal study on corresponding GV-26 and GV-24 points was found to increase brain GABA levels.[752]

An integrative approach to pediatric seizure disorder can combine Western neurologic examination and laboratory evaluations for diagnosis. Since acupuncture has minimal or no side-effects, it can be administered concomitantly with seizure medications. Tapering of medications, however, should be carried out carefully with close coordination with the neurologist. According to Chinese medicine, epileptic convulsions are internal Wind disturbances that can be due to both external and internal causes.

Generalized Seizures

Grand mal generalized seizures can be due to external pathogenic invasion or to internal imbalances.

External Pathogenic Invasion: Wind-Cold and Wind-Heat

Seizures are acute manifestations of the Jue Yin stage of Wind-Cold invasion and the Blood Level of Wind-Heat invasion—the sepsis and meningitis of Western diagnoses. The extreme Heat in the Liver generates Wind, dries up Liver Yin, thus preventing Liver from moistening the sinews. Muscles become rigid. Wind and Heat can cloud the Mind and cause unconsciousness. Both pathogens have penetrated to the deepest level of the child's body and have overcome the child's defense system. It is too late to expel the pathogens. The child is critically ill and most likely is already in the hospital on intravenous antibiotics. In those instances, acute seizure episodes are usually managed medically. However, the practitioner can try two classic acupuncture points that have been used to stop seizure and restore consciousness: GV-26 and KI-1. These points can be either needled or pinched very hard with the fingernail, so that parents can be taught to administer the treatment if the child progresses rapidly from mild febrile illness to convulsion. This is often seen in small infants who can progress from having mild symptoms to full blown sepsis in just a few hours.

Acupuncture can be used as a complementary treatment to dissipate Heat, subdue internal Wind, and tonify the child:

- GV-14 to dissipate Heat, to subdue Wind
- GV-16, GB-20 to subdue Wind
- LR-2 to clear Jue Yin Liver Heat
- LR-3 to subdue Liver Wind, nourish Liver Yin and Blood
- SI-3 to expel Wind from Governor Vessel channel
- GV-20 to increase Qi to the CNS.

Kidney Yin Deficiency/Liver Yin Deficiency

Yin deficiency in the Kidney and the Liver account for majority of the grand mal seizures in childhood: idiopathic form with strong genetic predisposition; CNS congenital anomalies or lesions; perinatal complications; or metabolic dysfunctions. Benign epilepsy of children and febrile convulsions may be milder forms of this imbalance, while infantile spasm is on the other end of the spectrum, being the most severe manifestation.

The majority of pediatric grand mal seizures are considered idiopathic, which indicates that Western medicine does not have a clear explanation of the etiology. Genetic predisposition correlates with Kidney Essence, which is Yin. Kidney Yin deficiency would rapidly result in Liver Yin deficiency because of the mother–child nurturing relationship between Kidney and Liver. Children are especially vulnerable because they are already constitutionally Yin deficient and Liver vulnerable. CNS congenital anomalies or lesions also correlate with Kidney, which is the foundation for marrow, the brain. Metabolic disorders are usually associated with the Liver.

Benign epilepsy of childhood and febrile convulsion probably represent milder forms of Kidney Yin/Liver Yin deficiency. Children in the Water phase of development—infancy and early childhood—are most vulnerable to Kidney imbalances and neurologic disorders. As the child matures, he moves out of the Water phase and therefore "outgrows" the epilepsy. Western medicine explains this as children having an immature brain which has a lower seizure threshold and is therefore vulnerable to developing epilepsy. A febrile seizure characteristically occurs within hours of onset of illness and therefore does not correlate with the Jue Yin stage or Blood level of pathogenic invasion. The predilection in infancy and early childhood again correlates with the Water phase of brain vulnerability. A strong genetic predisposition again suggests deficiency of pre-Heaven Essence, of Kidney Yin deficiency. During an acute illness with high fever, the intense internal Heat rapidly depletes Yin at the same time agitates internal Wind. Those with mild forms of deficiency would have one or two episodes. Those with more severe forms would progress to chronic epilepsy.

The pathophysiology of grand mal seizures is due to the direct effect of Liver Yin deficiency and the resultant Liver Yang excess. Liver Yin or Blood nourishes muscles and sinews. When Liver Yin/Blood is deficient, the emptiness in the Blood vessels is "filled" by internal Wind. Liver Yin deficiency causes Liver Yang rising, which stirs up Wind. Similarly, Heat from fever agitates Wind, both causing tonic–clonic movements in the extremities. The loss of consciousness or the Mind indicates involvement of Heart Yin, which is directly affected by Liver Yin via the mother–child relationship and by Kidney Yin, which is the foundation of all Yin, but especially of Liver and Heart. Infantile spasm is the most severe form of Kidney and Liver Yin deficiency, when there is not even enough Yin in the muscles and sinews for convulsive movements and the child becomes "stiff" in spasm.

There is general agreement between Western and Chinese medicine that the more severe forms of grand mal seizures need to be vigorously treated to prevent further neurologic injury. However, whereas Western medicine determines that benign childhood epilepsy and febrile convulsions do not need treatment, Chinese medicine posits that Kidney/Liver Yin of any degree of imbalance needs to be treated in order to prevent future disorders that may have other manifestations. For example, Western medicine has determined that epileptic children have a higher incidence of psychiatric disorders,[723] which in TCM represents imbalance of the Mind, of Shen. Since Western medicine operates on a different paradigm, there is no study that examines the correlation between febrile convulsion or childhood seizures and stroke in later years, both of which have the common TCM etiology in Liver Yin deficiency. Finally, whereas Western medicine must weigh the risk of medication side-effects with risk of seizure recurrence with nontreatment, acupuncture is safe and has the ability to "tonify" the child. There is no risk of "overdosing" the child with treatment, as no child can have too much Kidney Yin or Liver Yin.

Treatment

- Treatment for acute seizure: GV-26, KI-1
- Prophylactic treatment to prevent recurrence:
  - GV-14, LI-11 to clear Heat from the system
  - GV-16, GB-20 subdues Wind
- Tonify Kidney Yin and Liver Yin
- KI-6 tonifies Kidney Yin, an important point for seizures[753]
- LR-8 tonifies Liver Yin
- LR-3 subdues Liver Yang and Liver Wind, tonifies Liver Yin
- SP-6, KI-6 tonifies Yin
- BL-18 tonifies Liver Yin, also subdues Liver Yang
- SP-6, KI-3, BL-17, BL-20, BL-23 tonifies Blood.

LiverYin/HeartYin Deficiency—Absence Seizures

The major manifestations of absence seizures are brief loss of consciousness, staring vacantly, and lack of motor movements. These are suggestive of brief loss of Shen and Ethereal Soul. Shen, or Mind, resides in the Heart Yin while the Ethereal Soul, Hun, resides in the Liver Yin. The Mind controls consciousness. The Hun pertains to the Mind and is the coming and going of the Mind. The eyes, the external orifices of Liver, reflect the state of the Ethereal Soul, as in the Western saying: "the eyes are windows to the soul." During that brief moment when the child stares blankly, the Mind and the Soul are temporarily "gone." A genetic predisposition indicates that there is inheritance of both Liver and Heart Yin deficiency, or inheritance of Liver Yin deficiency that leads to Heart Yin deficiency via the mother–child relationship in the nurturing cycle. The course of this disorder is also compatible with the Five-Element Developmental Theory since children tend to "outgrow" this type of seizure in adolescence, the Fire phase of development, when the Heart is stronger. Liver Yin deficiency results in Liver Yang excess, which can stir up internal Wind.

However, unlike the grand mal seizures in Kidney Yin/Liver Yin deficiency, Liver Wind in this case carries excess Phlegm—which is usually abundant in children with constitutional Spleen deficiency. The Phlegm clouds the Heart, prevents the Heart from housing the Mind, and obstructs circulation to the eyes and an absence seizure ensues. The unpredictability and brevity of the attacks are characteristic of the coming-and-going of Wind.

This puzzling childhood disorder, therefore, can be explained by TCM theories. Emergency treatment is not necessary or possible since the attacks usually last only a few seconds. Treatment is directed toward prevention of recurrence, focusing on tonification of Heart and Liver Yin, calming the Shen, settling the Hun; and clearing Phlegm.

- GV-14, -16, GB-20 to subdue internal Wind
- ST-40 to dispel Phlegm
- PC-6 to resolve Phlegm from the Heart and clear orifices
- KI-6 to tonify Kidney Yin, the basis of all Yin
- HT-7 to tonify Heart Yin, calms the Mind
- BL-44 Shentang to calm Shen
- LR-3 to tonify Liver Yin, subdue Liver Yang
- BL-47 Hunman to settle the Ethereal Soul
- SP-6 to tonify Yin, dispel Phlegm
- Avoid excess sour and bitter foods (which would include bitter medications and herbs).

Spleen Yang Deficiency

Children are constitutionally Spleen deficient. Numerous factors can contribute to further Spleen deficiency: diet rich in Phlegm-producing foods, sweets, and greasy foods; living in a Damp environment; excess mental activities, as with academic overload; excess worrying and stress. Spleen deficiency can be responsible for both generalized convulsions and for absence seizures. Since Wood controls Earth, a weak Spleen is often associated with excess Liver Yang, which can stir up internal Wind. Phlegm can obstruct sensory orifices and invade channels and collaterals. Phlegm obstructs the Heart orifices and "mists the Mind," causing unconsciousness. Whereas insufficient Liver Yin is the basis of the Yin deficiency seizures, the Phlegm in Spleen Yang impedes the available Liver Yin or Blood from lubricating the sinews, resulting in generalized tonic–clonic seizures. Gurgling noises or foaming at the mouth during acute attacks are pathognomonic of the presence of Phlegm.

Treatment is directed toward tonifying Spleen, resolving Phlegm, and opening orifices:

- Acute tonic–clonic seizures can be treated with GV-26 and KI-1
- Prophylactic treatment: decrease Phlegm-producing, sweet and greasy foods
- Vigorously tonify Spleen using the Five-Element four-point protocol: tonify SP-2, HT-8; sedate SP-1, LR-1
- ST-40, SP-6 resolves Phlegm
- PC-5 resolves Phlegm from the Heart
- PC-6, HT-9 clears Heart, opens orifices
- ST-25 important point for Phlegm misting the Mind: regulates the Stomach, opens the Mind's orifices

- BL-15, BL-44 tonifies Heart, tonifies Shen
- GV-20 clears Mind
- LI-4, LU-7 regulate ascending of Clear Qi, descending of turbid Qi in the head, thus clearing the Mind
- GV-16, GB-20 to subdue Wind
- Modify lifestyle to decrease excess mental activities, to achieve a balance between rest and study, to minimize stressful situations that cause worry and anxiety.

Partial/Focal Seizures

Focal seizures are most often due to head trauma causing localized Blood stasis. Whereas Western medicine focuses on significant head trauma as the potential cause for focal seizures, Chinese medicine posits that any injury to the head—including a minor "bump" of the head which is usually forgotten—can result in localized Blood stasis. Athletic children participate in contact sports and often sustain mild head trauma on the field that would be unnoticed among all the kicks and bruises. Some children, especially boys, do not want to appear "wimpy" by complaining about a "hit" on the head. Since acupuncture treatment tonifies the child without side-effects, it would, in fact, be advisable to routinely treat young athletes to prevent Blood stasis. When there is focal seizure, treatment is indicated to move Blood and to calm the Mind.

Treatment

- Emergency treatment with GV-26, KI-1
- SP-6, BL-17 to move Blood
- PC-6 moves Blood, calms Mind
- HT-7 calms the Mind
- LR-14, BL-18 Liver Mu-Shu points to move Liver Blood (see Bibliography for further reading on this topic).

UPPER RESPIRATORY TRACT INFECTION

The common cold is the most frequent infection in children in the US and throughout the industrialized world. A preschool-aged child has an average of 4 to 10 colds per year. Upper respiratory tract infection (URI) is the major cause of absences from school.[754]

The clinical symptoms vary greatly without any correlation with specific viruses.[756] The majority of the symptoms are mild, consisting of rhinorrhea, sneezing, nasal congestion and obstruction, postnasal drip, and cough. There may often be additional symptoms of low-grade fever, sore throat, clear eye discharge, digestive discomfort, and general malaise.[756,757] Some common viruses that cause URI include rhinovirus, coronavirus, adenovirus, RSV, influenza and parainfluenza virus.[755,758,759] Transmission varies with different viruses. For example, RSV spreads primarily through contact with symptomatic children and contaminated objects; influenza mainly via airborne droplets. The precise route of transmission for rhinovirus remains controversial.[758]

The virulence of rhinovirus is maximum in infants before 1 year of age (median age is 6.5 months)[760] and in immune compromised children.[761] Wheezing is associated with RSV in children younger than 2 years of age and with rhinovirus in those over age 2.[762] Simultaneous infection by more than one virus, such as RSV and adenovirus together, can also occur frequently in the pediatric population.[760] Many children can also have associated bacterial infection, such as *Haemophilus influenzae* conjunctivitis.[760]

The viruses gain entry into host cells through specific viral surface proteins, which cause tissue injury and result in clinical disease.[763] Recent studies suggest that it is the host's response to the virus, not the virus itself, that determines the pathogenesis and severity of the common cold. Pro-inflammatory mediators, especially the cytokines, appear to be the central component of the response by infected epithelial cells.[764,765] Specific viral diagnosis is not necessary, both because of the benign, self-limiting nature of the disease,[766] and also because the prevalence of different viruses overlaps from fall to spring, so that it is very difficult to determine precisely which virus or viruses are causing the symptoms.[755] Current medical management of URI remains symptomatic, controversial, and in most cases, ineffective. Fluid, rest, a humidifier, and saline nose drops constitute the mainstay of nonpharmacologic treatment. The role of vitamin C both in prevention and in treatment of the common cold remains controversial[767,768] Topical adrenergic agents do not have systemic side-effects, but overuse can result in rebound congestion.[769]

Systemic medications are primarily used for symptomatic relief of congestion and cough, and most have limited efficacy.[765] Antihistamine and combinations of antihistamine with decongestants are the ingredients in at least 800 over-the-counter (OTC) cold remedies. The majority of studies have concluded that antihistamines are of marginal or no benefit in treating cold symptoms.[757,769–773] Dextromethorphan is an antitussive that is abundant in OTC formulations. Although this medication is reportedly safe when taken in the recommended dosages, there have been cases of "recreational" use by teenagers and deaths by overdose have been reported.[772] Codeine is ineffective in controlling URI cough.[773] Antibiotics are not indicated for the common cold,[757] but are often overprescribed, leading not only to higher health care costs[774] increased risk of side-effects, but also to the emergence of more resistant strains of bacteria.[775]

Research for new medical therapies for the common cold is directed toward increasing resistance to or immunity against the viruses. Interferons are proteins that can induce a nonspecific resistance to viral infection. However, the usual route of administration is by intramuscular injection, usually given on a daily basis because its blood concentration decreases sharply within 24 hours. In view of the self-limiting nature of URI, and the trauma of daily injections, it is unlikely that interferon would be used to treat URI in children.[776] Histamine antagonists are not indicated in the common cold.[777] Anti-inflammatory mediators[764] and specific antiviral agents[778] may be promising. Development of an effective vaccine against the common cold is unlikely because of the large number of viral serotypes.[756] Rhinovirus, for example, has at least 100 different immunotypes.[765]

Although viral URI is a benign illness of short duration, it can lead to bacterial complications, such as otitis media, sinusitis and lower respiratory tract infections, or even mastoiditis and meningitis that have much more significant consequences in children.[761,779] Antibiotics are appropriate for otitis and sinusitis.[780] Younger infants are especially susceptible to development of more serious bacterial infections. A 3-week-old baby with low-grade fever and congestion may warrant a full septic workup to rule out sepsis and meningitis, whereas a school-aged child is simply kept home from school and given symptomatic treatment for congestion and antipyretics for fever.

CHINESE MEDICINE

URI correlates to Wind-Cold invasion, discussed in detail in Chapter 6. The Chinese and Western medicine concepts of the etiology of URI are similar: virus infection is the external "Cold" pathogen transmitted via "Wind" or "airborne droplets." While Chinese medicine also prescribes symptomatic treatment and home management, its therapeutic principle focuses simultaneously on "eliminating the pathogenic factors by supporting the healthy energy"[781] which translates in biochemical terms as improving the immunity and general health of the child. This is especially important in URI because the host response is of primary importance in pathogenesis of URI, and because recurrent URIs are more likely to lead to complications.

Current reports support the efficacy of acupuncture for treating the common cold.[782–785] URI is at the Tai Yang level of illness, the most superficial stage of Wind-Cold invasion. Treatment of Bladder points can be beneficial, even in infants.[786] Symptomatic improvement can be substantiated by positive physiologic changes: acupuncture stimulation of LI-20 and LI-4 has been shown to increase the velocity of the nasal mucociliary transport in chronic rhinitis patients;[783] a pilot study showed change in nasal airway resistance, although the results were not statistically significant.[787]

Several reports indicate that acupuncture affects the immune system in URI. When acupuncture was pasted with Chinese herbs for treating rhinitis and bronchitis in infants, serum IgM, IgG, Complement C3, and especially IgA levels increased.[413] Needling general Wind-Cold points—Dazhui (GV-14), Fengchi (GB-13), and Quchi (LI-11)—resulted in decrease in temperature, respiratory rate, pulse and blood pressure with a simultaneous increase in the percentage of T-lymphocytes.[411] Even massaging local acupoints was effective in relieving symptoms and in enhancing immune functions with increasing in immune indices that persisted for at least 6 months.[781] One report of acumassage of Yingxiang LI-20 for just 30 seconds resulted in clinical relief from nasal congestion, even though there was no change in nasal airway resistance (NAR) or airflow.[788] These reports are encouraging for parents, since acupressure can be easily learned by nonprofessionals; is well tolerated by children of all ages, including infants; it has no side-effects and costs nothing. While Western medicine has acknowledged that most medications for the common cold are ineffective for symptom relief, none of the preparations has been demonstrated to affect immunity.

Acupuncture can be used to treat URI complications, such as otitis media or sinusitis. In a clinical study of chronic maxillary sinusitis that included children as young as 3 years of age, acupuncture treatment resulted in significant improvement of symptoms. However, because of the danger of rapid progression to more serious sequelae, the author recommends that antibiotics should still be considered for acute sinusitis.[789]

Treatment Protocol

- Increase fluid intake
- Decrease Cold energy foods
- General treatment to Dispel Wind—major points BL-12, GB-20
- Local points for rhinitis: LI-20, Yintang, ST-2
- Connect with ion pumping cord black on LI-20 or ST-2 and red on distal point, BL-60
- If using magnets, place bionorth (–) pole facing down on LI-20 or ST-2 and biosouth (+) pole facing down on BL-60 and connect with ion pumping cord as above
- Treat Tai Yang stage of Wind-Cold: use the Five-Element four-point Cold therapy to eliminate Cold from the Bladder channel: tonify BL-60, SI-5; sedate BL-66
- ST-40 to transform Phlegm
- GV-14, LI-11 to clear Heat if there is fever
- Tonify immune system
- Auriculopoints: Shenmen, Point Zero, Nose, Lung, Spleen
- Home massage program:
  - Teach parents to massage LI-20 for symptomatic relief
  - Massage Bladder meridian for general tonification and improvement of immunity.

URINARY CYSTITIS ("BLADDER INFECTION")

Urinary tract infections (UTI in this section refers only to urinary cystitis and bladder infection) occur frequently in the pediatric population.[790–792] Approximately 5% of all girls and 0.5% of all boys have at least one UTI urinary tract infection from infancy until their late teenage years. While boys have the highest incidence of UTI in the first year of life and show decreasing episodes of infection with age, girls remain vulnerable until adolescence.[791] UTI in children is often underdiagnosed.[793] Both diagnosis and treatment, especially in infants and young children, are challenging to the general pediatrician.

The risk factors for developing UTI vary according to the age of the child. Congenital anomalies that cause obstruction and reflux are the major factors that predispose infants and young children to UTI. School-aged children often hold back urine and delay urination for an extended period of time, especially when they are on the playground. Sexual activity is often associated with UTI in the adolescent.[794] Local immunologic impairment of the urinary tract—such as presence of the P1-blood-group antigen, increased urothelial colonization—also contribute to development of UTI.[791]

The overall health and defense of the child is also important in determining the severity of infection.[795] The highest incidence for first-time UTI is found in infants below 1 year of age.[796] Urinary tract infection in infants and young children up to 2 years of age is a special challenge for several reasons: (1) the manifestations of UTI in this age group tend to be nonspecific, and often present as unexplained high fever,[397] so that the diagnosis can be easily missed and prevalence underestimated;[795,796] (2) it is difficult to obtain a clean, midstream urine in the diaper population; and (3) the young kidney is most vulnerable to infection,[797] so that the early infections often rapidly progress to pyelonephritis.[796] Circumcision[797,798] and breast feeding[797] seem to offer some protection against UTI in babies.

The classic signs and symptoms of urinary cystitis in older children include dysuria—a burning sensation or pain with urination; increased frequency; nocturnal enuresis, abdominal and suprapubic pain, urgency, cloudy (pyuria) or bloody urine (hematuria).[394]

The Urinary Tract Subcommittee of the American Academy of Pediatrics Committee on Quality Improvement recommends that a culture needs to be performed on an adequately collected, clean-catch urine specimen. In children under age 2, invasive techniques, such as transurethral catheterization or suprapubic bladder tap, are needed to obtain an uncontaminated urine specimen.[799] Greater than 100 000 colonies of bacteria is diagnostic for UTI. The most common organism in children is *Escherichia coli*,[797] accounting for 90% of first episodes of acute cystitis in children and 75% of recurrent infections.[394] The pathogenic virulence of *E. coli* in UTI is in its ability to adhere to uroepithelial cells and red blood cells.[394] Other enteric bacteria, such as *Enterobacter*, *Klebsiella*, and *Proteus* may also cause pediatric UTI. Adolescent girls are susceptible to *Staphylococcus saprophyticus*.[394] The Subcommittee also recommends that all 2–24-month-olds should undergo complete imaging studies to include ultrasonography and voiding cystourethrogram,[799] in order to assess the abnormalities that predispose children to reflux and pyelonephritis and to assess the extent of renal involvement during infection.[795,800] There is no agreement on the most appropriate combination of studies in older children,[798] since subjecting the child to an invasive procedure is weighed against the low possibility of finding a congenital anomaly.[791]

Prompt diagnosis and treatment are important in order to prevent pyelonephritic scarring, especially in the first year of life.[801] Renal scarring is associated with development of hypertension in about 10% of children and accounts for approximately 20% of children with end-stage renal disease requiring dialysis or even renal transplant.[796,802] The severity of renal scarring is directly related to delay in diagnosis.[803]

Acute infection is managed with antibiotics for 7–14 days if an appropriate clinical response is observed.[799] A repeat microbiologic examination 48–72 hours after institution of treatment, and a follow-up culture within a week after cessation of therapy are recommended.[394,793] Prophylaxis is also important in pediatric UTI. Children who are found to have vesicoureteric reflux are managed with a single, daily dose of antibiotics for 3–6 months in order to prevent recurrence.[394,797,802] Children with underlying genitourinary abnormalities, such as congenital anomalies, obstructive uropathy, need to be treated for at least 1 year.[394] High-risk children, such as siblings, should be investigated for reflux.[802,803] Adolescents should be counseled about the relationship between sexual activities and the development of UTI.[794]

Asymptomatic bacteriuria has been a topic of concern for pediatricians. At this time, there does not appear to be any need for general screening for bacteriuria in healthy infants and children. Although bacteriuria may be found in 1–2% of the pediatric population, asymptomatic children have a very high rate of spontaneous clearing of the bacteriuria,[796] which in itself does not destroy the renal parenchyma.[791]

CHINESE MEDICINE

There is no data at this time on acupuncture treatment of UTI in children. In a three-armed study from Scandinavia that included real acupuncture, sham acupuncture, and an untreated control group, acupuncture was found to significantly prevent recurrent lower urinary tract infection in adult women.[804]

Because of scarring and renal complications, an integrative approach to urinary cystitis would be important, especially in infants and young children. Western laboratory confirmation should be used both for making a definitive diagnosis and for follow-up evaluation. Acupuncture can be an adjunctive therapy with antibiotics for acute episodes and as prophylaxis to prevent recurrences.

TCM defines urinary cystitis primarily as Damp Heat in the Bladder. This can occur as an acute Damp Heat invasion, or can be a chronic, recurrent condition due to Spleen deficiency, Liver and Gallbladder Heat, or Kidney Yin deficiency. The acute infections are due to invasion of Heat combined with Dampness in the Bladder. Spleen deficiency predisposes the child to chronic, recurrent infections.

Acute Urinary Cystitis—Damp Heat Invasion

Urine cultures have demonstrated that Bladder infections are caused by bacteria, most often by *E. coli*. Bacterial infections correlate to external Heat invasion in Chinese medicine. Whereas Wind-Heat invasion has a predilection for the upper parts of the body and causes respiratory symptoms, the source of bacteria for UTI is the gastrointestinal tract.[394] Since the female urethra is anatomically close to the rectum, the gastrointestinal bacteria ascend upward to the bladder, causing urinary bladder infection. The inflammation of Heat from bacteria normally rises, so the presence of Dampness would retain the Heat in the Lower Energizer. External Dampness can easily enter the body by penetrating the leg channels, then flowing upwards to settle in the Bladder. Children contract external Dampness when they sit on damp grass, walk in the rain, or sit by the pool with their feet dangling in water, etc. Adolescent girls are especially prone to invasion of Dampness during their menstrual periods.

With accumulation of Damp Heat in the Bladder, the water pathways become unregulated, giving rise to such symptoms as frequent, urgent, and painful urination, back pain, and restlessness. Heat may injure the blood vessels in the urinary tract and cause hematuria (blood in the urine).

Treatment

The Damp Heat in the urinary system obstructs the water passages, so that the treatment for all Bladder infections needs to expel Heat and dispel Dampness from the Bladder and open water passages.

- Increase fluid intake, encourage the child to empty the bladder whenever it feels full
- Decrease energetically Hot foods, Phlegm-producing foods
- ST-40 to disperse Dampness

- Expel Heat from Bladder using the Five-Element four-point protocol: tonify BL-66; sedate BL-60, SI-5
- Treat CV-3, BL-28 Mu and Shu points of Bladder, to clear Heat and drain Dampness
- BL-22 back Shu of the Triple Energizer, promotes the transformation of fluids and the separation of clear from turbid in the Lower Energizer, drains Dampness from the Lower Energizer
- SP-9 drains Damp Heat from the Lower Energizer
- BL-63 stops pain in the Bladder channel
- LU-7 is the confluent point of the Conception Vessel, and regulates Water passages, especially in descending fluids to the Bladder
- Tonify Spleen with either SP-3, meridian tonification, or Five-Element four-point protocol: tonify SP-2, HT-8; sedate SP-1, LR-1
- After the acute infection clears, strengthen the child with the immune protocol.

Chronic, Recurrent Cystitis

Spleen Qi Deficiency

Children are constitutionally Spleen Qi deficient. They may become more Spleen deficient due to inheritance of weak pre-Heaven Spleen Qi, such as a strong family of Spleen Qi deficiency, Spleen deficiency in both parents during conception, in the mother during pregnancy, due to a diet with excessive sweets, dairy and greasy foods, due to a Damp living environment, and due to chronic illnesses. Spleen Qi deficiency results in Dampness accumulation. Chronic Dampness would in turn further injure the Spleen. When external pathogenic Heat enters the Lower Energizer, Dampness combines with the Heat and tends to settles as Damp Heat in the urinary system since it is the more external Tai Yang channel. Spleen corresponds with the emotions worry and obsession, and with excess mental activities. A careful history would uncover any situations that would predispose to worry, and academic overload or lack of rest due to school or extracurricular activities.

Treatment

Since both acute and chronic cases of urinary cystitis have Damp Heat in the Bladder, the acute treatments are also applicable for chronic cystitis.

- Avoid artificially sweetened foods
- Vigorously tonify Spleen with the four-point protocol
- Modify lifestyle to allow the child to feel less pressure from school work and other activities, to minimize worry.

Liver and Gallbladder Heat

This condition is rarely seen in babies and very young children, and tends to affect children in the Wood phase of development when Liver and Gallbladder are vulnerable. Heat can accumulate in the Liver and Gallbladder when there is lingering pathogenic Heat, such as with previous Wind-Heat illnesses; from taking excess medications that are metabolized in the Liver; consuming excess greasy foods; or from excess Wood emotion such as frustration, irritability, anger. Most children have some degree of internal Dampness because of constitutional Spleen deficiency aggravated by diet and lifestyle that are injurious to the Spleen, excess Liver Heat is "pulled" downward by the Dampness, and becomes Damp Heat in the Bladder.

Treatment

- Treatment listed for acute UTI
- Avoid greasy or sour foods
- LR-3 and LR-13 to move Liver Qi
- Disperse Heat in the Liver and Gallbladder channels with four-point protocol:
  - Liver Heat: tonify LR-8, KI-10; sedate LR-2, HT-8
    - Two points: tonify LR-8; sedate LR-2
  - Gallbladder Heat: tonify GB-43, BL-66; sedate GB-38, SI-5
    - Two points: tonify GB-43; sedate GB-38
- Modify lifestyle to diminish stress that causes frustration and irritability
- Decrease medications, especially excessive over-the-counter medications
- Tonify Spleen.

Kidney Deficiency

Since Kidney is the foundation of all the Yin and Yang in the body, and since Kidney and Bladder are coupled Yin–Yang organs, Kidney Yin deficiency can easily lead to Bladder Yin deficiency and Bladder Heat accumulation. Since Kidney Yang holds in urine, deficiency in Kidney Yang would therefore lead to increased frequency. Kidney corresponds to the emotion fear. A careful history can uncover any situations that can precipitate fear in the child, such as fear of failure in school, fear of domestic disharmony, and even violence.

Western medicine is especially concerned that infants and young children with congenital anomalies frequently develop pyelonephritis that can lead to renal scarring, and therefore treat these children with prophylactic antibiotics for a prolonged period of time. Congenital anomalies in Chinese medicine are due to Kidney Yin, specifically Kidney Essence deficiency, and also Kidney Yang deficiency. Although acupuncture cannot correct the anatomic anomalies, which often need to have surgical intervention, acupuncture treatment can "modify" the Bladder "environment" to minimize Damp Heat accumulation.

Treatment

- Treatment listed for acute UTI
- Avoid salty foods
- Tonify Kidney Yin and Kidney Yang: KI-3 tonifies Kidney Yin, Essence and Kidney Yang
- Overall Kidney tonification with four-point protocol: tonify KI-7, LU-8; sedate KI-3, SP-3
- Modify lifestyle to minimize fearful situations. Family or individual therapy may be needed if there is a great deal of family dysfunction or other factors that precipitate fear in the child.

REFERENCES

1. Antonson D.L. (1994) Abdominal pain. *Gastrointestinal Endoscopy Clinics of North America* 4(1), 1–21.
2. Reynolds S.L. & Jaffe D.M. (1992) Diagnosing abdominal pain in a pediatric emergency department. *Pediatric Emergency Care* 8, 126–128.
3. Ruddy R.M. (1993) Pain-Abdomen. In Fleisher G.R. & Ludwig S. (eds) *Textbook of Pediatric Emergency Medicine*, 3rd edition. Baltimore, Williams & Wilkins, pp 340–347.
4. Crady S.K., Jones J.S., Wyn T. *et al.* (1993) Clinical validity of ultrasound in children with suspected appendicitis. *Annals of Emergency Medicine* 22, 1125–1128.
5. Quillin S.P. & Siegel M.J. (1993) Color Doppler US of children with acute lower abdominal pain. *Radiographics* 13, 1281–1293.
6. Laing F.C. (1992) Ultrasonography of the acute abdomen. *Radiology Clinics of North America* 30, 389– 404.
7. Rubin S.Z. & Martin D.J. (1990) Ultrasonography in the management of possible appendicitis in childhood. *Journal of Pediatric Surgery* 25, 737–740.
8. Siegel M.J., Carel C. & Surratt S. (1991) Ultrasonography of acute abdominal pain in children. *Journal of the American Medical Association* 266, 1987–1989.
9. Sivit C.J., Newman K.D., Boenning D.A. *et al.* (1992) Appendicitis: usefulness of ultrasound in a pediatric population. *Radiology* 185, 549–552.
10. Swischuk L.E. (1992) Abdominal pain and anorexia. *Pediatric Emergency Care* 8, 45–46.
11. Zheng X.L., Chen C. & Wu X.Z. (1985) Acupuncture therapy in acute abdomen. *American Journal of Chinese Medicine* 13(1–4), 127–131.
12. Li C.K., Nauck M., Loser C., Folsch U.R. & Creutzfeldt W. (1991) Acupuncture to alleviate pain during colonoscopy. *Deutsche Medizinische Wochenschrift* 116(10), 367–370. [Abstract. Article in German]
13. Ho R.T., Jawan B., Fung S.T., Cheung H.K. & Lee J.H. (1990) Electro-acupuncture and postoperative emesis. *Anaesthesia* 45(4), 327–329.
14. Chu H., Zhao S.Z. & Huang Y.Y. (1987) Application of acupuncture to gastroscopy using a fiberoptic endoscope. *Journal of Traditional Chinese Medicine* 7(4), 279.
15. Cheng Y.Q., Wang Z.Q., Zhang S.Y., Wu J.J. & Wu W.Y. (1984) The use of needling Zusanli in fiberoptic gastroscopy. *Journal of Traditional Chinese Medicine* 4(2), 91–92.
16. Sodipo J.O. & Ogunbiyi T.A. (1981) Acupuncture analgesia for upper gastrointestinal endoscopy: a Lagos experience. *American Journal of Chinese Medicine* 9(2), 171–173.
17. Cahn A.M., Carayon P., Hill C. & Flamant R. (1978) Acupuncture in gastroscopy. *Lancet* 1(8057), 182–183.
18. Belman A.B. (1991) Ureteropelvic junction obstruction as a cause for intermittent abdominal pain in children. *Pediatrics* 88, 1066–1069.
19. Ross A.J. (1994) Intestinal obstruction in the newborn. *Pediatrics in Review* 15, 338–347.
20. Swischuk L.E. (1992) Acute abdomen with right lower quadrant pain. *Pediatric Emergency Care* 8, 241–242.
21. Swischuk L.E. (1994) Sudden onset right side abdominal pain. *Pediatric Emergency Care* 8, 51–53.
22. Axon A.T., Long D.E. & Jones S.C. (1991) Editorial. Abdominal migraine: does it exist? *Journal of Clinical Gastroenterology* 13, 615–616.
23. Mason J.D. (1996) The Evaluation of Acute Abdominal Pain In Children. Gastrointestinal Emergencies, Part I. *Emergency Medicine Clinics of North America* Volume 14 Number 3, 629–643.
24. Singer H.S. (1994) Migraine headaches in children. *Pediatrics in Review* 15, 94–101.
25. Macarthur C., Saunders N. & Feldman W. (1995) *Helicobacter pylori*, gastroduodenal disease, and recurrent abdominal pain in children. *Journal of the American Medical Association* 273, 729–734.
26. Salvi E., Pistilli A., Romiti P., Bedogni G. & Pedrazzoli C. (1983) Duodenal ulcer. Gastroscopic aspects before and after acupuncture treatment. *Minerva Medica* 74(42), 2541–2546. [Abstract. Article in Italian]
27. Boyle T.J. (1997) Recurrent Abdominal Pain: An Update. *Pediatrics in Review* 18, 310–321.
28. Qi Q.H., Xue C.R. & Wang P.Z. (1995) Analysis of treatment in 84 cases of severe pancreatitis. *Zhongguo Zhong Xi Yi Jie He Za Zhi* 15(1), 28–30. [Abstract. Article in Chinese]

29. Ballegaard S., Christophersen S.J., Dawids S.G., Hesse J. & Olsen N.V. (1985) Acupuncture and transcutaneous electric nerve stimulation in the treatment of pain associated with chronic pancreatitis. A randomized study. *Scandinavian Journal of Gastroenterology* 20(10), 1249–1254.

30. Xu Y. (1992) Treatment of acute pain with auricular pellet pressure on ear Shenmen as the main point. *Journal of Traditional Chinese Medicine* 12(2), 114–115.

31. Rothrock S.G., Skeoch G., Rush J.J. *et al.* (1991) Clinical features of misdiagnosed appendicitis in children. *Annals of Emergency Medicine* 20, 45–73.

32. Cobb L.M. & Lelli J.L. (1993) Appendicitis. In Reisdorff E.J., Roberts M.R. & Wiegenstein J.G. (eds) *Pediatric Emergency Medicine*. Philadelphia, WB Saunders, pp 314–321.

33. Harberg F. (1989) The acute abdomen in childhood. *Pediatric Annals* 18, 169–178.

34. Rappaport W.D., Peterson M. & Stanton C. (1989) Factors responsible for the high perforation rate seen in early childhood appendicitis. *American Surgery* 55, 602–605.

35. Rasmussen O. & Hoffman J. (1991) Assessment of the reliability of the symptoms and signs of acute appendicitis. *Journal of the Royal College of Surgeons of Edinburgh (Scotland)* 36, 372–377.

36. Folkman J. & First L.R. (1995) Abdominal pain. Audio-Digest: *Pediatrics* 41(5).

37. Gilchrist B.F., Lobe T.E., Schropp K.P. *et al.* (1992) Is there a role for laparoscopic appendectomy in pediatric surgery? *Journal of Pediatric Surgery* 27, 209–214.

38. Maciocia G. (1994) *The Practice of Chinese Medicine, The Treatment of Diseases with Acupuncture and Chinese Herbs*. London, Churchill Livingstone.

39. Deadman P. & Al-Khafaji M. (1998) *A Manual of Acupuncture*. East Sussex, England, Journal of Chinese Medicine Publications.

40. Levy J.H. & Texidor M.S. (1988) The lack of importance of Lanwei point in the diagnosis of acute appendicitis. *Pain* 33(1), 79–80.

41. Gu Y. (1992) Treatment of acute abdomen by electro-acupuncture—a report of 245 cases. *Journal of Traditional Chinese Medicine* 12(2), 110–113.

42. Fan Y.K. & Zhang C.C. (1983) 20 years' acupuncture in 461 acute appendicitis cases. *Chinese Medicine Journal (England)* 96(7), 491–494.

43. Tang H. & Fu Y.D. (1981) Helium–neon laser irradiation of acupuncture points in treatment of 50 cases of acute appendicitis. *Journal of Traditional Chinese Medicine* 1(1), 43–44.

44. Chen H. (1993) Recent studies on auriculoacupuncture and its mechanism. *Journal of Traditional Chinese Medicine* 13(2), 129–143.

45. Sun P., Li L. & Si M. (1992) Comparison between of acupuncture and epidural anesthesia in appendectomy. *Zhen Ci Yan Jiu* 17(2), 87–89. [Abstract. Article in Chinese]

46. Chen P. & Chen Y. (1990) Clinical approaches to improvement of appendectomy effects under acupuncture anesthesia. *Zhen Ci Yan Jiu* 15(3), 167–169. [Abstract. Article in Chinese]

47. Luks F.I., Yazbeck S., Perreault G. *et al.* (1992) Changes in the presentation of intussusception. *American Journal of Emergency Medicine* 10, 574–576.

48. Losek J.D. (1991) Intussusception and the diagnostic value of testing stool for occult blood. *American Journal of Emergency Medicine* 9, 1.

49. Alford B.A. & McIlhenny J. (1992) The child with acute abdominal pain and vomiting. *Radiology Clinics of North America* 30, 441–453.

50. Bhisitkul D.M., Listernick R., Shkolnik A. *et al.* (1992) Clinical application of ultrasonography in the diagnosis of intussusception. *Journal of Pediatrics* 121, 182–186.

51. Lam A.H. & Firman K. (1992) Value of sonography including color Doppler in the diagnosis and management of long standing intussusception. *Pediatric Radiology* 22, 112–114.

52. Everarts P., Clapuyt P., Claus D. & Ninane J. (1994) The role of ultrasonography in abdominal pain in children in the emergency room. *Journal Belge Radiologie* 77(5), 201–203. [Abstract. Article in French]

53. Ong N.-T. & Beasley D.W. (1990) The leadpoint in intussusception. *Journal of Pediatric Surgery* 25, 640–643.

54. Choong C.K. & Beasley S.W. (1998) Intra-abdominal manifestations of Henoch–Schonlein purpura. *Journal of Pediatric Child Health* 34(5), 405–409.

55. Wan Y.G. & Yu L.Y. (1981) Volvulus of the stomach successfully treated with acupuncture report of 9 cases. *Journal of Traditional Chinese Medicine* 1(1), 39–42.

56. Ross J.H. (1994) Urologic concerns. Audio-Digest: *Pediatrics* 40(1).

57. Qian L.W. & Lin Y.P. (1993) Effect of electroacupuncture at zusanli (ST36) point in regulating the pylorus peristaltic function. *Zhongguo Zhong Xi Yi Jie He Za Zhi* 13(6), 336–339, 324. [Abstract. Article in Chinese]

58. Singer J. (1996) Acute abdominal conditions that may require surgical intervention. In Strange G.R., Ahrens W., Lelyveld S. *et al.* (eds) *Pediatric Emergency Medicine: A Comprehensive Study Guide.* New York, McGraw-Hill, pp 311–319.

59. Sun Z.F. (1987) Herniorrhaphy under electro-acupuncture anesthesia—a clinical investigation. *Zhen Ci Yan Jiu* 12(2), 94–98. [Article in Chinese. No Abstract]

60. Reif S., Sloven D.G. & Lebenthal E. (1993) Gallstones in children: abdominal pain unrelated to trauma. *Pediatrics in Review* 14, 302–311.

61. Turck D. (1998) Chronic abdominal pain in children. *Rev Prat* 48(4), 369–375. [Abstract. Article in French]

62. Lake A.M. (1999) Chronic abdominal pain in childhood: diagnosis and management. *American Family Physician* 59(7), 1823–1830.

63. Scott R.B. (1994) Recurrent abdominal pain during childhood. *Canadian Family Physician* 40, 539–542, 545–547.

64. Croffie J.M., Fitzgerald J.F. & Chong S.K. (2000) Recurrent abdominal pain in children—a retrospective study of outcome in a group referred to a pediatric gastroenterology practice. *Clinical Pediatrics (Philadelphia)* 39(5), 267–274.

65. Oymar K., Fluge G. & Rosendahl K. (1993) Recurrent abdominal pain. A prospective study of 68 children. *Tidsskrift For Den Norske Laegeforening* 113(20), 2566–2568. [Abstract. Article in Norwegian]

66. Buller H.A. (1997) Problems in diagnosis of IBD in children. *Netherlands Journal of Medicine* 50(2), S8–S11.

67. Gremse D.A. & Shakoor S. (1993) Symptoms of acid-peptic disease in children. *Southern Medical Journal* 86(9), 997–100.

68. Salky B.A. & Edye M.B. (1998) The role of laparoscopy in the diagnosis and treatment of abdominal pain syndromes. *Surgical Endoscopy* 12(7), 911–914.

69. Hyams J.S. (1999) Functional gastrointestinal disorders. *Current Opinions in Pediatrics* 11(5), 375–378.

70. Thompson W.G., Longstreth G.F., Drossman D.A., Heaton K.W., Irvine E.J. & Muller-Lissner S.A. (1999) Functional bowel disorders and functional abdominal pain. *Gut* 45 Suppl 2, II43–II47.

71. Oberlander T.F. & Rappaport L.A. (1993) Recurrent abdominal pain during childhood. *Pediatrics in Review* 14, 313–323.

72. Forbes D. (1994) Abdominal pain in childhood. *Australian Family Physician* 23(3), 347–348, 351, 354–357.

73. Silverberg M. (1991) Chronic abdominal pain in adolescents. *Pediatric Annals* 20(4), 179–185.

74. Krowchuk D.P. (2000) Managing acne in adolescents. *Pediatric Clinics of North America* 47(4), 841–857.

75. Krowchuk D.P. (2000) Treating acne. A practical guide. *Medical Clinics of North America* 84(4), 811–828.

76. Goodman G.J. (2001) Post-acne scarring, a short review of its pathophysiology. *Australian Journal of Dermatology* 42(2), 84–90.

77. Nelson W.E. *et al.* (eds) (1996) *Nelson's Textbook of Pediatrics,* 15th edition. Philadelphia, WB Saunders, Co.

78. Jacob C.I., Dover J.S. & Kaminer M.S. (2001) Acne scarring: a classification system and review of treatment options. *Journal of the American Academy of Dermatology* 45(1), 109–117.

79. Fyrand O. (1997) Treatment of acne. *Tidsskrift For Den Norske Laegeforening* 117(20), 2985–2987. [Abstract. Article in Norwegian]

80. Usatine R.P. & Quan M.A. (2000) Pearls in the management of acne: an advanced approach. *Primary Care* 27(2), 289–308.

81. Shalita A.R. (1998) Clinical aspects of acne. *Dermatology* 196(1), 93–94.

82. Xu Y. (1990) Treatment of facial skin diseases with acupuncture. *Journal of Traditional Chinese Medicine* 10(1), 22–25.

83. Dai G.Q. (1997) Advances in the acupuncture treatment of acne. *Journal of Traditional Chinese Medicine* 17(1), 65–72.

84. Liu J. (1993) Treatment of adolescent acne with acupuncture. *Journal of Traditional Chinese Medicine* 13(3), 187–188.

85. Oleson T.D. (1992) *Auriculotherapy Manual, Chinese and Western Systems of Ear Acupuncture.* Los Angeles, Health Care Alternatives.

86. Werner H.A. (2001) Status asthmaticus in children: a review. *Chest* 119(6), 1913–1929.

87. National Center for Health Statistics (1990) Asthma—United States, 1980–1987. *MMWR Morbidity and Mortality Weekly Report* 39, 493–497.

88. Warner J.O. (1999) Worldwide variations in the prevalence of atopic symptoms: what does it all mean? *Thorax* 54, S46–S51.

89. Asthma mortality and hospitalization among children and young adults— United States, 1980–1993. *Morbidity and Mortality Weekly Report* 1996; 45, 350–353.

90. Sly R.M. (1999) Changing prevalence of allergic rhinitis and asthma. *Annals of Allergy, Asthma, and Immunology* 82, 233–248.

91. Blessing-Moore J. Asthma affects all age groups but requires special consideration in the pediatric age group especially in children less than five years of age. *Journal of Asthma* 31(6), 415–418.

92. Neville R.G., McCowan C., Hoskins G. & Thomas G. (2001) Cross-sectional observations on the natural history of asthma. *British Journal of General Practice* 51(466), 361–365.

93. Asthma–United States, 1980–1987. *Morbidity and Mortality Weekly Report* 1990; 39, 493–497.

94. Mannino D.M., Homa D.M., Pertowski C.A. *et al.* (1998) Surveillance for asthma—United States, 1960–1995. *Morbidity and Mortality Weekly Report CDC Surveillance* 47, 1–27.

95. Crane J., Pearce N., Flatt A. *et al.* (1989) Prescribed fenoterol and death from asthma in New Zealand, 1981–83: case control study. *Lancet* 1, 917–922.

96. Spitzer W.O., Suissa S., Ernst P. *et al.* (1992) The use of β-agonists and the risk of death and near death from asthma. *New England Journal of Medicine* 326, 501–506.

97. Chung K.F. (1999) Non-invasive biomarkers of asthma. *Pediatric Pulmonology Supplement* 18, 41–44.

98. Gaston B. (1998) Managing asthmatic airway inflammation: what is the role of expired nitric oxide measurement? *Current Problems in Pediatrics* 28, 245–252.

99. Szefler S.J. & Nelson H.S. (1998) Alternative agents for anti-inflammatory treatment of asthma. *Journal of Allergy and Clinical Immunology* 102(4 Pt 2), S23–S35.

100. Weisberg S.C. (2000) Pharmacotherapy of asthma in children, with special reference to leukotriene receptor antagonists. *Pediatric Pulmonology* 29(1), 46–61.

101. Kemp J.P. (2000) Role of leukotriene receptor antagonists in pediatric asthma. *Pediatric Pulmonology* 30(2), 177–182.

102. Larsen G.L. (2001) Differences between adult and childhood asthma. *Dis Mon* 47(1), 34–44.

103. Martinez F.D. (2001) Links between pediatric and adult asthma. *Journal of Allergy and Clinical Immunology* 107(5 Suppl), 449S–455S.

104. Bisgaard H. (2001) Pathophysiology of the cysteinyl leukotrienes and effects of leukotriene receptor antagonists in asthma. *Allergy* 56(S66), 7–11.

105. Laitinen L.A., Heino M., Laitinen A. *et al.* (1985) Damage of airway epithelium and bronchial reactivity in patients with asthma. *American Review of Respiratory Diseases* 131, 599–606.

106. Platts-Mills T.A., Rakes G. & Heymann P.W. (2000) The relevance of allergen exposure to the development of asthma in childhood. *Journal of Allergy and Clinical Immunology* 105(2 pt 2), 503–508.

107. Pilotto L.S., Smith B.J., Nitschke M. *et al.* (1999) Industry, air quality, cigarette smoke and rates of respiratory illness in Port Adelaide. *Australia and New Zealand Journal of Public Health* 23, 657–660.

108. Wahlgren D.R., Hovell M.F., Meltzer E.O. *et al.* (2000) Involuntary smoking and asthma. *Current Opinion in Pulmonary Medicine* 6, 31–36.

109. Avital A., Springer C., Bar-Yishay E. *et al.* (1995) Adenosine, methacholine, and exercise challenges in children with asthma or paediatric chronic obstructive pulmonary disease. *Thorax* 50, 511–516. [Abstract.]

110. Vamos M. & Kolbe J. (1999) Psychological factors in severe chronic asthma. *Australian and New Zealand Journal of Psychiatry* 33, 538–544.

111. Dubus J.C., Bosdure E., Mates M. & Mely L. (2001) Virus and respiratory allergy in children. *Allergy and Immunology (Paris)* 33(2), 78–81. [Abstract. Article in French]

112. Cohen N.H., Eigen H. & Shaughnessy T.E. (1997) Status asthmaticus. *Critical Care Clinic* 13, 459–476.

113. Helfaer M.A., Nichols D.G. & Rogers M.C. (1996) Lower airway disease: bronchiolitis and asthma. In Rogers M., Nichols D. (eds) *Textbook of Pediatric Intensive Care*, 3rd edition. Baltimore, Williams & Wilkins, pp 127–164.

114. Woodcock A. & Custovic A. (2000) Allergen avoidance: does it work? *British Medical Bulletin* 56(4), 1071–1086.

115. Bibi H., Shoychet E., Shoseyov D., Armoni M., Chai E. & Ater D. (1999) Evaluation of asthmatic children presenting at emergency rooms. *Harefuah* 137(9), 383–387, 430. [Abstract. Article in Hebrew]

116. Johnston S.L. (1999) The role of viral and atypical bacterial pathogens in asthma pathogenesis. *Pediatric Pulmonology* Suppl 18, 141–143.

117. Laurie S. & Khan D. (2001) Inhaled corticosteroids as first-line therapy for asthma. Why they work—and what the guidelines and evidence suggest. *Postgraduate Medicine* 109(5), 44–46, 49–52, 55–56.

118. Chipps B.E. & Chipps D.R. (2001) A review of the role of inhaled corticosteroids in the treatment of acute asthma. *Clinical Pediatrics (Philadelphia)* 40(4), 185–189.

119. Zorc J.J. & Pawlowski N.A. (2000) Prevention of asthma morbidity: recent advances. *Current Opinions in Pediatrics* 12(5), 438–443.

120. Skoner D.P. (2001) Management and treatment of pediatric asthma: update. *Allergy Asthma Proceedings* 22(2), 71–74.

121. Chen K., Li S., Shi Z., Liu S. & Zhao L. (2000) Two hundred and seventeen cases of winter diseases treated with acupoint stimulation in summer. *Journal of Traditional Chinese Medicine* 20(3), 198–201.

122. Personal observation. (1999) TCM Pediatric Ward, Xinhua Hospital, Shanghai, China.

123. Yan S. (1998) 14 cases of child bronchial asthma treated by auricular plaster and meridian instrument. *Journal of Traditional Chinese Medicine* 18(3), 202–204.

124. Hossri C.M. (1976) The treatment of asthma in children through acupuncture massage. *Journal of the American Society of Psychosomatic Dentistry and Medicine* 23(1), 3–16.

125. Haidvogl M. (1990) Alternative treatment possibilities of atopic diseases. *Padiatric Pädologie* 25(6), 389–396. [Abstract. Article in German]

126. Fung K.P., Chow O.K. & So S.Y. (1986) Attenuation of exercise-induced asthma by acupuncture. *Lancet* 2(8521–22), 1419–1422.

127. Yu D.Y. & Lee S.P. (1976) Effect of acupuncture on bronchial asthma. *Clinical Science and Molecular Medicine* 51(5), 503–509.

128. Zhou R.L. & Zhang J.C. (1997) An analysis of combined desensitizing acupoints therapy in 419 cases of allergic rhinitis accompanying asthma. *Zhongguo Zhong Xi Yi Jie He Za Zhi* 17(10), 587–589. [Article in Chinese]

129. Chen L.L., Li A.S. & Tao J.N. (1996) Clinical and experimental studies on preventing and treating anaphylactic asthma with Zusanli point immunotherapy. *Zhongguo Zhong Xi Yi Jie He Za Zhi* 16(12), 709–712. [Article in Chinese]

130. Zang J. (1990) Immediate antiasthmatic effect of acupuncture in 192 cases of bronchial asthma. *Journal of Traditional Chinese Medicine* 10(2), 89–93.

131. Rogers P.A., Schoen A.M. & Limehouse J. (1992) Acupuncture for immune-mediated disorders. Literature review and clinical applications. *Problems in Veterinary Medicine* 4(1), 162–193.

132. Sato T., Yu Y., Guo S.Y., Kasahara T. & Hisamitsu T. (1996) Acupuncture stimulation enhances splenic natural killer cell cytotoxicity in rats. *Japan Journal of Physiology* 46(2), 131–136.

133. Dong L., Yuan D., Fan L., Su L. & Fu Z. (1996) [Effect of HE-NE laser acupuncture on the spleen in rats]. *Zhen Ci Yan Jiu* 21(4), 64–67. [Abstract. Article in Chinese]

134. Sakic B., Kojic L., Jankovic B.D. & Skokljev A. (1989) Electro-acupuncture modifies humoral immune response in the rat. *Acupuncture Electrotherapy Research* 14(2), 115–120.

135. Joos S., Schott C., Zou H., Daniel V. & Martin E. (2000) Immunomodulatory effects of acupuncture in the treatment of allergic asthma: a randomized controlled study. *Journal of Alternative and Complementary Medicine* 6(6), 519–525.

136. Okumura M., Toriizuka K., Iijima K., Haruyama K., Ishino S. & Cyong J.C. (1999) Effects of acupuncture on peripheral T lymphocyte subpopulation and amounts of cerebral catecholamines in mice. *Acupuncture Electrotherapy Research* 24(2), 127–139.

137. Ma Z., Wang Y. & Fan Q. (1992) [The influence of acupuncture on interleukin 2 interferon-natural killer cell regulatory network of kidney-deficiency mice]. *Zhen Ci Yan Jiu.* 17(2), 139–142. [Abstract. Article in Chinese]

138. Yan W.X., Wang J.H. & Chang Q.Q. (1991) [Effect of leu-enkephalin in striatum on modulating cellular immune during electropuncture]. *Sheng Li Xue*

Bao. 43(5), 451–456. [Abstract. Article in Chinese]

139. Sato T., Yu Y., Guo S.Y., Kasahara T. & Hisamitsu T. (1996) Acupuncture stimulation enhances splenic natural killer cell cytotoxicity in rats. *Japanese Journal of Physiology* 46(2), 131–136.

140. Petti F., Bangrazi A., Liguori A., Reale G. & Ippoliti F. (1998) Effects of acupuncture on immune response related to opioid-like peptides. *Journal of Traditional Chinese Medicine* 18(1), 55–63.

141. Bianchi M., Jotti E., Sacerdote P. & Panerai A.E. (1991) Traditional acupuncture increases the content of beta-endorphin in immune cells and influences mitogen induced proliferation. *American Journal of Chinese Medicine* 19(2), 101–104.

142. Hu J. (1998) Clinical observation on 25 cases of hormone dependent bronchial asthma treated by acupuncture. *Journal of Traditional Chinese Medicine* 18(1), 27–30.

143. Sun Y. (1995) External approach to the treatment of pediatric asthma. *Journal of Traditional Chinese Medicine* 15(4), 290–291.

144. Shaywitz B.A., Fletcher J.M. & Shaywitz S.E. (1997) Attention-deficit/ hyperactivity disorder. *Advances in Pediatrics* 44, 331–367.

145. Kidd P.M. (2000) Attention deficit/hyperactivity disorder (ADHD) in children: rationale for its integrative management. *Alternative Medicine Review* 5(5), 402–428.

146. Schweitzer J.B., Cummins T.K. & Kant C.A. (2001) Attention-deficit/ hyperactivity disorder. *Medical Clinics of North America* 85(3), 757–777.

147. Richardson A.J. & Ross M.A. (2000) Fatty acid metabolism in neurodevelopmental disorder: a new perspective on associations between attention-deficit/hyperactivity disorder, dyslexia, dyspraxia and the autistic spectrum. *Prostaglandins, Leukotrienes and Essential Fatty Acids* 63(1–2), 1–9.

148. Schneider S.C. & Tan G. (1997) Attention-deficit hyperactivity disorder. In pursuit of diagnostic accuracy. *Postgraduate Medicine* 101(4), 231–232, 235–240.

149. Modigh K., Berggren U. & Sehlin S. (1998) High risk for children with DAMP/ADHD to become addicts later in life. *Lakartidningen* 95(47), 5316–5319. [Article in Swedish]

150. Arnold L.E. (1996) Sex differences in ADHD: conference summary. *Journal of Abnormal Child Psychology* 24(5), 555–569.

151. Shelley-Tremblay J.F. & Rosen L.A. (1996) Attention deficit hyperactivity disorder: an evolutionary perspective. *Journal of Genetic Psychology* 157(4), 443–453.

152. Bradley J.D. & Golden C.J. (2001) Biological contributions to the presentation and understanding of attention-deficit/hyperactivity disorder: a review. *Clinical Psychology Review* 21(6), 907–929.

153. Biederman J. (1998) Attention-deficit/hyperactivity disorder: a life-span perspective. *Journal of Clinical Psychiatry* 59 Suppl 7, 4–16.

154. Taylor M.A. (1999) Attention-deficit hyperactivity disorder on the frontlines: management in the primary care office. *Comprehensive Therapy* 25(6–7), 313–325.

155. Hechtman L. (2000) Assessment and diagnosis of attention-deficit/ hyperactivity disorder. *Child and Adolescent Psychiatric Clinics of North America* 9(3), 481–498.

156. Faraone S.V., Biederman J., Spencer T., Wilens T., Seidman L.J., Mick E. & Doyle A.E. (2000) Attention-deficit/ hyperactivity disorder in adults: an overview. *Biological Psychiatry* 48(1), 9–20.

157. Zuddas A., Ancilletta B., Muglia P. & Cianchetti C. (2000) Attention-deficit/hyperactivity disorder: a neuropsychiatric disorder with childhood onset. *European Journal of Paediatric Neurology* 4(2), 53–62.

158. Williams C., Wright B. & Partridge I. (1999) Attention deficit hyperactivity disorder—a review. *British Journal for the General Practitioner* 49(444), 563–571.

159. Buitelaar J.K. & Kooij J.J. (2000) Attention deficit hyperactivity disorder (ADHD): etiology, diagnosis and treatment. *Nederlands Tijdschrift voor Geneeskunde* 2, 144(36), 1716–1723. [Abstract. Article in Dutch]

160. Denney C.B. (2001) Stimulant effects in attention deficit hyperactivity disorder: theoretical and empirical issues. *Journal of Clinical Child Psychology* 30(1), 98–109.

161. Eisenberg J., Zohar A., Mei-Tal G., Steinberg A., Tartakovsky E., Gritsenko I., Nemanov L. & Ebstein R.P. (2000) A haplotype relative risk study of the dopamine D4 receptor (DRD4) exon III repeat polymorphism and attention deficit hyperactivity disorder (ADHD). *American Journal of Medical Genetics* 96(3), 258–261.

162. Faraone S.V. & Doyle A.E. (2000) Genetic influences on attention deficit hyperactivity disorder. *Current Psychiatry Report* 2(2), 143–146.

163. Levy F., Barr C. & Sunohara G. (1998) Directions of aetiologic research on attention deficit hyperactivity disorder. *Australian and New Zealand Journal of Psychiatry* 32(1), 97–103.

164. Lou H.C. (1996) Etiology and pathogenesis of attention-deficit hyperactivity disorder (ADHD): significance of prematurity and perinatal hypoxic-haemodynamic encephalopathy. *Acta Pediatrica* 85(11), 1266–1271.

165. Mercugliano M. (1999) What is attention-deficit/hyperactivity disorder? *Pediatric Clinics of North America* 46(5), 831–843.

166. Faraone S.V. & Biederman J. (1998) Neurobiology of attention-deficit hyperactivity disorder. *Biological Psychiatry* 44(10), 951–958.

167. Barkley R.A. (1998) *Attention Deficit Hyperactivity Disorder, a Handbook for Diagnosis and Treatment*. New York, The Guilford Press.

168. Baird J., Stevenson J.C. & Williams D.C. (2000) The evolution of ADHD: a disorder of communication? *Quarterly Review of Biology* 75(1), 17–35.

169. Niedermeyer E. & Naidu S.B. (1997) Attention-deficit hyperactivity disorder (ADHD) and frontal-motor cortex disconnection. *Clinical Electroencephalography* 28(3), 130–136.

170. Cameron J. (2000) U.S. temperament researcher. Personal communications.

171. Breakey J. (1997) The role of diet and behaviour in childhood. *Journal of Pediatric Child Health* 33(3), 190–194.

172. Boris M. & Mandel F.S. (1994) Foods and additives are common causes of the attention deficit hyperactive disorder in children. *Annals of Allergy* 72(5), 462–468.

173. Max J.E., Lindgren S.D., Knutson C., Pearson C.S., Ihrig D. & Welborn A. (1998) Child and adolescent traumatic brain injury: correlates of disruptive behaviour disorders. *Brain Injury* 12(1), 41–52.

174. Accardo P. (1999) A rational approach to the medical assessment of the child with attention-deficit/hyperactivity disorder. *Pediatric Clinics of North America* 46(5), 845–856, v.

175. Blackman J.A. (1999) Attention-deficit/hyperactivity disorder in preschoolers. Does it exist and should we treat it? *Pediatric Clinics of North America* 46(5), 1011–1025.

176. American Psychological Association (1994) *Diagnostic and Statistical Manual of Mental Disorders (DSM-IV)*, 4th edition. Washington, DC, American Psychiatric Press.

177. Pliszka S.R. (2000) Patterns of psychiatric comorbidity with attention-deficit/hyperactivity disorder. *Child and Adolescent Psychiatric Clinics of North America* 9(3), 525–540, vii.

178. Searight H.R., Rottnek F. & Abby S.L. (2001) Conduct disorder: diagnosis and treatment in primary care. *American Family Physician* 63(8), 1579–1588.

179. Faraone S.V. & Biederman J. (1997) Do attention deficit hyperactivity disorder and depression share familial risk factors? *Journal of Nervous and Mental Disorders* 185(9), 533–541.

180. Spencer T., Biederman J. & Wilens T. (1999) Attention-deficit/hyperactivity disorder and comorbidity. *Pediatric Clinics of North America* 46(5), 915–927, vii.

181. Vance A.L. & Luk E.S. (1998) Attention deficit hyperactivity disorder and anxiety: is there an association with neurodevelopmental deficits? *Australian and New Zealand Journal of Psychiatry* 32(5), 650–657.

182. Lorch E.P., Milich R. & Sanchez R.P. (1998) Story comprehension in children with ADHD. *Clinical Child and Family Psychology Review* 1(3), 163–178.

183. Shaywitz B.A., Fletcher J.M. & Shaywitz S.E. (1995) Defining and classifying learning disabilities and attention-deficit/hyperactivity disorder. *Journal of Child Neurology* 10 Suppl 1, S50–S57.

184. Chermak G.D., Hall J.W. 3rd & Musiek F.E. (1999) Differential diagnosis and management of central auditory processing disorder and attention deficit hyperactivity disorder. *Journal of American Academy of Audiology* 10(6), 289–303.

185. Damico J.S., Damico S.K. & Armstrong M.B. (1999) Attention-deficit

hyperactivity disorder and communication disorders. Issues and clinical practices. *Child and Adolescent Psychiatric Clinics of North America* 8(1), 37–60, vi.

186. Blondis T.A. (1999) Motor disorders and attention-deficit/hyperactivity disorder. *Pediatric Clinics of North America* 46(5), 899–913, vi–vii.

187. Pineda D., Ardila A., Rosselli M., Cadavid C., Mancheno S. & Mejia S. (1998) Executive dysfunctions in children with attention deficit hyperactivity disorder. *International Journal of Neuroscience* 96(3–4), 177–196. [Colombia.]

188. Janzen T., Graap K., Stephanson S. *et al.* (1995) Differences in baseline EEG measures for ADD and normally achieving preadolescent males. *Biofeedback and Self Regulation* 20(1), 65.

189. Comings D.E. (1993) Serotonin and the biochemical genetics of alcoholism: lessons from studies of attention deficit hyperactivity disorder (ADHD) and Tourette syndrome. *Alcohol* Suppl 2, 237–241.

190. Stratton J. & Gailfus D. (1998) A new approach to substance abuse treatment. Adolescents and adults with ADHD. *Journal of Substance Abuse and Treatment* 15(2), 89–94.

191. DiScala C., Lescohier I., Barthel M. & Li G. (1998) Injuries to children with attention deficit hyperactivity disorder. *Pediatrics* 102(6), 1415–1421.

192. Wilens T.E. & Spencer T.J. (2000) The stimulants revisited. *Child and Adolescent Psychiatric Clinics of North America* 9(3), 573–603, viii.

193. Greenhill L.L. (1992) Pharmacologic treatment of attention deficit hyperactivity disorder, pediatric psychopharmacology. *Psychiatric Clinics of North America* 15, 1.

194. Bennett F.C., Brown R.T., Craver J. & Anderson D. (1999) Stimulant medication for the child with attention-deficit/hyperactivity disorder. *Pediatric Clinics of North America* 46(5), 929–944, vii.

195. Biederman J. *et al.* (1989) A double-blind placebo controlled study of desipramine in the treatment of ADD. I. Efficacy. *Journal of American Academy of Child and Adolescent Psychiatry* 28, 777.

196. Casat C.D., Pleasants D.Z., Schroeder D.H. & Parler D.W. (1989) Bupropion in children with attention deficit disorder. *Psychopharmacology Bulletin* 25(2), 198.

197. Chen S.W. & Vidt D.G. (1989) Patient acceptance of transdermal clonidine: a retrospective review of 25 patients. *Cleveland Clinical Journal of Medicine* 56(10), 21.

198. Dulcan M.K. (1990) Using psychostimulants to treat behavioral disorders of children and adolescents. *Journal of Child and Adolescent Psychopharmacology* 1, 7.

199. Ghuman J.K., Ginsburg G.S., Subramaniam G., Ghuman H.S., Kau A.S. & Riddle M.A. (2001) Psychostimulants in preschool children with attention-deficit/hyperactivity disorder: clinical evidence from a developmental disorders institution. *Journal of American Academy of Child and Adolescent Psychiatry* 40(5), 516–524.

200. Shevell M. & Schreiber R. (1997) Pemoline-associated hepatic failure: a critical analysis of the literature. *Pediatric Neurology* 16(1), 14–16.

201. Kappagoda C., Schell D.N., Hanson R.M. & Hutchins P. (1998) Clonidine overdose in childhood: implications of increased prescribing. *Journal of Pediatric and Child Health* 34(6), 508–512.

202. Connor D.F., Fletcher K.E. & Swanson J.M. (1999) A meta-analysis of clonidine for symptoms of attention-deficit hyperactivity disorder. *Journal of American Academy of Child and Adolescent Psychiatry* 38(12), 1551–1559.

203. Abikoff H. (1991) Cognitive training in ADHD children: less to it than meets the eye. *Journal of Learning Disabilities* 24, 205.

204. Abikoff H. & Gittleman R. (1985) Hyperactive children treated with stimulants: is cognitive training a useful adjunct? *Archives of General Psychiatry* 42, 953.

205. Brown R.T., Wynne M.E. & Medenis R. (1985) Methylphenidate and cognitive therapy: a comparison of treatmet approaches with hyperactive boys. *Journal of Abnormal Child Psychology* 13, 69.

206. Ialongo N.S. *et al.* (1993) The effects of a multimodal intervention with attention deficit hyperactivity disorder children: a 9-month follow-up. *Journal of American Academy of Child and Adolescent Psychiatry* 32(1), 182.

207. Jensen P.S., Hinshaw S.P., Swanson J.M. et al. (2001) Findings from the NIMH Multimodal Treatment Study of ADHA (MTA): implications and applications for primary care providers. *Journal of Developmental and Behavioral Pediatrics* 22(1), 60–73.

208. Lawrence J.D., Lawrence D.B. & Carson B.S. (1997) Optimizing ADHD therapy with sustained release methylphenidate. *American Family Physician* 55(5), 1705.

209. Bennett D.S., Power T.J., Rostain A.L. & Carr D.E. (1996) Parent acceptability and feasibility of ADHD intervention, assessment, correlates, and predictive validity. *Journal of Pediatric Psychiatry* 21, 643.

210. Power T.J., Hess L.E. & Bennett D.S. (1995) The acceptability of interventions for attention deficit hyperactivity disorder among elementary and middle school teachers. *Journal of Developmental and Behavioral Pediatrics* 16, 238.

211. Sun Y., Wang Y., Qu X., Wang J., Fang J. & Zhang L. (1994) Clinical observation and treatment of hyperkinesia in children by traditional Chinese medicine. *Journal of Traditional Chinese Medicine* 14(2), 105–109.

212. Zhang H. & Huang J. (1990) Preliminary study of traditional Chinese medicine treatment of minimal brain dysfunction: analysis of 100 cases. *Zhong Xi Yi Jie He Za Zhi* 10(5), 278–279, 260. [Article in Chinese]

213. Arnold L.E. (2001) Alternative treatments for adults with attention-deficit hyperactivity disorder (ADHD). *Annals of New York Academy of Science* 931, 310–341.

214. Loo M., Naeser M.A., Hinshaw S. & Bay R.B. Laser acupuncture treatment for ADHD. NIH grant #1 RO3 MH56009–01.

215. Pinyerd B.J. (1992) Strategies for consoling the infant with colic: fact or fiction? *Journal of Pediatric Nursing* 7(6), 403–411.

216. Barr R.G. (1998) Crying in the first year of life: good news in the midst of distress. *Child Care Health and Development* 24(5), 425–439.

217. Jordan N.B. & Lugo C.E. (1990) Infant Colic. [Abstract. Article in Spanish] *Boletin—Asociacion Medica de Puerto Rico.* 82(7), 302–306.

218. Colon A.R. & DiPalma J.S. (1989) Colic. Removal of cows' milk protein from the diet eliminates colic in 30% of infants. *American Family Physician* 40(6), 122–124.

219. James-Roberts I.S., Conroy S. & Wilsher K. (1996) Bases for maternal perceptions of infant crying and colic behavior. *Archives of Diseases of Children* 75(5), 375–384.

220. Keefe M.R., Kotzer A.M., Froese-Fretz A. & Curtin M. (1996) A longitudinal comparison of irritable and nonirritable infants. *Nursing Research* 45(1), 4–9.

221. Hewson P., Oberklaid F. & Menahem, S. (1987) Infant colic, distress, and crying. *Clinical Pediatrics* 26(92), 69–76.

222. Walker A.M. & Menahem S. (1994) Normal early infant behavior patterns. *Journal of Pediatric and Child Health* 30(3), 260–262.

223. Canivet C., Jakobsson I. & Hagander B. (2000) Infantile colic. Follow-up at four years of age: still more "emotional". *Acta Paediatrica* 89(1), 13–17.

224. Stagnara J., Blanc J.P., Danjou G., Simon-Ghediri M.J. & Durr F. (1997) Clinical data on the diagnosis of colic in infants. Survey in 2773 infants aged 15–119 days. *Archives of Pediatrics* 4(10), 959–966.

225. Lehtonen L., Korvenranta H. & Eerola E. (1994) Intestinal microflora in colicky and noncolicky infants: bacterial cultures and gas-liquid chromatography. *Journal of Pediatric Gastroenterology and Nutrition* 19(3), 310–314.

226. Newman J. (1990) Breastfeeding problems associated with the early introduction of bottles and pacifiers. *Journal of Human Lactation* 6(2), 59–63.

227. Jakobsson I. & Lindberg T. (1978) Cows' milk as a cause of infantile colic in breast-fed infants. *Lancet* 2(8087), 437–439.

228. Jakobsson I. & Lindberg T. (1983) Cows' milk proteins cause infantile colic in breast-fed infants: a double-blind crossover study. *Pediatrics* 71(2), 268–271.

229. Jenkins G.H. (1981) Milk-drinking mothers with colicky babies. *Lancet* 2(8240), 261.

230. Gerrard J.W. (1984) Allergies in breastfed babies to foods ingested by the mother. *Clinical Reviews on Allergy* 2(2), 143–149.

231. Jacobson D. & Melvin N. (1995) A comparison of temperament and maternal bother in infants with and without colic. *Journal of Pediatric Nursing* 10(3), 181–188.

232. Lehtonen L., Korhonen T. & Korvenranta H. (1994) Temperament and sleeping patterns in colicky infants during the first year of life. *Journal of Developmental and Behavioral Pediatrics* 15(6), 416–420.

233. Miller A.R., Barr R.G. & Eaton W.O. (1993) Crying and motor behavior of six-week-old infants and postpartum maternal mood. *Pediatrics* 92(4), 551–558.

234. Crowcroft N.S. & Strachan D.P. (1997) The social origins of infantile colic: questionnaire study covering 76 747 infants. *British Medical Journal* 314(7090), 1325–1328.

235. McKenzie S. (1991) Troublesome crying in infants: effect of advice to reduce stimulation. *Archives of Diseases of Children* 66(12), 1416–1420.

236. Stifter C.A. & Bono M.A. (1998) The effect of infant colic on maternal self-perceptions and mother–infant attachment. *Child Care Health Development* 24(5), 339–351.

237. Menahem S. (1978) The crying baby—why colic? *Australian Family Physician* 7(10), 1262–1266.

238. Pauli-Pott U., Becker K., Mertesacker T. & Beckmann D. (2000) Infants with "colic"—mothers' perspectives on the crying problem. *Journal of Psychosomatic Research* 48(2), 125–132.

239. Levitzky S. & Cooper R. (2000) Infant colic syndrome—maternal fantasies of aggression and infanticide. *Clinical Pediatrics* 39(7), 395–400.

240. Rautava P., Helenius H. & Lehtonen L. (1993) Psychosocial predisposing factors for infantile colic. *British Medical Journal* 307(6904), 600–604.

241. Raiha H., Lehtonen L., Korhonen T. & Korvenranta H. (1997) Family functioning 3 years after infantile colic. *Journal of Developmental and Behavioral Pediatrics* 18(5), 290–294.

242. Cao J. et al. (1990) *Essentials of Traditional Chinese Pediatrics*. Beijing, Foreign Language Press.

243. Diagnosis and Treatment of Gynecology and Pediatrics. In *China Zhenjiuology, A Series of Teaching Videotapes,* coproduced by Chinese Medical Audio-Video Organization and Meditalent Enterprises Ltd.

244. Flaws B. (1997) *A Handbook of TCM Pediatrics, A Practitioner's Guide to the Care and Treatment of Common Childhood Diseases*. Denver, Blue Poppy Press.

245. Scott J. (1991) *Acupuncture in the Treatment of Children*. London, Eastland Press.

246. Friedlaender M.H. (1995) A review of the causes and treatment of bacterial and allergic conjunctivitis. *Clinical Therapeutics* 17(5), 800–810, discussion 779.

247. Howes D.S. (1988) The red eye. *Emergency Medical Clinics of North America* 6(1), 43–56.

248. Joss J.D. & Craig T.J. (1999) Seasonal allergic conjunctivitis: overview and treatment update. *Journal of American Osteopathic Association* 99(7 Suppl), S13–S18.

249. Perdomo de Ponce D., Uribe M. & Wolff I. (1990) Allergic and nonallergic rhinitis: their characterization in a tropical environment. *Investigacion Clinica* 31(3), 129–138. [Abstract. Article in Italian]

250. Nezabudkin S.N., Kachan A.T., Fedoseev G.B. & Gamaiunov K.P. (1992) The reflexotherapy of patients with respiratory allergoses. *Teraperticheskii Arkhiv* 64(1), 64–67. [Article in Russian]

251. Deng S.F. (1985) Treatment and prevention of fulminant red-eye by acupuncture and bloodletting. *Journal of Traditional Chinese Medicine* 5(4), 263–264.

252. Ellis E., Wiseman N. & Boss K. (1991) *Fundamentals of Chinese Acupuncture*, revised edition. Brookline, Paradigm Publications.

253. Maciocia G. (1989) *The Foundations of Chinese Medicine, a Comprehensive Text for Acupuncturists and Herbalists*. London, Churchill Livingstone.

254. Baker S.S., Liptak G.S., Colletti R.B., Croffie J.M., Di Lorenzo C., Ector W. & Nurko S. (1999) Constipation in infants and children: evaluation and treatment. A medical position statement of the North American Society for Pediatric Gastroenterology and Nutrition. *Journal of Pediatric Gastroenterology and Nutrition* 29(5), 612–626.

255. Roy C.C., Silverman A. & Alagille D. (1995) *Pediatric Clinical Gastroenterology*, 4th edition. New York, Mosby.

256. Loening-Baucke V. (1994) Management of chronic constipation in infants and toddlers. *American Family Physician* 49(2), 397–400, 403–406, 411–413.

257. Messina M., Meucci D., Di Maggio G., Garzi A., Lagana C. & Tota G. (2000) Idiopathic constipation in children, 10-year experience. *Pediatria Medica Chirugira* 21(4), 187–191. [Abstract. Article in Italian]

258. Nurko S. (2000) Advances in the management of pediatric constipation. *Current Gastroenterology Reports* 2(3), 234–240.

259. LaFranchi S. (1987) Diagnosis and treatment of hypothyroidism in children. *Comprehensive Therapy* 13(10), 20–30.

260. Hirschman G.H., Rao D.D., Oyemade O. & Chan J.C. (1976) Renal tubular acidosis: practical guides to diagnosis and treatment. *Clinical Pediatrics (Philadelphia)* 15(7), 645–650.

261. Loening-Baucke V. (1996) Encopresis and soiling. *Pediatric Clinics of North America* 43(1), 279–298.

262. Brooks R.C., Copen R.M., Cox D.J., Morris J., Borowitz S. & Sutphen J. (2000) Review of the treatment literature for encopresis, functional constipation, and stool-toileting refusal. *Annals of Behavioral Medicine* 22(3), 260–267.

263. Loening-Baucke V. (1995) Functional constipation. *Seminars in Pediatric Surgery* 4(1), 26–34.

264. Koletzko S. (1993) Constipation in childhood—from the pediatric viewpoint. *Kinderarztliche Praxis* 61(7–8), 245–249. [Abstract. Article in German]

265. Loening-Baucke V. (1994) Constipation in children. *Current Opinion in Pediatrics* 6(5), 556–561.

266. Marty T.L., Seo T., Matlak M.E., Sullivan J.J., Black R.E. & Johnson D.G. (1995) Gastrointestinal function after surgical correction of Hirschsprung's disease: long-term follow-up in 135 patients. *Journal of Pediatric Surgery* 30(5), 655–658.

267. Griffin G.C., Roberts S.D. & Graham G. (1999) How to resolve stool retention in a child. Underwear soiling is not a behavior problem. *Postgraduate Medicine* 105(1), 159–161, 165–166, 172–173.

268. Broide E., Pintov S., Portnoy S., Barg J., Klinowski E. & Scapa E. (2001) Effectiveness of acupuncture for treatment of childhood constipation. *Digestive Diseases and Sciences* 46(6), 1270–1275.

269. Khasaev K.M., Svarich V.G. & Kopylov S.M. (1993) A rehabilitative method for children operated on for Hirschsprung's disease. *Vestnik Khirurgii Imeni II Grekova* 150(1–2), 71–73. [Abstract. Article in Russian]

270. *English-Chinese Encyclopedia of Practical Traditional Chinese Medicine*, volumes 1–14, 1990. Beijing, Higher Education Press.

271. Helms J. (1995) *Acupuncture Energetics, A Clinical Approach for Physicians.* Berkeley, Medical Acupuncture Publishers.

272. Loo M. (1999) Alternative therapies in children. In Spencer *et al. Complementary/Alternative Medicine, An Evidence-Based Approach.* St Louis, Mosby.

273. *Nei Ching, The Yellow Emperor's Classic of Internal Medicine,* translated by Ilza Veith (1949) Berkeley, University of California Press.

274. O'Connor J. & Bensky, D (eds) (1981) *Acupuncture, A Comprehensive Text.* Seattle, Eastland Press.

275. Scowen P. (2000) Nappy rash: let's give mothers more help. *Professional Care of Mother and Child.* 10(1), 26–28, 30.

276. Boiko S. (1999) Treatment of diaper dermatitis. *Dermatology Clinic.* 17(1), 235–240.

277. Odio M. & Friedlander S.F. (2000) Dermatitis and advances in diaper technology. *Current Opinions in Pediatrics.* 12(4), 342–346.

278. Chosidow O., Lebrun-Vignes B. & Bourgault-Villada I. (1999) Local corticosteroid therapy in dermatology. *Presse Medicale* 28(37), 2050–2056. [Abstract. Article in French]

279. Singleton J.K. (1997) Pediatric dermatoses, three common skin disruptions in infancy. *Nurse Practitioner* 22(6), 32–33, 37, 43–44.

280. Northrup R.S. & Flanigan T.P. (1994) Gastroenteritis. *Pediatrics in Review* 15, 461–472.

281. Marbet U.A. (1994) Diagnosis and therapy of diarrhea. *Schweizerische Medizinische Wochenschrift* 124(11), 439–451. [Abstract. Article in German]

282. Guerrant R.L. *et al.* (2001) Practice guidelines for the management of infectious diarrhea. Infectious Diseases Society of America. *Clinical Infectious Diseases* 32, 331–350.

283. Oguz F., Sidal M., Uzel N., Ugur S., Suoglu O., Kartoglu U. & Nezyi O. (1994) The impact of systematic use of oral rehydration therapy on outcome in acute diarrheal disease in children. *Pediatric Emergency Care* 10(6), 326–329.

284. Thompson S.C. (1994) Infectious diarrhoea in children: controlling transmission in the child care setting. *Journal of Pediatric Child Health* 30(3), 210–219.

285. Laney D.W. Jr, & Cohen M.B. (1993) Approach to the pediatric patient with diarrhea. *Gastroenterology Clinics of North America* 22(3), 499–516.

286. Walter J.E. & Mitchell D.K. (2000) Role of astroviruses in childhood diarrhea. *Current Opinion in Pediatrics* 12(3), 275–279.

287. DeWitt T.G. (1989) Acute diarrhea in children. *Pediatrics in Review* 11(1), 6–13.

288. Koutkia P., Mylonakis E. & Flanigan T. (1997) Enterohemorrhagic *Escherichia coli* O157: H7—an emerging pathogen. *American Family Physician* 56(3), 853–856, 859–861.

289. Trachtman H. & Christen E. (1999) Pathogenesis, treatment, and therapeutic trials in hemolytic uremic syndrome. *Current Opinion in Pediatrics* 11(2), 162–168.

290. Hart C.A., Batt R.M. & Saunders J.R. (1993) Diarrhoea caused by *Escherichia coli*. *Annals of Tropical Pediatrics* 13(2), 121–131.

291. Hjelt K., Paerregaard A. & Krasilnikoff P.A. (1993) Giardiasis in children with chronic diarrhea. Incidence, growth, clinical symptoms and changes in the small intestine. *Ugeskr Laeger* 155(50), 4083–4086. [Abstract. Article in Danish]

292. Liebelt E.L. (1998) Clinical and laboratory evaluation and management of children with vomiting, diarrhea, and dehydration. *Current Opinions in Pediatrics* 10(5), 461–469.

293. Gracey M. (1999) Nutritional effects and management of diarrhoea in infancy. *Acta Pediatria* Suppl 88(430), 110–126.

294. Schmitz J. (1999) Anti-rotavirus vaccinations. *Archives of Pediatrics* 6(9), 979–984. [Abstract. Article in French]

295. Meyers A. (1995) Modern management of acute diarrhea and dehydration in children. *American Family Physician* 51(5), 1103–1118.

296. Roncoroni A.J. Jr, de Cortigianni M.R. & Garcia Damiano M.C. (1989) Cost and effectiveness of fecal culture in the etiologic diagnosis of acute diarrhea. *Boletin de la Oficina Sanitaria Panamericana* 107(5), 381–387. [Abstract. Article in Spanish]

297. de Sousa J.S. (1996) Acute infectious diarrhea in children. *Acta Medica Portuguesa* 9(10–12), 347–352. [Abstract. Article in Portuguese]

298. Bernstein D.I., Glass R.I., Rodgers G. et al. (1995) Evaluation of rhesus rotavirus monovalent and tetravalent reassortant vaccines in US children. *Journal of the American Medical Association* 273, 1191–1196.

299. McFarland L.V. (1999) Microecologic approaches for traveler's diarrhea, antibiotic-associated diarrhea, and acute pediatric diarrhea. *Current Gastroenterology Reports* 1(4), 301–307.

300. Paerregaard A., Hjelt K. & Krasilnikoff P.A. (1990) Vitamin B12 and folic acid absorption and hematological status in children with postenteritis enteropathy. *Journal of Pediatrics Gastroenterology and Nutrition* 11(3), 351–355.

301. Stern M. (1989) Secondary carbohydrate and protein intolerances following gastroenteritis. *Monatsschrift fur Kinderheilkde* 137(9), 585–589. [Abstract. Article in German]

302. Davidson G.P. & Robb T.A. (1985) Value of breath hydrogen analysis in management of diarrheal illness in childhood: comparison with duodenal biopsy. *Journal of Pediatric Gastroenterology and Nutrition* 4(3), 381–387.

303. Davidson G.P., Robb T.A. & Kirubakaran C.P. (1984) Bacterial contamination of the small intestine as an important cause of chronic diarrhea and abdominal pain: diagnosis by breath hydrogen test. *Pediatrics* 74(2), 229–235.

304. Fenton T.R., Harries J.T. & Milla P.J. (1983) Disordered small intestinal motility: a rational basis for toddlers' diarrhoea. *Gut* 24(10), 897–903.

305. Hugot J.P. & Cezard J.P. (1998) Diarrhea in children. *Rev Prat* 48(4), 382–388. [Article in French]

306. Mehta D.I. & Blecker U. (1998) Chronic diarrhea in infancy and childhood. *Journal of the Louisiana State Medical Society* 150(9), 419–429.

307. Leung A.K. & Robson W.L. (1996) Evaluating the child with chronic diarrhea. *American Family Physician* 53(2), 635–643.

308. Baldassano R.N. & Liacouras C.A. (1991) Chronic diarrhea. A practical approach for the pediatrician. *Pediatric Clinics of North America* 38(3), 667–686.

309. Rudolph J.A. & Cohen M.B. (1999) New causes and treatments for infectious diarrhea in children. *Current Gastroenterology Reports* 1(3), 238–244.

310. Cervetto J.L., Ramonet M., Nahmod L.H. & Gallardo F. (1987) Giardiasis. Functional, immunological and histological study of the small bowel. Therapeutic trial with a single dose of tinidazole. *Arquives de Gastroenterologia* 24(2), 102–112. [Abstract]

311. Ansaldi N., Villata L., Santini B., Fantino N., Robazza V., Ciervo T., Barbera C., Elia G. & Oderda G. (1987) Irritable bowel syndrome in children. *Pediatria Medica Chirugica* 9(4), 453–459. [Abstract. Article in Italian]

312. Hambidge K.M. (1992) Zinc and diarrhea. *Acta Paediatrica* Suppl 381, 82–86.

313. Poole S.R. (1982) Irritable colon syndrome of infancy. *American Family Physician* 26(3), 127–131.

314. Bonamico M., Culasso F., Colombo C. & Giunta A.M. (1995) Irritable bowel syndrome in children: an Italian multicentre study. Collaborating Centres. *Italian Journal of Gastroenterology* 27(1), 13–20. [Abstract. Article in Italian]

315. Greene H.L. & Ghishan F.K. (1983) Excessive fluid intake as a cause of chronic diarrhea in young children. *Journal of Pediatrics* 102(6), 836–840.

316. Kneepkens C.M. & Hoekstra J.H. (1996) Chronic nonspecific diarrhea of childhood: pathophysiology and management. *Pediatric Clinics of North America*. 43(2), 375–390.

317. Rasquin-Weber A., Hyman P.E., Cucchiara S., Fleisher D.R., Hyams J.S., Milla P.J. & Staiano A. (1999) Childhood functional gastrointestinal disorders. *Gut* 45 Suppl 2, II60–II68. Review.

318. Montes R.G. & Perman J.A. (1991) Lactose intolerance: Pinpointing the source of nonspecific gastrointestinal symptoms. *Postgraduate Medicine* 89, 175–184.

319. Hoekstra J.H., van den Aker J.H., Ghoos Y.F., Hartemink R. & Kneepkens C.M. (1995) Fluid intake and industrial processing in apple juice induced chronic non-specific diarrhoea. *Archives of Diseases of Children* 73(2), 126–130.

320. Dennison B.A. (1996) Fruit juice consumption by infants and children: a review. *Journal of the American College of Nutrition* 15 (5 Suppl), 4S–11S.

321. Smith M.M. & Lifshitz F. (1994) Excess fruit juice consumption as a contributing factor in nonorganic failure to thrive. *Pediatrics* 93(3), 438–443.

322. Ament M.E. (1996) Malabsorption of apple juice and pear nectar in infants and children: clinical implications. *Journal of the American College of Nutrition* 15 (5 Suppl), 26S–29S.

323. Panizon F. (1987) Food allergy and psychosomatic medicine. New frontiers. *Pediatria Medica Chirugica* 9(6), 671–677. [Abstract. Article in Italian]

324. Perlmutter D.H., Leichtner A.M., Goldman H. & Winter H.S. (1985) Chronic diarrhea associated with hypogammaglobulinemia and enteropathy in infants and children. *Digestive Diseases and Sciences* 30(12), 1149–1155.

325. Boehm P., Nassimbeni G. & Ventura A. (1998) Chronic non-specific diarrhoea in childhood: how often is it iatrogenic? *Acta Pediatrica* 87(3), 268–271.

326. Lin Y.C. (1987) Observation of the therapeutic effects of acupuncture treatment in 170 cases of infantile diarrhea. *Journal of Traditional Chinese Medicine* 7(3), 203–204.

327. Feng W.L. (1989) Acupuncture treatment for 30 cases of infantile chronic diarrhea. *Journal of Traditional Chinese Medicine* 9(2), 106–107.

328. Jiang R. (1990) Analgesic effect of acupuncture on acute intestinal colic in 190 cases. *Journal of Traditional Chinese Medicine* 10(1), 20–21.

329. Su Z. (1992) Acupuncture treatment of infantile diarrhea: a report of 1050 cases. *Journal of Traditional Chinese Medicine* 12(2), 120–121.

330. Xu J.H., Lin L.H. & Zhang P.Y. (1996) [Treatment of infantile diarrhea with anisodamine by the injection method of Zu San Li acupuncture points.] *Zhonghua Hu Li Za Zhi* 31(6), 345–346. [Abstract. Article in Chinese]

331. Lin Y., Zhou Z. *et al.* (1993) Clinical and experimental studies on shallow needling technique for treating childhood diarrhea. *Journal of Traditional Chinese Medicine* 13(2), 107–114.

332. Fan, Y.L. (1994) *Chinese Pediatric Massage Therapy, A Parent's and Practitioner's Guide to the Treatment*

and Prevention of Childhood Disease. Denver, Blue Poppy Press.

333. O'Dwyer T.P. & Conlon B.J. (1997) The surgical management of drooling—a 15 year follow-up. Clinical Otolaryngology 22(3), 284–287.

334. Sochaniwsky A.E., Koheil R.M., Bablich K., Milner M. & Kenny D.J. (1986) Oral motor functioning, frequency of swallowing and drooling in normal children and in children with cerebral palsy. Archive of Physical Medicine and Rehabilitation 67(12), 866–874.

335. Lespargot A., Langevin M.F., Muller S. & Guillemont S. (1993) Swallowing disturbances associated with drooling in cerebral-palsied children. Developmental Medicine and Child Neurology 35(4), 298–304.

336. Shott S.R., Myer C.M. 3rd & Cotton R.T. (1989) Surgical management of sialorrhea. Otolaryngology, Head and Neck Surgery 101(1), 47–50.

337. Talmi Y.P., Finkelstein Y., Zohar Y. & Laurian N. (1988) Reduction of salivary flow with Scopoderm TTS. Annals of Otorhinolaryngology 97(2 Pt 1), 128–130.

338. O'Dwyer T.P., Timon C. & Walsh M.A. (1989) Surgical management of drooling in the neurologically damaged child. Journal of Laryngology and Otology 103(8), 750–752.

339. Colbert A. (2001) Magnet Treatments. 1999 American Academy of Medical Acupuncture (AAMA), and personal communications.

340. Wong V., Sun J.G. & Wong W. (2001) Traditional chinese medicine (tongue acupuncture) in children with drooling problems. Pediatric Neurology 25(1), 47–54.

341. Thestrup-Pedersen K. (2000) Clinical aspects of atopic dermatitis. Clinical Experimental Dermatology 25(7), 535–543. [Article in Danish]

342. Fennessy M., Coupland S., Popay J. & Naysmith K. (2000) The epidemiology and experience of atopic eczema during childhood: a discussion paper on the implications of current knowledge for health care, public health policy and research. Journal of Epidemiology and Community Health 54(8), 581–589.

343. Kay A.B. & Lessof M.H. (1992) Allergy. Conventional and alternative concepts. A report of the Royal College of Physicians Committee on Clinical Immunology and Allergy. Clinical and Experimental Allergy 22 Suppl 3, 1–44.

344. Warner J.A. & Warner J.O. (2000) Early life events in allergic sensitisation. British Medical Bulletin 56(4), 883–893.

345. Kramer M.S. (2000) Maternal antigen avoidance during lactation for preventing atopic disease in infants of women at high risk. Cochrane Database Systematic Review (2), CD000132.

346. Lewis-Jones S. (2001) Atopic dermatitis in childhood. Hospital Medicine 62(3), 136–143.

347. Chosidow O., Lebrun-Vignes B. & Bourgault-Villada I. (1999) [Local corticosteroid therapy in dermatology]. Presse Medicale 28(37), 2050–2056. [Abstract. Article in French]

348. Lun X. & Rong L. (2000) Twenty-five cases of intractable cutaneous pruritus treated by auricular acupuncture. Journal of Traditional Chinese Medicine 20(4), 287–288.

349. Sun Y. & Wang D. (1996) Acupuncture treatment of dermopathies and pediatric diseases. Journal of Traditional Chinese Medicine 16(3), 214–217.

350. Lu S. (1993) Acupuncture and moxibustion in the treatment of dermatoses. Journal of Traditional Chinese Medicine 13(1), 69–75.

351. Liao S.J. (1988) Acupuncture for poison ivy contact dermatitis. A clinical case report. Acupuncture Electrotherapy Research 13(1), 31–39.

352. Caione P., Nappo S., Capozza N., Minni B. & Ferro F. (1994) Primary enuresis in children. Which treatment today. Minerva Pediatrica 46(10), 437–443. [Abstract. Article in Italian]

353. Chao S.M., Yap H.K., Tan A., Ong E.K., Murugasu B., Low E.H. & Tan S.P. (1997) Primary monosymptomatic nocturnal enuresis in Singapore—parental perspectives in an Asian community. Annals of the Academy of Medicine Singapore 26(2), 179–183.

354. Bhatia M.S., Dhar N.K., Rai S. & Malik S.C. (1990) Enuresis: an analysis of 82 cases. Indian Journal of Medical Sciences 44(12), 337–342.

355. Miller K. (1993) Concomitant nonpharmacologic therapy in the treatment of primary nocturnal enuresis. Clinical Pediatrics (Philadelphia) Spec No, 32–37.

356. Chiozza M.L. (1997) An update on clinical and therapeutic aspects of nocturnal enuresis. Pediatria Medica Chirugira 19(5), 385–390. [Abstract. Article in Italian]

357. Djurhuus J.C. & Rittig S. (1998)
Current trends, diagnosis, and treatment
of enuresis. *European Urology* 33 Suppl
3, 30–33.

358. Alon U.S. (1995) Nocturnal enuresis.
Pediatric Nephrology 9(1), 94–103.

359. Schwobel M. & Bodmer C. (1998)
Urodynamic studies in the child with
urinary incontinence. *Wien Medizinische
Wochenschrift* 148(22), 508–510.
[Abstract. Article in German]

360. Von Gontard A. & Lehmkuhl G. (1997)
Enuresis nocturna—new studies of
genetic, pathophysiologie and psychiatric
correlations. *Praxis der
Kinderpsychologie und
Kinderpsychiatrie* 46(10), 709–726.
[Abstract. Article in German]

361. Kelleher R.E. (1997) Daytime and
nighttime wetting in children: a review
of management. *Journal of Social
Pediatric Nursing* 2(2), 73–82.

362. MacKeith R. (1969) A frequent factor in
the etiology of enuresis. Fear in the third
year of life. *Casopis Lekaru Ceskych*
108(2), 36–37. [Article in Czech]

363. Guilleminault C. & Anders T.F. (1976)
The pathophysiology of sleep disorders
in pediatrics. Part II. Sleep disorders in
children. *Advances in Pediatrics* 22,
151–174.

364. Kales A., Soldatos C.R. & Kales J.D.
(1987) Sleep disorders: insomnia,
sleepwalking, night terrors, nightmares,
and enuresis. *Annals of Internal
Medicine* 106(4), 582–592.

365. Koff S.A. (1996) Cure of nocturnal
enuresis: why isn't desmopressin very
effective? *Pediatric Nephrology* 10(5),
667–670.

366. Maizels M., Gandhi K., Keating B. &
Rosenbaum D. (1993) Diagnosis and
treatment for children who cannot
control urination. *Current Problems in
Pediatrics* 23(10), 402–450.

367. Djurhuus J.C. (1999) Definitions of
subtypes of enuresis. *Scandinavian
Journal of Urology and Nephrology,
Supplement* 202, 5–7.

368. Brueziere J. (1992) Enuresis. *Annales de
Urologie (Paris)* 26(4), 218–224.
[Abstract. Article in French]

369. Heiliczer J.D., Canonigo B.B., Bishof
N.A. & Moore E.S. (1987) Noncalculi
urinary tract disorders secondary to
idiopathic hypercalciuria in children.
Pediatric Clinics of North America
34(3), 711–718.

370. Lettgen B. (1998) Differential diagnosis
of enuresis nocturna. *Wiener
Medizinische Wochenschrift* 148(22),
515–516. [Article in German]

371. Robson W.L. & Leung A.K. (2000)
Secondary nocturnal enuresis. *Clinical
Pediatrics (Philadelphia)* 39(7),
379–385.

372. Diamond J.M. & Stein J.M. (1983)
Enuresis: a new look at stimulant
therapy. *Canadian Journal of Psychiatry*
28(5), 395–397.

373. Hjalmas K. (1999) Desmopressin
treatment: current status. *Scandinavian
Journal of Urology and Nephrology*
Supplement 202, 70–72.

374. Kong D.S. (1995) Psychiatric disorders
in pre-schoolers. *Singapore Medical
Journal* 36(3), 318–321.

375. Hara H. (1994) Diagnosis and drug
treatment in hyperactive children. *No To
Hattatsu* 26(2), 169–174. [Abstract.
Article in Japanese]

376. Eidlitz-Markus T., Shuper A. & Amir J.
(2000) Secondary enuresis, post-
traumatic stress disorder in children after
car accidents. *Israel Medical Association
Journal* 2(2), 135–137.

377. Nowak K.C. & Weider D.J. (1998)
Pediatric nocturnal enuresis secondary to
airway obstruction from cleft palate
repair. *Clinical Pediatrics (Philadelphia)*
37(11), 653–657.

378. Warzak W.J. (1993) Psychosocial
implications of nocturnal enuresis.
Clinical Pediatrics (Philadelphia) Spec
No, 38–40.

379. Wiener J.M. (1984)
Psychopharmacology in childhood
disorders. *Psychiatric Clinics of North
America* 7(4), 831–843.

380. Roje-Starcevic M. (1990) The treatment
of nocturnal enuresis by acupuncture.
Neurologija 39(3), 179–184. [Abstract.
Text in Romanian]

381. Huo J.S. (1988) Treatment of 11 cases of
chronic enuresis by acupuncture and
massage. *Journal of Traditional Chinese
Medicine* 8(3), 195–196.

382. Yang C.P. (1988) Acupuncture of
guanyuan (Ren 4) and Baihui (Du 20) in
the treatment of 500 cases of enuresis.
Journal of Traditional Chinese Medicine
8(3), 197.

383. Chen Z. & Chen L. (1991) The
treatment of enuresis with scalp
acupuncture. *Journal of Traditional
Chinese Medicine* 11(1), 29–30.

384. Xu B. (1991) 302 cases of enuresis
treated with acupuncture. *Journal of
Traditional Chinese Medicine* 11(2),
121–122.

385. Serel T.A., Perk H., Koyuncuoglu H.R., Kosar A., Celik K. & Deniz N. (2001) Acupuncture therapy in the management of persistent primary nocturnal enuresis—preliminary results. *Scandinavican Journal of Urology and Nephrology* 35(1), 40–43.

386. Hu J. (2000) Acupuncture treatment of enuresis. *Journal of Traditional Chinese Medicine* 20(2), 158–160.

387. Bjorkstrom G., Hellstrom A.L. & Andersson S. (2000) Electro-acupuncture in the treatment of children with monosymptomatic nocturnal enuresis. *Scandinavian Journal of Urology and Nephrology* 34(1), 21–26.

388. Capozza N., Creti G., De Gennaro M., Minni B. & Caione P. (1991) The treatment of nocturnal enuresis. A comparative study between desmopressin and acupuncture used alone or in combination. *Minerva Pediatria* 43(9), 577–582. [Abstract. Article in Italian]

389. Tret'iakova E.E. & Komissarov V.I. (1990) Characteristics of the electric activity of the projection areas of the large hemispheres in children with enuresis. *Zhurnal Nevropatologii i Psikhiatrii Imeni S S Korsakova* 90(8), 41–44. [Article in Russian]

390. Minni B., Capozza N., Creti G., De Gennaro M., Caione P. & Bischko J. (1990) Bladder instability and enuresis treated by acupuncture and electro-therapeutics: early urodynamic observations. *Acupuncture Electrotherapy Research* 15(1), 19–25. [Abstract. Article in Italian]

391. Kachan A.T., Trubin M.I., Skoromets A.A. & Shmushkevich A.I. (1993) Acupuncture reflexotherapy of neurogenic bladder dysfunction in children with enuresis. *Zhurnal Nevropatologii i Psikhiatrii Imeni S S Korsakova* 93(5), 40–42. [Abstract. Article in Russian]

392. Tuzuner F., Kecik Y., Ozdemir S. & Canakci N. (1989) Electro-acupuncture in the treatment of enuresis nocturna. *Acupuncture Electrotherapy Research* 14(3–4), 211–215. [Abstract]

393. Bartocci C. & Lucentini M. (1981) Acupuncture and micro-massage in the treatment of idiopathic nocturnal enuresis. *Minerva Medica* 72(33), 2237. [Abstract. Article in Italian]

394. Feigin R.D. & Cherry J.D. (1992) *Textbook of Pediatric Infectious Diseases*, 3rd edition. Philadelphia, WB Saunders Co.

395. Cranston W.I. (1992) Central mechanisms of fever. In Feigin R.D., Cherry J.D. (eds) *Textbook of Pediatric Infectious Diseases*, 3rd edition. Philadelphia, WB Saunders Co.

396. Rajadhyaksha S. & Shah K.N. (2000) Controversies in febrile seizures. *Indian Journal of Pediatrics* 67(1 Suppl), S71–S79.

397. Bourrillon A. (1999) Management of prolonged fever in infants. *Archives of Pediatrics* 6(3), 330–335. [Abstract. Article in French]

398. Crocetti M., Moghbeli N. & Serwint J. (2001) Fever phobia revisited: have parental misconceptions about fever changed in 20 years? *Pediatrics* 107(6), 1241–1246.

399. McErlean M.A., Bartfield J.M., Kennedy D.A., Gilman E.A., Stram R.L. & Raccio-Robak N. (2001) Home antipyretic use in children brought to the emergency department. *Pediatric Emergency Care* 17(4), 249–251.

400. Li S.F., Lacher B. & Crain E.F. (2000) Acetaminophen and ibuprofen dosing by parents. *Pediatric Emergency Care* 16(6), 394–397.

401. Stamm D. (1994) Paracetamol and other antipyretic analgesics: optimal doses in pediatrics. *Archives of Pediatrics* 1(2), 193–201. [Abstract. Article in French]

402. Plaisance K.I., Kudaravalli S., Wasserman S.S., Levine M.M. & Mackowiak P.A. (2000) Effect of antipyretic therapy on the duration of illness in experimental influenza A, *Shigella sonnei*, and *Rickettsia rickettsii* infections. *Pharmacotherapy* 20(12), 1417–1422.

403. Knudsen F.U. (2001) Febrile convulsions, treatment and prognosis. *Ugeskrift for Laeger* 163(8), 1098–1102. [Abstract. Article in Danish]

404. Fang J.Q., Guo S.Y., Asano K., Yu Y., Kasahara T. & Hisamitsu T. (1998) Antipyretic action of peripheral stimulation with electroacupuncture in rats. *In Vivo* 12(5), 503–510.

405. Rogers P.A., Schoen A.M. & Limehouse J. (1992) Acupuncture for immune-mediated disorders. Literature review and clinical applications. *Problems in Veterinary Medicine* 4(1), 162–193.

406. Nezhentsev M.V. & Aleksandrov S.I. (1992) The problem of fever and its elimination in children.

Eksperimentalnaia I Klinicheskaia Farmakologiia 55(1), 58–61. [Abstract. Article in Russian]

407. Nezhentsev M.V. & Aleksandrov S.I. (1994) The current concepts of the humoral mechanisms of the analgetic and antipyretic actions of acupuncture (a review of the literature). *Sprava* (3–4), 39–42. [Abstract. Article in Russian]

408. Nezhentsev M. & Aleksandrov S. (1993) Effect of naloxone on the antipyretic action of acupuncture. *Pharmacology* 46(5), 289–293. [Abstract. Article in Russian]

409. Lin M.T., Chandra A., Chen-Yen S.M. & Chern Y.F. (1981) Stimulation of acupuncture loci Chu-Chih (LI-11) and Ho-Ku (LI-4) hypothermia effects and analgesia in normal adults. *Journal of Traditional Chinese Medicine* 9(1), 74–83.

410. Nezhentsev M.V. & Aleksandrov S.I. (1993) Evaluation of the antipyretic action of psychotropic drugs and their effect on the antipyretic effect of acupuncture therapy. *Biulleten Eksperimentalnoi Biologii I Meditsiny* 115(3), 262–264. [Abstract. Article in Russian]

411. Tan D. (1992) Treatment of fever due to exopathic wind-cold by rapid acupuncture. *Journal of Traditional Chinese Medicine* 12(4), 267–271.

412. Kuang X., Liang C., Liang Z., Lu C. & Zhong G. (1992) The effect of acupuncture on rabbits with fever caused by endotoxin. *Ci Yan Jiu* 17(3), 212–216. [Abstract. Article in Chinese]

413. Yu P., Hao X., Zhao R. & Qin M. (1992) Pasting acupoints with Chinese herbs applying in infant acute bronchitis and effect on humoral immune substances. *Zhen Ci Yan Jiu* 17(2), 110–112. [Abstract. Article in Chinese]

414. O'Neill-Murphy K., Liebman M. & Barnsteiner J.H. (2001) Fever education: does it reduce parent fever anxiety? *Pediatric Emergency Care* 17(1), 47–51.

415. Swaiman K.F. (1989) *Pediatric Neurology, Principles and Practice.* St. Louis, Mosby.

416. Szczepanik E. (2000) [Idiopathic headache in children]. *Medycyny Wieku Rozwojowego* 4(2), 185–195. [Abstract. Article in Polish]

417. Cano A. *et al.* (2000) Migraine without aura and migrainous disorder in children; International Headache Society (IHS) and revised IHS criteria. *Cephalalgia* 20(7), 617–620.

418. Winner P., Martinez W., Mate L. & Bello L. (1995) Classification of pediatric migraine: proposed revision to the IHS criteria. *Headache* 35(7), 407–410.

419. Wober-Bingol C., Wober C., Wagner-Ennsgraber C., Karwautz A., Vesely C., Zebenhoizer K. & Geldner J. (1996) IHS criteria for migraine and tension-type headache in children and adolescents. *Headache* 36(4), 231–238.

420. Metsahonkala L. & Sillanpaa M. (1994) Migraine in children—an evaluation of the IHS criteria. *Cephalalgia* 14(4), 285–290.

421. Seshia S.S., Wolstein J.R., Adams C., Booth F.A. & Reggin J.D. (1994) International headache society criteria and childhood headache. *Developmental Medicine Child Neurology* 36(5), 419–428.

422. Sanin L.C., Mathew N.T., Bellmeyer L.R. & Ali S. (1994) The International Headache Society (IHS) headache classification as applied to a headache clinic population. *Cephalalgia* 14(6), 443–446.

423. Burton L.J., Quinn B., Pratt-Cheney J.L. & Pourani M. (1997) Headache etiology in a pediatric emergency department. *Pediatric Emergency Care* 13(1), 1–4.

424. Kan L., Nagelberg J. & Maytal J. (2000) Headaches in a pediatric emergency department: etiology, imaging, and treatment. *Headache* 40(1), 25–29.

425. Wober-Bingol C., Wober C., Karwautz A. *et al.* (1995) Diagnosis of headache in childhood and adolescence: a study in 437 patients. *Cephalalgia* 15(1), 13–21.

426. Abbas A. (1989) Headache. *Practitioner* 233(1473), 1081–1082, 1084.

427. Zebenholzer K., Wober C., Kienbacher C. & Wober-Bingol C. (2000) Migrainous disorder and headache of the tension-type not fulfilling the criteria: a follow-up study in children and adolescents. *Cephalalgia* 20(7), 611–616.

428. Niczyporuk-Turek A. (1997) Factors contributing to so-called idiopathic headaches. *Neurologia i Neurochirugia Polska* 31(5), 895–904. [Abstract. Article in Polish]

429. Gervil M. (1997) Headache in children. *Ugeskrift for Laeger* 159(18), 2680–2685. [Article in Danish]

430. Silberstein S.D. (1990) Twenty questions about headaches in children and adolescents. *Headache* 30(11), 716–724.

431. Lipton R.B., Goadsby P. & Silberstein S.D. (1999) Classification and epidemiology of headache. *Clinical Cornerstone* 1(6), 1–10.

432. Wober C. & Wober-Bingol C. (2000) Clinical management of young patients presenting with headache. *Functional Neurology* 15 Suppl 3, 89–105.

433. Winner P.K. (1997) Headaches in children. When is a complete diagnostic workup indicated? *Postgraduate Medicine* 101(5), 81–85, 89–90.

434. Fichtel A. & Larsson B. (2001) Does relaxation treatment have differential effects on migraine and tension-type headache in adolescents? *Headache* 41(3), 290–296.

435. Bischko J.J. (1978) Acupuncture in headache. *Research Clinical Studies in Headache* 5, 72–85.

436. Melchart D., Linde K., Fischer P., Berman B., White A., Vickers A. & Allais G. (2001) Acupuncture for idiopathic headache (Cochrane Review). *Cochrane Database* 1, CD001218.

437. Dowson D.I., Lewith G.T. & Machin D. (1985) The effects of acupuncture versus placebo in the treatment of headache. *Pain* 21(1), 35–42.

438. Loh L., Nathan P.W., Schott G.D. & Zilkha K.J. (1984) Acupuncture versus medical treatment for migraine and muscle tension headaches. *Journal of Neurology, Neurosurgery, and Psychiatry* 47(4), 333–337.

439. Vesnina V.A. (1980) Current methods of migraine reflexotherapy. *Zhurnal Nevropatologii i Psikhiatrii Imeni SS Korsakova* 80(5), 703–709. [Article in Russian]

440. White A.R., Resch K.L., Chan J.C., Norris C.D., Modi S.K., Patel J.N. & Ernst E. (2000) Acupuncture for episodic tension-type headache: a multicentre randomized controlled trial. *Cephalalgia* 20(7), 632–637.

441. Tavola T., Gala C., Conte G. & Invernizzi G. (1992) Traditional Chinese acupuncture in tension-type headache: a controlled study. *Pain* 48(3), 325–329.

442. Wright M.S. (1995) Update on pediatric trauma care. *Current Opinion in Pediatrics* 7(3), 292–296.

443. Savitsky E.A. & Votey S.R. (2000) Current controversies in the management of minor pediatric head injuries. *American Journal of Emergency Medicine* 18(1), 96–101.

444. Mitchell K.A., Fallat M.E., Raque G.H., Hardwick V.G., Groff D.B. & Nagaraj H.S. (1994) Evaluation of minor head injury in children. *Journal of Pediatric Surgery* 29(7), 851–854.

445. Reece R.M. & Sege R. (2000) Childhood head injuries: accidental or inflicted? *Archives of Pediatric and Adolescent Medicine* 154(1), 11–15.

446. Gruskin K.D. & Schutzman S.A. (1999) Head trauma in children younger than 2 years: are there predictors for complications? *Archives of Pediatric and Adolescent Medicine* 153(1), 15–20.

447. Vera M., Fleisher G.R., Barnes P.D., Bjornson B.H., Allred E.N. & Goldmann D.A. (1993) Computed tomography imaging in children with head trauma: utilization and appropriateness from a quality improvement perspective. *Infection Control and Hospital Epidemiology* 14(8), 491–499.

448. Gallai V., Sarchielli P., Carboni F., Benedetti P., Mastropaolo C. & Puca F. (1995) Applicability of the 1988 IHS criteria to headache patients under the age of 18 years attending 21 Italian headache clinics. Juvenile Headache Collaborative Study Group. *Headache* 35(3), 146–153.

449. Annequin D., Dumas C., Tourniaire B. & Massiou H. (2000) [Migraine and chronic headache in children]. *Revue Neurologique (Paris)* 156, 4S68–4S74. [Abstract. Article in French]

450. Annequin D., Tourniaire B. & Dumas C. (2000) Migraine, misunderstood pathology in children. *Archives of Pediatrics* 7(9), 985–990. [Abstract. Article in French]

451. Peroutka S.J. (1997) Dopamine and migraine. *Neurology* 49(3), 650–656.

452. Spierings E.L. (2001) Mechanism of migraine and action of antimigraine medications. *Medical Clinics of North America* 85(4), 943–958, vi–vii.

453. Del Zompo M. (2000) Dopaminergic hypersensitivity in migraine: clinical and genetic evidence. *Functional Neurology* 15 Suppl 3, 163–170.

454. Di Piero V., Bruti G., Venturi P., Talamonti F., Biondi M., Di Legge S. & Lenzi G.L. (2001) Aminergic tone correlates of migraine and tension-type headache: a study using the tridimensional personality questionnaire. *Headache* 41(1): 63–71.

455. Markelova V.F., Tauleuv A.M., Belitskaia R.A. & Kozina G.S. (1982) Effect of reflexotherapy on catecholamine excretion in migraine.

Soviet Medicine (2), 59–63. [Abstract. Article in Russian]

456. Markelova V.F., Vesnina V.A., Malygina S.I. & Dubovskaia L.A. (1984) Changes in blood serotonin levels in patients with migraine headaches before and after a course of reflexotherapy *Zhurnal Nevropatologii Psikhiatrii i Imeni S S Korsakova* 84(9), 1313–1316. [Abstract. Article in Russian]

457. Peroutka S.J. (1998) Beyond monotherapy: rational polytherapy in migraine. *Headache* 38(1), 18–22.

458. Ferrari M.D. (1992) Biochemistry of migraine. *Pathologie Biologie (Paris)* 40(4), 287–292.

459. Mascia A., Afra J. & Schoenen J. (1998) Dopamine and migraine: a review of pharmacological, biochemical, neurophysiological, and therapeutic data. *Cephalalgia* 18(4), 174–182.

460. Fanciullacci M., Alessandri M. & Del Rosso A. (2000) Dopamine involvement in the migraine attack. *Functional Neurology* 15 Suppl 3, 171–181.

461. Barth N., Riegels M., Hebebrand J. & Remschmidt H. (2000) "Cyclic vomiting" in childhood and adolescence. *Zeitschrift fur Kinder- und Jugendpsychiatrie und Psychotherapie* 28(2), 109–117. [Abstract. Article in German]

462. Rashed H., Abell T.L., Familoni B.O. & Cardoso S. (1999) Autonomic function in cyclic vomiting syndrome and classic migraine. *Digestive Diseases and Sciences* 44(8 Suppl), 74S–78S.

463. Guitera V., Gutierrez E., Munoz P., Castillo J. & Pascual J. (2001) Personality changes in chronic daily headache: a study in the general population. *Neurologia* 16(1), 11–16. [Abstract. Article in Spanish]

464. Schafer M.L., Lautenbacher S. & Postberg-Flesch C. (2000) New investigations on the melancholic type personality structure in migraine patients. *Nervenarzt* 71(7), 573–579. [Abstract. Article in German]

465. Hassinger H.J., Semenchuk E.M. & O'Brien W.H. (1999) Appraisal and coping responses to pain and stress in migraine headache sufferers. *Journal of Behavioral Medicine* 22(4), 327–340.

466. Guillem E., Pelissolo A. & Lepine J.P. (1999) Mental disorders and migraine: epidemiologic studies. *Encephale* 25(5), 436–442. [Abstract. Article in French]

467. Lanzi G., Zambrino C.A., Ferrari-Ginevra O., Termine C., D'Arrigo S.,

Vercelli P., De Silvestri A. & Guglielmino C.R. (2001) Personality traits in childhood and adolescent headache. *Cephalalgia* 21(1), 53–60.

468. Linder S.L. & Winner P. (2001) Pediatric headache. *Medical Clinics of North America*. 85(4), 1037–1053.

469. Riederer P., Tenk H., Werner H., Bischko J., Rett A. & Krisper H. (1975) Manipulation of neurotransmitters by acupuncture (?) (A preliminary communication). *Journal of Neural Transmission* 37(1), 81–94.

470. Pintov S., Lahat E., Alstein M., Vogel Z. & Barg J. (1997) Acupuncture and the opioid system: implications in management of migraine. *Pediatric Neurology* 17(2), 129–133.

471. Yu S., Kuang P., Zhang F. & Liu J. (1995) Anti-inflammatory effects of tianrong acupoint on blood vessels of dura mater. *Journal of Traditional Chinese Medicine* 15(3), 209–213.

472. Duo X. (1999) 100 cases of intractable migraine treated by acupuncture and cupping. *Journal of Traditional Chinese Medicine* 19(3), 205–206.

473. Reilly R. (1994) Acute and prophylactic treatment of migraine. *Nursing Times* 90(29), 35–36.

474. Massiou H. (2000) Prophylactic treatments of migraine. *Revue Neurologique (Paris)* 156 Suppl 4, 4S79–4S86.

475. Hesse J., Mogelvang B. & Simonsen H. (1994) Acupuncture versus metoprolol in migraine prophylaxis: a randomized trial of trigger point inactivation. *Journal of Internal Medicine* 235(5), 451–456.

476. Baischer W. (1995) Acupuncture in migraine: long-term outcome and predicting factors. *Headache* 35(8), 472–474.

477. Gao S., Zhao D. & Xie Y. (1999) A comparative study on the treatment of migraine headache with combined distant and local acupuncture points versus conventional drug therapy. *American Journal of Acupuncture* 27(1–2), 27–30.

478. Vincent C.A. (1989) A controlled trial of the treatment of migraine acupuncture, *Clinical Journal of Pain* 5, 305.

479. Liguori A., Petti F., Bangrazi A., Camaioni D., Guccione G., Pitari G.M., Bianchi A. & Nicoletti W.E. (2000) Comparison of pharmacological treatment versus acupuncture treatment for migraine without aura—analysis of

socio-medical parameters. *Journal of Traditional Chinese Medicine* 20(3), 231–240.

480. Johnson G.D. (1998) Medical management of migraine-related dizziness and vertigo. *Laryngoscope* 108(1 Pt 2), 1–28.

481. Baischer W. (1993) Psychological aspects as predicting factors for the indication of acupuncture in migraine patients. *Wiener Klinische Wochenschrift* 105(7), 200–203. Review. [Abstract. Article in German]

482. Chrubasik S., & Kress W. (1995) Value of acupuncture in treatment of migraine. *Anesteziologiia Reanimatologia* 20(6), 150–152. Review. [Abstract. Article in German]

483. Hu J. (1998) Acupuncture treatment of migraine in Germany. *Journal of Traditional Chinese Medicine* 18(2), 99–101.

484. Seiden A.M. & Martin V.T. (2001) Headache and the frontal sinus. *Otolaryngology Clinics of North America* 34(1), 227–241.

485. Diener H.C., Dichgans J., Scholz E., Geiselhart S., Gerber W.D. & Bille A. (1989) Analgesic-induced chronic headache: long-term results of withdrawal therapy. *Journal of Neurology* 236(1), 9–14. [Abstract]

486. Hu J. (1994) Headache. *Journal of Traditional Chinese Medicine* 14(3), 237–240.

487. Gao S., Zhao D. & Xie Y. (1999) A comparative study on the treatment of migraine headache with combined distant and local acupuncture points versus conventional drug therapy. *American Journal of Acupuncture* 27(1–2), 27–30.

488. Zhu Z. & Wang X. (1998) Clinical observation on the therapeutic effects of wrist-ankle acupuncture in treatment of pain of various origins. *Journal of Traditional Chinese Medicine* 18(3), 192–194.

489. Zhang X., Li Y., Ren S., Kuang P., Wu W., Zhang F. & Liu J. (2000) Efficacy and effect of SI17 therapy on pancreatic polypeptide in vascular and tension-type headache. *Journal of Traditional Chinese Medicine* 20(3), 206–209.

490. Rao X. (2000) Clinical application of Taichong acupoint. *Journal of Traditional Chinese Medicine* 20(1), 38–39, 2000.

491. Lin B. (1991) Treatment of frontal headache with acupuncture on

zhongwan—a report of 110 cases. *Journal of Traditional Chinese Medicine* 11(1), 7–8.

492. Liu H. (1998) Illustrative cases treated by the application of the extra point sishencong. *Journal of Traditional Chinese Medicine* 18(2), 111–114.

493. Brouillette R.T., Thach B.T., Abu-Osba Y.K. & Wilson S.L. (1980) Hiccups in infants: characteristics and effects on ventilation. *Journal of Pediatrics* 96(2), 219–225.

494. Federspil P.A. & Zenk J. (1999) Hiccup. *HNO* 47(10), 867–875. [Article in German]

495. Johnson B.R. & Kriel R.L. (1996) Baclofen for chronic hiccups. *Pediatric Neurology* 15(1), 66–67.

496. Lewis J.H. (1985) Hiccups: causes and cures. *Journal of Clinical Gastroenterology* 7(6), 539–552.

497. Lipps D.C., Jabbari B., Mitchell M.H. & Daigh J.D. Jr. (1990) Nifedipine for intractable hiccups. *Neurology* 40(3 Pt 1), 531–532.

498. Johnson D.L. (1993) Intractable hiccups: treatment by microvascular decompression of the vagus nerve. Case Report. *Journal of Neurosurgery* 78(5), 813–816.

499. Yan L.S. (1988) Treatment of persistent hiccupping with electro-acupuncture at "hiccup-relieving" point. *Journal of Traditional Chinese Medicine* 8(1), 29–30.

500. Zhao C.X. (1989) Acupuncture and moxibustion treatment of hiccup. *Journal of Traditional Chinese Medicine* 9(3), 182–183.

501. Cui S. (1992) Clinical application of acupoint tianshu. *Journal of Traditional Chinese Medicine* 12(1), 52–54.

502. Oleson T.D. (1992) *Auriculotherapy Manual, Chinese and Western Systems of Ear Acupuncture*. Los Angeles, Health Care Alternatives.

503. Li X., Yi J. & Qi B. (1990) Treatment of hiccough with auriculo-acupuncture and auriculo-pressure—a report of 85 cases. *Journal of Traditional Chinese Medicine* 10(4), 257–259.

504. Li F., Wang D. & Ma X. (1991) Treatment of hiccoughs with auriculoacupuncture. *Journal of Traditional Chinese Medicine* 11(1), 14–16.

505. Yoo T.W. (1977) *Koryo Hand Acupuncture*, Vol. I. Seoul, Korea, Eum Yang Mek Jin Publishing Co.

506. Schlager A. (1998) Korean hand acupuncture in the treatment of chronic hiccups. *American Journal of Gastroenterology* 93(11), 2312–2313.

507. Qi Y. (1993) Treatment of hiccough with acupuncture on middle sifeng. *Journal of Traditional Chinese Medicine* 13(3), 202.

508. Jiang Y.G. (1986) Clinical applications of point futu. *Journal of Traditional Chinese Medicine* 6(1), 6–8.

509. Herrod H.G. (1997) Follow-up of pediatric patients with recurrent infection and mild serologic immune abnormalities. *Annals of Allergy, Asthma and Immunology* 79(5), 460–464.

510. Gross T.G., Steinbuch M., DeFor T., Shapiro R.S., McGlave P., Ramsay N.K., Wagner J.E. & Filipovich A.H. (1999) B cell lymphoproliferative disorders following hematopoietic stem cell transplantation: risk factors, treatment and outcome. *Bone Marrow Transplant* 23(3), 251–258.

511. Jorissen M. (2000) Differential diagnosis of local defense mechanism diseases in ENT. *Acta Otorhinolaryngolia Belgica* 54(3), 413–415.

512. Chandra R.K. (1999) Nutrition and immunology: from the clinic to cellular biology and back again. *Proceedings of Nutrition Society* 58(3), 681–683.

513. Beisel W.R. (1996) Nutrition in pediatric HIV infection: setting the research agenda. Nutrition and immune function: overview. *Journal of Nutrition* 126(10 Suppl), 2611S–2615S.

514. Bhaskaram P. (1992) Nutritional modulation of immunity to infection. *Indian Journal of Pathology and Microbiology* 35(4), 392–400.

515. Martin T.R. (1987) The relationship between malnutrition and lung infections. *Clinical Chest Medicine* 8(3), 359–372.

516. Keusch G.T. (1991) Nutritional effects on response of children in developing countries to respiratory tract pathogens: implications for vaccine development. *Review of Infectious Diseases* 13 Suppl 6, S486–S491.

517. Dhur A., Galan P. & Hercberg S. (1989) Iron status, immune capacity and resistance to infections. *Comparative Biochemistry and Physiology A* 94(1), 11–19.

518. Oppenheimer S.J. (2001) Iron and its relation to immunity and infectious disease. *Journal of Nutrition* 131(2S–2), 616S–633S; discussion 633S–635S.

519. Harris B.H. & Gelfand J.A. (1995) The immune response to trauma. *Seminars in Pediatric Surgery* 4(2), 77–82.

520. Koller M., Wick M. & Muhr G. (2001) Decreased leukotriene release from neutrophils after severe trauma: role of immature cells. *Inflammation* 25(1), 53–59.

521. Crowe J.E. Jr. (1998) Immune responses of infants to infection with respiratory viruses and live attenuated respiratory virus candidate vaccines. *Vaccine* 16(14–15), 1423–1432.

522. Bot A. (2000) DNA vaccination and the immune responsiveness of neonates. *International Reviews of Immunology* 19(2–3), 221–245.

523. Dekaris D. (1998) [Characteristics of immunoreactivity in neonates and young children. Review of the literature]. *Lijecnicki Vjesnik* 120(3–4), 65–72. [Abstract. Article in Romanian]

524. Wolach B. (1997) Neonatal sepsis: pathogenesis and supportive therapy. *Seminars in Perinatology* 21(1), 28–38.

525. Haeney M. (1994) Infection determinants at extremes of age. *Journal of Antimicrobial Chemotherapy* 34 Suppl A, 1–9.

526. Fleer A., Gerards L.J. & Verhoef J. (1988) Host defence to bacterial infection in the neonate. *Journal of Hospital Infection* 11 Suppl A, 320–327.

527. Sakkas L.I. & Platsoucas C.D. (1995) Immunopathogenesis of juvenile rheumatoid arthritis: role of T cells and MHC. *Immunology Research* 14(3), 218–236.

528. Tucker L.B. (1993) Juvenile rheumatoid arthritis. *Current Opinions in Rheumatology* 5(5), 619–628.

529. Kolbas V. (1990) [Immunology of cardiovascular diseases in children]. *Lijecnicki Vjesnik* 112(11–12), 404–407. [Article in Serbo-Croatian]

530. Fohlman J. & Friman G. (1993) Is juvenile diabetes a viral disease? *Annals of Medicine* 25(6), 569–574.

531. Rogers P.A., Schoen A.M. & Limehouse J. (1992) Acupuncture for immune-mediated disorders. Literature review and clinical applications. *Problems in Veterinary Medicine* 4(1), 162–193.

532. Pahwa S. & Morales M. (1998) Interleukin-2 therapy in HIV infection. *AIDS Patient Care STDS* 12(3), 187–197.

533 Bellanti J.A. (1997) Recurrent respiratory tract infections in paediatric patients. *Drugs* 54 Suppl 1, 1–4.

534. Seki S., Habu Y., Kawamura T., Takeda K., Dobashi H., Ohkawa T. & Hiraide H. (2000) The liver as a crucial organ in the first line of host defense: the roles of Kupffer cells, natural killer (NK) cells and NK1.1 Ag+ T cells in T helper 1 immune responses. *Immunology Review* 174, 35–46.

535. Sato T., Yu Y., Guo S.Y., Kasahara T. & Hisamitsu T. (1996) Acupuncture stimulation enhances splenic natural killer cell cytotoxicity in rats. *Japan Journal of Physiology* 46(2), 131–136.

536. Dong L., Yuan D., Fan L., Su L. & Fu Z. (1996) [Effect of HE-NE laser acupuncture on the spleen in rats]. *Zhen Ci Yan Jiu* 21(4), 64–67. [Abstract. Article in Chinese]

537. Ketiladze E.S., Krylov V.F., Ershov F.I., Kniazeva L.D. & Umanskaia A.A. (1987) [Interferon and other immunological indices of influenza patients undergoing different methods of treatment]. *Voprosy Virusologii* 32(1), 35–39. [Article in Russian]

538. Liu W.G. & Zhao J.C. (1989) Relationship between acupuncture-induced immunity and the regulation of central neurotransmitters in the rabbit: VI. The influence of NDR stimulation on acupuncture regulation of immune function in rabbit. *Acupuncture Electrotherapy Research* 14(3–4), 197–203.

539. Sakic B., Kojic L., Jankovic B.D. & Skokljev A. (1989) Electro-acupuncture modifies humoral immune response in the rat. *Acupuncture Electrotherapy Research* 14(2), 115–120.

540. Joos S., Schott C., Zou H., Daniel V. & Martin E. (2000) Immunomodulatory effects of acupuncture in the treatment of allergic asthma: a randomized controlled study. *Journal of Alternative and Complementary Medicine* 6(6), 519–525.

541. Okumura M., Toriizuka K., Iijima K., Haruyama K., Ishino S. & Cyong J.C. (1999) Effects of acupuncture on peripheral T lymphocyte subpopulation and amounts of cerebral catecholamines in mice. *Acupuncture Electrotherapy Research* 24(2), 127–139.

542. Liu X., Sun L., Xiao J., Yin S., Liu C., Li Q., Li H. & Jin B. (1993) Effect of acupuncture and point-injection treatment on immunologic function in rheumatoid arthritis. *Journal of Traditional Chinese Medicine* 13(3), 174–178.

543. Zhai D., Din B., Liu R., Hua X. & Chen H. (1996) [Regulation on ACTH, beta-EP and immune function by moxibustion on different acupoints]. *Zhen Ci Yan Jiu* 21(2), 77–81. [Abstract. Article in Chinese]

544. Du L., Jiang J. & Cao X. (1995) [Time course of the effect of electroacupuncture on immunomodulation of normal rat]. *Zhen Ci Yan Jiu* 20(1), 36–39. [Abstract. Article in Chinese]

545. Zhao R., Ma C., Tan L., Zhao X. & Zhuang D. (1994) [The effect of acupuncture on the function of macrophages in rats of immunodepression]. *Zhen Ci Yan Jiu* 19(2), 66–68. [Abstract. Article in Chinese]

546. Petti F., Bangrazi A., Liguori A., Reale G. & Ippoliti F. (1998) Effects of acupuncture on immune response related to opioid-like peptides. *Journal of Traditional Chinese Medicine* 18(1), 55–63.

547. Yu Y., Kasahara T., Sato T., Guo S.Y., Liu Y.A., Asano K. & Hisamitsu T. (1997) Enhancement of splenic interferon-gamma, interleukin-2, and NK cytotoxicity by S36 acupoint acupuncture in F344 rats. *Japanese Journal of Physiology* 47(2), 173–178.

548. Deng Y., Zeng T., Zhou Y. & Guan X. (1996) [The influence of electroacupuncture on the mast cells in the acupoints of the stomach meridian]. *Zhen Ci Yan Jiu* 21(3), 68–70. [Abstract. Article in Chinese]

549. Cheng X.D., Wu G.C., He Q.Z. & Cao X.D. (1997) Effect of continued electroacupuncture on induction of interleukin-2 production of spleen lymphocytes from the injured rats. *Acupuncture Electrotherapy Research* 22(1), 1–8.

550. Yuan D., Fu Z. & Li S. (1992) [Effect of He–Ne laser acupuncture on lymph-nodes in ras]. *Zhen Ci Yan Jiu* 17(1), 54–58. [Abstract. Article in Chinese]

551. Zhao J.C. & Liu W.G. (1988) Relationship between acupuncture-induced immunity and the regulation of central neurotransmitters in the rabbit: I. Effect of central catecholaminergic neurons in regulating acupuncture-induced immune function. *Acupuncture Electrotherapy Research* 13(2–3), 79–85.

552. Zhao J.C. & Liu W.Q. (1989) Relationship between acupuncture-induced immunity and the regulation of

central neurotransmitter system in rabbits—II. Effect of the endogenous opioid peptides on the regulation of acupuncture-induced immune reaction. *Acupuncture Electrotherapy Research* 14(1), 1–7.

553. Lundeberg T., Eriksson S.V. & Theodorsson E. (1991) Neuroimmunomodulatory effects of acupuncture in mice. *Neuroscience Letter* 128(2), 161–164.

554. Zhao J. (1996) [The effects of C-fibers of primary afferent on immune responses regulated by EA in mice]. *Zhen Ci Yan Jiu* 21(3), 36–41. [Abstract. Article in Chinese]

555. Fujiwara R., Tong Z.G., Matsuoka H., Shibata H., Iwamoto M. & Yokoyama M.M. (1991) Effects of acupuncture on immune response in mice. *International Journal of Neuroscience* 57(1–2), 141–150.

556. Ma Z., Wang Y. & Fan Q. (1992) [The influence of acupuncture on interleukin 2 interferon-natural killer cell regulatory network of kidney-deficiency mice]. *Zhen Ci Yan Jiu* 17(2), 139–142. [Abstract. Article in Chinese]

557. Yan W.X., Wang J.H. & Chang Q.Q. (1991) [Effect of leu-enkephalin in striatum on modulating cellular immune during electropuncture]. *Sheng Li Xue Bao* 43(5), 451–456. [Abstract. Article in Chinese]

558. Bianchi M., Jotti E., Sacerdote P. & Panerai A.E. (1991) Traditional acupuncture increases the content of beta-endorphin in immune cells and influences mitogen induced proliferation. *American Journal of Chinese Medicine* 19(2), 101–104.

559. Janssens L.A., Rogers P.A. & Schoen A.M. (1988) Acupuncture analgesia: a review. *Veterinary Record* 122(15), 355–358.

560. Gollub R.L., Hui K.K. & Stefano G.B. (1999) Acupuncture: pain management coupled to immune stimulation. *Zhongguo Yao Li Xue Bao* 20(9), 769–777.

561. Zhao X. (1995) [Effect of HC-3 on electroacupuncture-induced immunoregulation]. *Zhen Ci Yan Jiu* 20(2), 59–62. [Abstract. Article in Chinese]

562. Sternfeld M., Fink A., Bentwich Z. & Eliraz A. (1989) The role of acupuncture in asthma: changes in airways dynamics and LTC4 induced LAI. *American Journal of Chinese Medicine* 17(3–4), 129–134.

563. Shen D., Wei D., Liu B. & Zhang F. (1995) [Effects of electroacupuncture on gastrin, mast cell and gastric mucosal barrier in the course of protecting rat stress peptic ulcer]. *Zhen Ci Yan Jiu* 20(3), 46–49. [Abstract. Article in Chinese]

564. Fang J. (1994) [The influence of acupuncture at zusanli on cyclic nucleotide contents of plasma, different brain regions and spleen in rats]. *Zhen Ci Yan Jiu* 19(1), 42–45. [Abstract. Article in Chinese]

565. Wu B., Zhou R.X. & Zhou M.S. (1996) [Effect of acupuncture on immunomodulation in patients with malignant tumors]. *Zhongguo Zhong Xi Yi Jie He Za Zhi* 16(3), 139–141. [Abstract. Article in Chinese]

566. Liu L.J., Guo C.J. & Jiao X.M. (1995) [Effect of acupuncture on immunologic function and histopathology of transplanted mammary cancer in mice]. *Zhongguo Zhong Xi Yi Jie He Za Zhi* 15(10), 615–617. [Abstract. Article in Chinese]

567. Yuan J. & Zhou R. (1993) [Effect of acupuncture on T-lymphocyte and its subsets from the peripheral blood of patients with malignant neoplasm]. *Zhen Ci Yan Jiu* 18(3), 174–177. [Abstract. Article in Chinese]

568. Du L.N., Jiang J.W., Wu G.C. & Cao X.D. (1998) Naloxone and electroacupuncture (EA) improve the immune function of traumatized rats. *Sheng Li Xue Bao* 50(6), 636–642.

569. Yang J., Zhao R., Yuan J., Chen G., Zhang L., Yu M., Lu A. & Zhang Z. (1994) [The experimental study of prevention and treatment of the side-effects of chemotherapy with acupuncture (comparison among the effect of acupuncture at different acupoint)]. *Zhen Ci Yan Jiu* 19(1), 75–78. [Abstract. Article in Chinese]

570. Baldassano R.N. & Piccoli D.A. (1999) Inflammatory bowel disease in pediatric and adolescent patients. *Gastroenterology Clinics of North America* 28(2), 445–458.

571. Farmer R.G. & Michener W.M. (1979) Prognosis of Crohn's Disease with onset in childhood or adolescence. *Digestive Diseases and Sciences* 24, 752. [Abstract]

572. Buller H.A. (1997) Problems in diagnosis of IBD in children. *Netherlands Journal of Medicine* 50(2), S8–S11. [Article in Dutch]

573. Scholmerich J. (2000) Future developments in diagnosis and treatment of inflammatory bowel disease. *Hepatogastroenterology* 47(31), 101–114. [Abstract]

574. Mendeloff A.I. & Calkins B.M. (1988) The epidemiology of idiopathic Inflammatory Bowel Disease. In Kirsner J.B. & Shorter R.G. (eds): *Inflammatory Bowel Disease*. Philadelphia, Lea & Febiger, pp 3–34.

575. Calkins B.M., Lilienfield A.M. & Garland C.G. *et al.* (1984) Trends in incidence rates of ulcerative colitis and Crohn's Disease. *Digestive Diseases and Sciences* 29, 913. [Abstract]

576. Andres P.G. & Friedman L.S. (1999) Epidemiology and the natural course of inflammatory bowel disease. *Gastroenterology Clinics of North America* 28(2), 255–281, vii.

577. Tysk C., Lindberg E., Jarnerot G. *et al.* (1988) Ulcerative colitis and Crohn's disease in an unselected population of monozygotic and dizygotic twins: A study of heritability and the influence of smoking. *Gut* 29, 990–996. [Abstract]

578. Duerr R.H., Barmada M.M., Zhang L., Davis S., Preston R.A., Chensny L.J., Brown J.L., Ehrlich G.D., Weeks D.E. & Aston C.E. (1998) Linkage and association between inflammatory bowel disease and a locus on chromosome 12. *American Journal of Human Genetics* 63(1), 95–100.

579. Duerr R.H., Barmada M.M., Zhang L., Pfutzer R. & Weeks D.E. (2000) High-density genome scan in Crohn disease shows confirmed linkage to chromosome 14q11–12. *American Journal of Human Genetics* 66(6), 1857–1862.

580. Devroede G.J., Taylor W.F., Sauer J. *et al.* (1973) Cancer risk and life expectancy of children with ulcerative colitis. *New England Journal of Medicine* 289, 491. [Citation]

581. Casati J. & Toner B.B. (2000) Psychosocial aspects of inflammatory bowel disease. *Biomedical Pharmacotherapy* 54(7), 388–393.

582. Lee J.C. & Lennard-Jones J.E. (1996) Inflammatory bowel disease in 67 families each with three or more affected first-degree relatives. *Gastroenterology* 111(3), 587–596.

583. Markowitz J., Daum F., Algar M. *et al.* (1984) Perianal Disease in children and adolescents with Crohn's Disease. *Gastroenterology* 86, 829. [Abstract]

584. Griffiths A.M. (1992) Crohn's Disease. *Recent Advances in Pediatrics* 10, 145ff.

585. Goulet O. (1998) Inflammatory bowel disease in children. *Revue Pratique* 48(4), 403–409. [Abstract. Article in French]

586. Booth I.W. (1991) The nutritional consequences of gastrointestinal disease in adolescence. *Acta Pediatrica Scandinavica* 373(suppl), 91–102.

587. Hildebrand H., Karlberg J. & Kristiansson B. (1994) Longitudinal growth in children and adolescents with Inflammatory Bowel Disease. *Journal of Pediatric Gastroenterology and Nutrition* 18, 165–173. [Abstract]

588. O'Gorman M. & Lake A.M. (1993) Chronic inflammatory bowel disease in childhood. *Pediatrics Review* 14, 475–480.

589. Langholz E., Munkholm P. & Krasilnikoff P.A. (1997) Inflammatory Bowel Disease with onset in childhood. *Scandinavian Journal of Gastroenterology* 32, 139–147. [Abstract]

590. Grand R.J. & Homer D.R. (1975) Inflammatory Bowel Disease in childhood and adolescence. *Pediatric Clinics of North America* 22, 835. [Citation]

591. Binder S.C., Patterson J.F. & Glotzer D.J. (1974) Toxic megacolon in ulcerative colitis. *Gastroenterology* 66, 1088. [Citation]

592. Ekbom A., Helmick C., Zack M. *et al.* (1990) Ulcerative colitis and colorectal cancer: A population-based study. *New England Journal of Medicine* 323, 1228–1233. [Abstract]

593. Griffiths A.M. & Sherman P.M. (1997) Colonoscopic surveillance for cancer in ulcerative colitis: A critical review. *Journal of Pediatric Gastroenterology and Nutrition* 24, 202–210. [Citation]

594. Danzi J.T. (1988) Extraintestinal manifestations of idiopathic Inflammatory Bowel Disease. *Archives of Internal Medicine* 148, 297. [Abstract]

595. Gryboski J.D. & Spiro H.M. (1978) Prognosis in children with Crohn's Disease. *Gastroenterology* 74, 807. [Abstract]

596. Winesett M. (1997) Inflammatory bowel disease in children and adolescents. *Pediatric Annals* 26(4), 227–234.

597. Hassall E., Barclay G.N. & Ament M.E. (1984) Colonoscopy in childhood. *Pediatrics* 73, 594. [Abstract]

598. Hyams J.S., Ferry G.D., Mandel F.S. *et al.* (1991) Development and validation of a pediatric Crohn's Disease Activity Index. *Journal of Pediatric Gastroenterology and Nutrition* 12, 439. [Abstract]

599. Oliva M.M. & Lake A.M. (1996) Nutritional considerations and management of the child with inflammatory bowel disease. *Nutrition* 12(3), 151–158.

600. Belluzzi A., Brignola C., Campieri M. *et al.* (1996) Effect of enteric-coated fish oil preparation on relapses in Crohn's Disease. *New England Journal of Medicine* 334, 1557–1560. [Abstract]

601. Aranda R. & Horgan K. (1998) Immunosuppressive drugs in the treatment of inflammatory bowel disease. *Seminars in Gastrointestinal Diseases* 9(1), 2–9.

602. Haller C. & Markowitz J. (2001) A perspective on inflammatory bowel disease in the child and adolescent at the turn of the millennium. *Current Gastroenterology Report* 3(3), 263–271.

603. Kozarek R.A. (1993) Review article: immunosuppressive therapy for inflammatory bowel disease. *Alimentary Pharmacologic Therapy* 7(2), 117–123.

604. Lofberg R., Rutgeerts P., Malchow H. *et al.* (1996) Budesonide prolongs time to relapse in ileal ileocecal Crohn's Disease: A placebo controlled one year study. *Gut* 39, 82–86. [Abstract]

605. Stotland B.R. & Lichtenstein G.R. (1996) Newer treatments for inflammatory bowel disease. *Primary Care* 23(3), 577–608.

606. Choi P.M. & Targan S.R. (1994) Immunomodulator therapy in inflammatory bowel disease. *Digestive Diseases and Sciences* 39(9), 1885–1892.

607. Hilsden R.J., Scott C.M. & Verhoef M.J. (1998) Complementary medicine use by patients with inflammatory bowel disease. *American Journal of Gastroenterology* 93(5), 697–701.

608. Moum B. (2000) Medical treatment: does it influence the natural course of inflammatory bowel disease? *European Journal of Internal Medicine* 11(4), 197–203.

609. Wang B., Ren S., Feng W., Zhong Z. & Qin C. (1997) Kui jie qing in the treatment of chronic non-specific ulcerative colitis. *Journal of Traditional Chinese Medicine* 17(1), 10–13.

610. Diehl D. (1991) Acupuncture for gastrointestinal and hepatobiliary disorders. *Journal of Alternative and Complementary Medicine* 5(1), 27–45.

611. Zhang X. (1998) 23 cases of chronic nonspecific ulcerative colitis treated by acupuncture and moxibustion. *Journal of Traditional Chinese Medicine* 18(3), 188–191.

612. Yang C. & Yan H. (1999) Observation of the efficacy of acupuncture and moxibustion in 62 cases of chronic colitis. *Journal of Traditional Chinese Medicine* 19(2), 111–114.

613. Chen Z. (1995) Treatment of ulcerative colitis with acupuncture. *Journal of Traditional Chinese Medicine* 15(3), 231–233.

614. Proimos J. & Sawyer S. (2000) Obesity in childhood and adolescence. *Australian Family Physician* 29(4), 321–327.

615. Stettler N. (2000) Obesity in children and adolescents. *Therapeutische Umschau* 57(8), 532–536. [Abstract. Article in German]

616. Troiano R.P., Flegal K.M. & Kuczmarski R.J. (1995) Overweight prevalence and trends for children and adolescents. *Archives of Pediatric and Adolescent Medicine* 149, 1085–1091.

617. Goran M.I. (2001) Metabolic precursors and effects of obesity in children: a decade of progress, 1990–1999. *American Journal of Clinical Nutrition* 73(2), 158–171.

618. Perusse L. & Bouchard C. (1999) Role of genetic factors in childhood obesity and in susceptibility to dietary variations. *Annals of Medicine* 31 Suppl 1, 19–25.

619. Freedman D.S., Srinivasan S.R., Valdez R.A., Williamson D.F. & Berenson G.S. (1997) Secular increases in relative weight and adiposity among children over two decades: the Bogalusa Heart Study. *Pediatrics* 99, 420–426. [Abstract]

620. Rudloff L.M. & Feldmann E. (1999) Childhood obesity: addressing the issue. *Journal of American Osteopathic Association* 99(4 Suppl), S1–S6.

621. Strauss R. (1999) Childhood obesity. *Current Problems in Pediatrics* 29(1), 1–29.

622. Holtz C., Smith T.M. & Winters F.D. (1999) Childhood obesity. *Journal of American Osteopathic Association* 99(7), 366–371.

623. Moran R. (1999) Evaluation and treatment of childhood obesity. *American Family Physician* 59(4), 861–868, 871–873.

624. Klish W.J. (1995) Childhood obesity: pathophysiology and treatment. *Acta Paediatrica Japan* 37(1), 1–6.

625. Berenson G.S., Wattigney W.A., Tracy R.E. *et al.* (1992) Atherosclerosis of the aorta and coronary-arteries and cardiovascular risk-factors in persons aged 6 to 30 years and studied at necropsy (The Bogalusa Heart Study). *American Journal of Cardiology* 70, 851–858.

626. Dietz W. (1999) How to tackle the problem early? The role of education in the prevention of obesity. *International Journal of Obesity and Related Metabolic Disorders* 23 Suppl 4, S7–S9.

627. Whitaker R.C., Wright J.A., Pepe M.S., Seidel K.D. & Dietz W. (1997) Predicting obesity in young adulthood from childhood and parental obesity. *New England Journal of Medicine* 337, 869–873.

628. Wilding J. (1997) Science, medicine, and the future: obesity treatment. *British Medical Journal* 315, 997–1000 (18 October).

629. Andersen R.E., Crespo C.J., Bartlett S.J., Cheskin L.J. & Pratt M. (1998) Relationship of physical activity and television watching with body weight and level of fatness in among children. *Journal of the American Medical Association* 279, 938–942.

630. Feld L.G., Springate J.E. & Waz W.R. (1998) Special topics in pediatrics hypertension. *Seminars in Nephrology* 18(3), 295–303.

631. Bartosh S.M. & Aronson A.J. (1999) Childhood hypertension. An update on etiology, diagnosis, and treatment. *Pediatric Clinics of North America* 46(2), 235–252.

632. Bronfin D.R. & Urbina E.M. (1995) The role of the pediatrician in the promotion of cardiovascular health. *American Journal of Medicine and Science* 310 Suppl 1, S42–S47.

633. Pinhas-Hamericaniel O., Dolan L.M., Daniels S.R., Standiford D., Khoury P.R. & Zeitler P. (1996) Increased incidence of non-insulin-dependent diabetes mellitus among adolescents. *Journal of Pediatrics* 128, 608–615.

634. Libman I. & Arslanian S.A. (1999) Type II diabetes mellitus: no longer just adults. *Pediatric Annals* 28(9), 589–593.

635. Marcus C.L. & Loughlin G.M. (1996) Obstructive sleep apnea in children. *Seminars in Pediatric Neurology* 3(1), 23–28.

636. Macdonald I.A. (2000) Obesity: are we any closer to identifying causes and effective treatments? *Trends in Pharmacologic Science* 21(9), 334–336.

637. Keller C. & Stevens K.R. (1996) Assessment, etiology, and intervention in obesity in children. *Nurse Practitioner* 21(9), 31–36, 38, 41–42.

638. Liu Z.C., Sun F.M. & Wang Y.Z. (1995) Good regulation of acupuncture in simple obesity patients with stomach-intestine excessive heat type. *Zhongguo Zhong Xi Yi Jie He Za Zhi* 15(3), 137–140. [Article in Chinese]

639. Liu Z. (1995) Recent progress in the studies on weight reduction by acupuncture and moxibustion. *Journal of Traditional Chinese Medicine* 15(3), 224–230.

640. Zhan J. (1993) Observations on the treatment of 393 cases of obesity by semen pressure on auricular points. *Journal of Traditional Chinese Medicine* 13(1), 27–30.

641. Tang X. (1997) 75 cases of simple obesity treated with auricular and body acupuncture. *Journal of Traditional Chinese Medicine* 17(1), 55–56.

642. Shiraishi T., Onoe M., Kagey A.T., Saeshima Y., Kojima T., Konishi S., Yoshimatsu H. & Sakata T. (1995) Effects of auricular acupuncture stimulation on nonobese, healthy volunteer subjects. *Obesity Research* 3 Suppl 5, 667S–673S.

643. Liu Z., Sun F., Li J., Wang Y. & Hu K. (1993) Effect of acupuncture on weight loss evaluated by adrenal function. *Journal of Traditional Chinese Medicine* 13(3), 169–173.

644. Zhao M., Liu Z. & Su J. (2000) The time-effect relationship of central action in acupuncture treatment for weight reduction. *Journal of Traditional Chinese Medicine* 20(1), 26–29.

645. Liu Z. (1996) Effects of acupuncture on lipid, TXB2, 6-keto-PGF, alpha in simple obese patients complicated with hyperlipidemia. *Zhen Ci Yan Jiu* 21(4), 17–21. [Article in Chinese]

646. Liu Z. (1990) Effect of acupuncture and moxibustion on the high density lipoprotein cholesterol in simple obesity. *Zhen Ci Yan Jiu* 15(3), 227–231. [Article in Chinese]

647. Gadzhiev A.A., Mugarab-Samericanedicinei V.V., Isaev I.I. & Rafieva S.K. (1993) Acupuncture therapy of constitution-exogenous obesity in children. *Problemi*

Endokrinologii (Moskow) 39(3), 21–24. [Abstract. Article in Russian]

648. Sun Q. & Xu Y. (1993) Simple obesity and obesity hyperlipemia treated with otoacupoint pellet pressure and body acupuncture. *Journal of Traditional Chinese Medicine* 13(1), 22–26.

649. Zhao Y. (1992) Effect of acupuncture on carbohydrate metabolism in patients with simple obesity. *Journal of Traditional Chinese Medicine* 12(2), 129–132.

650. Sun F. (1996) The antiobesity effect of acupuncture and its influence on water and salt metabolism. *Zhen Ci Yan Jiu* 21(2), 19–24. [Abstract. Article in Chinese]

651. Liu Z., Sun F., Li J., Shi X., Hu L., Wang Y. & Qian Z. (1992) Prophylactic and therapeutic effects of acupuncture on simple obesity complicated by cardiovascular diseases. *Journal of Traditional Chinese Medicine* 12(1), 21–29.

652. Liu Z.C., Sun F.M. & Shen D.Z. (1991) Effect of acupuncture and moxibustion on antiobesity in the variation of plasma cyclic nucleotide and the function of vegetative nervous system. *Zhong Xi Yi Jie He Za Zhi* 11(2), 83–86, 67–68. [Abstract. Article in Chinese]

653. Mazzoni R., Mannucci E., Rizzello S.M., Ricca V. & Rotella C.M. (1999) Failure of acupuncture in the treatment of obesity: a pilot study. *Eating Weight Disorders* 4(4), 198–202.

654. Huang M.H., Yang R.C. & Hu S.H. (1996) Preliminary results of triple therapy for obesity. *International Journal of Obesity and Related Metabolism* 20(9), 830–836.

655. Zhang Z. (1990) Weight reduction by auriculo-acupuncture—a report of 110 cases. *Journal of Traditional Chinese Medicine* 10(1), 17–18.

656. Tang X. (1993) 75 cases of simple obesity treated with auricular and body acupuncture. *Journal of Traditional Chinese Medicine* 13(3), 194–195.

657. Gu Y.S., Zheng X.L., Cui S.G., Chu H. & Xu Z.Z. (1989) Clinical observations on weight reduction by pressing auricular points with semen vaccariae—a report of 473 cases. *Journal of Traditional Chinese Medicine* 9(3), 166.

658. Xu B. & Fei J.Z. (1985) Clinical observation of the weight-reducing effect of ear acupuncture in 350 cases of obesity. *Journal of Traditional Chinese Medicine* 5(2), 87–88.

659. Gellis S. & Kagan B.M. (1993) *Current Pediatric Therapy*, vol 14. Philadelphia, WB Saunders.

660. White C.B. & Foshee W.S. (2000) Upper respiratory tract infections in adolescents. *Adolescent Medicine* 11(2), 225–249.

661. Anderson L.J. (2000) Respiratory syncytial virus vaccines for otitis media. *Vaccine* 19 Suppl 1, S59–S65.

662. Hayden F.G. (2000) Influenza virus and rhinovirus-related otitis media: potential for antiviral intervention. *Vaccine* 19 Suppl 1, S66–S70.

663. Heikkinen T. (2000) The role of respiratory viruses in otitis media. *Vaccine* 19 Suppl 1, S51–S55.

664. Jund R. & Grevers G. (2000) Rhinitis, sore throat and otalgia... Benign common cold or dangerous infection? *Fortschritte der Medizin* 142(48), 32–36. [Abstract. Article in German]

665. Glezen W.P. (2000) Prevention of acute otitis media by prophylaxis and treatment of influenza virus infections. *Vaccine* 19 Suppl 1, S56–S58. Review.

666. Ruoff G. (1998) Upper respiratory tract infections in family practice. *Pediatric Infectious Diseases Journal* 17(8 Suppl), S73–S78.

667. Oh H.M. (1995) Upper respiratory tract infections—otitis media, sinusitis and pharyngitis. *Singapore Medical Journal* 36(4), 428–431.

668. Cappelletty D. (1998) Microbiology of bacterial respiratory infections. *Pediatric Infectious Diseases Journal* 17(8 Suppl), S55–S61.

669. St Geme J.W. 3rd. (2000) The pathogenesis of nontypable *Haemophilus influenzae* otitis media. *Vaccine* 19 Suppl 1, S41–S50. Review.

670. Pichichero M.E. (1998) Group A beta-hemolytic streptococcal infections. *Pediatrics in Review* 19(9), 291–302.

671. Rynnel-Dagoo B. & Agren K. (2000) The nasopharynx and the middle ear. Inflammatory reactions in middle ear disease. *Vaccine* 19 Suppl 1, S26–S31.

672. Park K. & Lim D.J. (1993) Development of secretory elements in murine tubotympanum: lysozyme and lactoferrin immunohistochemistry. *Annals of Otology, Rhinology, Laryngology* 102(5), 385–395.

673. Zimmerman R.K. (2001) Pneumococcal conjugate vaccine for young children. *American Family Physician* 63(10), 1991–1998.

674. Tuomanen E.I. (2000) Pathogenesis of pneumococcal inflammation: otitis media. *Vaccine* 19 Suppl 1, S38–S40.

675. Dunne A.A. & Werner J.A. (2001) [Status of the controversial discussion of the pathogenesis and treatment of chronic otitis media with effusion in childhood]. *Laryngorhinootologie* 80(1), 1–10. [Article in German]

676. Knight L.C. & Eccles R. (1993) The relationship between nasal airway resistance and middle ear pressure in subjects with acute upper respiratory tract infection. *Otolaryngology* 113(2), 196–200.

677. Lim D.J., Chun Y.M., Lee H.Y., Moon S.K., Chang K.H., Li J.D. & Andalibi A. (2000) Cell biology of tubotympanum in relation to pathogenesis of otitis media— a review. *Vaccine* 19 Suppl 1, S17–S25.

678. Krause P.J. *et al.* (1982) Penetration of amoxicillin, cefaclor, erythromycin-sulfisoxazole, and trimethoprim–sulfamethoxazole into the middle ear fluid of patients with chronic serous otitis media. *Journal of Infectious Diseases* 145(6), 815–821.

679. Klimek J.J. *et al.* (1977) Comparison of concentrations of amoxicillin and ampicillin in serum and middle ear fluid of children with chronic otitis media. *Journal of Infectious Diseases* 135(6), 999–1002.

680. Middleton D.B. (1996) Pharyngitis. *Primary Care* 23(4), 719–739.

681. Brook I. (1998) Microbial factors leading to recurrent upper respiratory tract infections. *Pediatric Infectious Diseases Journal* 17(8 Suppl), S62–S67.

682. Mogyoros M. (2001) Challenges of managed care organizations in treating respiratory tract infections in an age of antibiotic resistance. *American Journal of Managed Care* 7(6 Suppl), S163–S169.

683. Heinig M.J. (2001) Host defense benefits of breastfeeding for the infant. Effect of breastfeeding duration and exclusivity. *Pediatric Clinics of North America* 48(1), 105–123, ix.

684. Giebink G.S. (2000) Otitis media prevention: non-vaccine prophylaxis. *Vaccine* 19 Suppl 1, S129–S133.

685. Pelton S.I. (2000) Acute otitis media in the era of effective pneumococcal conjugate vaccine: will new pathogens emerge? *Vaccine* 19 Suppl 1, S96–S99.

686. Briles D.E., Hollingshead S.K., Nabors G.S., Paton J.C. & Brooks-Walter A. (2000) The potential for using protein vaccines to protect against otitis media caused by *Streptococcus pneumoniae*. *Vaccine* 19 Suppl 1, S87–S95.

687. Ledwith M. (2001) Pneumococcal conjugate vaccine. *Current Opinions in Pediatrics* 13(1), 70–74.

688. Cabenda S.I. *et al.* (1988) Serous otitis media (SOM). A bacteriological study of the ear canal and the middle ear. *International Journal of Pediatric Otolaryngology* 16(2), 119–124.

689. Maxim P.E. *et al.* (1977) Chronic serous otitis media: an immune complex disease. *Transactions of the American Academy of Ophthalmology and Otolaryngology* 84(2), 234–238.

690. Prellner K. *et al.* (1980) Complement and C1q binding substances in otitis media. *Annals of Otology, Rhinology and Laryngology* Supplement 89(3 Pt 2), 129–132.

691. Van der Baan S. *et al.* (1988) Serous otitis media and immunological reactions in the middle ear mucosa. *Acta Otolaryngologia* 106(5–6), 428–434.

692. Gundersen T. *et al.* (1984) Ventilating tubes in the middle ear. Long-term observations. *Archives of Otolaryngology* 110(12), 783–784.

693. Tian Z.M. (1985) Acupuncture treatment for aerotitis media. *Journal of Traditional Chinese Medicine* 5(4), 259–260.

694. Paulussen C., Claes J., Claes G. & Jorissen M. (2000) Adenoids and tonsils, indications for surgery and immunological consequences of surgery. *Acta Otorhinolaryngolia Belgica* 54(3), 403–408.

695. Rynnel-Dagoo B. & Agren K. (2000) The nasopharynx and the middle ear. Inflammatory reactions in middle ear disease. *Vaccine* 19 Suppl 1, S26–S31.

696. Bisno A.L., Gerber M.A., Gwaltney J.M. Jr, Kaplan E.L. & Schwartz R.H. (1997) Diagnosis and management of group A streptococcal pharyngitis: a practice guideline. *Clinical Infectious Diseases* 25(3), 574–583.

697. Peter J. & Ray C.G. (1998) Infectious mononucleosis. *Pediatrics Review* 19(8), 276–279.

698. White C.B. & Foshee W.S. (2000) Respiratory tract infections in adolescents. *Adolescent Medicine* 11(2), 225–249.

699. Cappelletty D. (1998) Microbiology of bacterial respiratory infections. *Pediatric Infectious Diseases Journal* 17(8 Suppl), S55–S61.

700. Hayes C.S. & Williamson H. Jr. (2001) A beta-hemolytic streptococcal pharyngitis. *Family Physician* 63(8), 1557–1564.

701. Olivier C. (2000) Rheumatic fever—is it still a problem? *Journal of Antimicrobial Chemotherapy* 45 Suppl, 13–21.

702. Olivier C. (1998) [Acute articular rheumatism in the child in 1997]. *Pathologie Biologie (Paris)* 46(10), 802–812. [Abstract. Article in French]

703. Tsevat J. & Kotagal U.R. (1999) Management of sore throats in children: a cost-effectiveness analysis. *Archives of Pediatric and Adolescent Medicine* 153(7), 681–688.

704. Guggenbichler J.P. (1994) Cefetamet pivoxil in the treatment of pharyngitis/tonsillitis in children and adults. *Drugs* 47 Suppl 3, 27–33; discussion 34.

705. Pichichero M.E. (1995) Group A streptococcal tonsillopharyngitis: cost-effective diagnosis and treatment. *Emergency Medicine* 25(3), 390–403.

706. Pichichero M.E., Green J.L., Francis A.B. et al. (1998) Recurrent group A streptococcal tonsillopharyngitis. *Pediatric Infectious Diseases Journal* 17(9), 809–815.

707. Pichichero M.E. (1997) Sore throat after sore throat after sore throat. Are you asking the critical questions? *Postgraduate Medicine* 101(1), 205–206, 209–212, 215–218.

708. Kiselica D. (1994) Group A beta-hemolytic streptococcal pharyngitis: current clinical concepts. *American Family Physician* 49(5), 1147–1154.

709. Ruoff G. (1998) Upper respiratory tract infections in family practice. *Pediatric Infectious Diseases Journal* 17(8 Suppl), S73–S78.

710. Hover A.R., Cornwell V., Stevenson S. & Sponenberg D. (2000) Evaluation of the American Academy of Pediatrics Principles on Management of Common Office Infections in a managed care setting. *Medicine* 97(12), 541–544.

711. Garcia-de-Lomas J. & Navarro D. (1997) New directions in diagnostics. *Pediatric Infectious Diseases Journal* 16(3 Suppl), S43–S48.

712. Oh H.M. (1995) Upper respiratory tract infections – otitis media, sinusitis and pharyngitis. *Singapore Medical Journal* 36(4), 428–431.

713. Bezold L.I. & Bricker J.T. (1994) Acquired heart disease in children. *Current Opinions in Cardiology* 9(1), 121–129.

714. Sanabria Gomez F., Cenjor Espanol C., Marquez Dorsch F. & Barrientos Augustinus J.C. (1993) [Acute pharyngo-tonsillitis. Penicillin, yes or no?] *Revista Clinica Espanola* 193(1), 31–34. [Abstract. Article in Spanish]

715. Dajani A.S. (1996) Adherence to physicians' instructions as a factor in managing streptococcal pharyngitis. *Pediatrics* 97(6 Pt 2), 976–980.

716. Gerber M.A. & Tanz R.R. (2001) Approaches to the treatment of group A streptococcal pharyngitis. *Opinions in Pediatrics* 13(1), 51–55.

717. Adam D. (2000) Short-course antibiotic therapy for infections with a single causative pathogen. *Internal Medicine Research* 28 Suppl 1, 13A–24A.

718. Wolter J.M. (1998) Management of a sore throat. Antibiotics are no longer appropriate. *Australian Family Physician* 27(4), 279–281.

719. Bicknell P.G. (1994) Role of adenotonsillectomy in the management of pediatric ear, nose and throat infections. *Pediatric Infectious Diseases Journal* 13(1 Suppl 1), S75–S78; discussion S78–S79.

720. Wu J.S. (1989) Observation on analgesic effect of acupuncturing the dazhui point. *Journal of Traditional Chinese Medicine* 9(4), 240–242.

721. Lu F. (1995) Experience in the clinical application of acupoint zhaohai (K 6). *Journal of Traditional Chinese Medicine* 15(2), 118–121.

722. Thiele E.A., Gonzalez-Heydrich J. & Riviello J.J. Jr. (1999) Epilepsy in children and adolescents. *Child and Adolescent Psychiatric Clinics of North America* 8(4), 671–694.

723. (No author listed) Managing childhood epilepsy. *Drug Therapy Bulletin* 2001 39(2), 11–16.

724. Arnold S.T. & Dodson W.E. (1996) Epilepsy in children. Baillières *Clinical Neurology* 5(4), 783–802.

725. Barron T. (1991) The child with spells. *Pediatric Clinics of North America* 38(3), 711–724.

726. Appleton R.E. (1995) Treatment of childhood epilepsy. *Pharmacologic Therapy* 67(3), 419–431.

727. Jensen F.E. (1999) Acute and chronic effects of seizures in the developing brain: experimental models. *Epilepsia* 40 Suppl 1, S51–S58; discussion S64–S66.

728. Engelborghs S., D'Hooge R. & De Deyn P.P. (2000) Pathophysiology of epilepsy. *Acta Neurologica Belgica* 100(4), 201–213.

729. Korinthenberg R. (1992) Grand mal epilepsy in childhood. *Monatsschrift Kinderheilkde* 140(9), 614–618. [Abstract. Article in German]

730. Dam M. (1990) Children with epilepsy: the effect of seizures, syndromes, and etiological factors on cognitive functioning. *Epilepsia* 31 Suppl 4, S26–S29.

731. Cavazzuti G.B. (1998) Discontinuing of antiepileptic therapy. *Pediatrica Medica Chirugica* 20(5), 317–322. [Abstract. Article in Italian]

732. Nordli D.R. Jr. & Kelley K.R. (2001) Selection and evaluation of children for epilepsy surgery. *Pediatric Neurosurgery* 34(1), 1–12.

733. Olson D.M. (2001) Evaluation of children for epilepsy surgery. *Pediatric Neurosurgery* 34(3), 159–165.

734. Wong M. & Trevathan E. (2001) Infantile spasms. *Pediatric Neurology* 24(2), 89–98.

735. Ormrod D. & McClellan K. (2001) Topiramate: a review of its use in childhood epilepsy. *Paediatric Drugs* 3(4), 293–319.

736. Dulac O. (2000) Benign epilepsies of childhood—distinct syndromes and overlap. *Epileptic Disorders* 2 Suppl 1, S41–S43.

737. Baumann R.J. & Duffner P.K. (2000) Treatment of children with simple febrile seizures: the AAP practice parameter. American Academy of Pediatrics. *Pediatric Neurology* 23(1), 11–17.

738. Rajadhyaksha S. & Shah K.N. (2000) Controversies in febrile seizures. *Indian Journal of Pediatrics* 67(1 Suppl), S71–S79.

739. Knudsen F.U. (2001) Febrile convulsions: Treatment and prognosis. *Ugeskrift for Laeger* 163(8), 1098–1102. [Article in Danish]

740. Bettis D.B. & Ater S.B. (1985) Febrile seizures: emergency department diagnosis and treatment. *Journal of Emergency Medicine* 2(5), 341–348.

741. Mirsky A.F., Duncan C.C. & Myslobodsky M.S. (1986) Petit mal epilepsy: a review and integration of recent information. *Journal of Clinical Neurophysiology* 3(3), 179–208.

742. Duncan J.S. (1997) Idiopathic generalized epilepsies with typical absences. *Journal of Neurology* 244(7), 403–411.

743. Porter R.J. (1993) The absence epilepsies. *Epilepsia* 34 Suppl 3, S42–S48.

744. Costeff H., Groswasser Z. & Goldstein R. (1990) Long-term follow-up review of 31 children with severe closed head trauma. *Journal of Neurosurgery* 73(5), 684–687.

745. Lai C.W. & Lai Y.H. (1991) History of epilepsy in Chinese traditional medicine. *Epilepsia* 32(3), 299–302.

746. Chen K.Y., Chen G.P. & Feng X. (1983) Observation of immediate effect of acupuncture on electroencephalograms in epileptic patients. *Journal of Traditional Chinese Medicine* 3(2), 121–124.

747. Liu A. (1999) Clinical application of moxibustion over point dazhui. *Journal of Traditional Chinese Medicine* 19(4), 283–286.

748. Kloster R., Larsson P.G., Lossius R., Nakken K.O., Dahl R., Xiu-Ling X., Wen-Xin Z., Kinge E. & Rossberg E. (1999) The effect of acupuncture in chronic intractable epilepsy. *Seizure* 8(3), 170–174.

749. Yang J. (1990) Treatment of status epilepticus with acupuncture. *Journal of Traditional Chinese Medicine* 10(2), 101–102.

750. Shi Z.Y., Gong B.T., Jia Y.W. & Huo Z.X. (1987) The efficacy of electro-acupuncture on 98 cases of epilepsy. *Journal of Traditional Chinese Medicine* 7(1), 21–22.

751. Xiang L., Wang H. & Li Z. (1996) TCD observation on cerebral blood flow dynamics inference of cerebral palsy with scalp therapy. *Zhen Ci Yan Jiu* 21(4), 7–9. [Article in Chinese]

752. Wu Y., Shen Q. & Zhang Q. (1992) The effect of acupuncture on high oxygen pressure-induced convulsion and its relationship to the brain GABA concentration in mice. *Zhen Ci Yan Jiu* 17(2), 104–109. [Article in Chinese]

753. Lu F. (1995) Experience in the clinical application of acupoint zhaohai (K 6). *Journal of Traditional Chinese Medicine* 15(2), 118–121.

754. Stickler G.B., Smith T.F. & Broughton D.D. (1985) The common cold. *European Journal of Pediatrics* 144(1), 4–8.

755. Freymuth F., Vabret A., Gouarin S., Petitjean J. & Campet M. (2001) Epidemiology of respiratory virus infections. *Allergy and Immunology (Paris)* 33(2), 66–69. [Abstract. Article in French]

756. Kirkpatrick G.L. (1996) The common cold. *Primary Care* 23(4), 657–675.

757. Middleton D.B. (1991) An approach to pediatric upper respiratory infections. *American Family Physician* 44(5 Suppl), 33S–40S, 46S–47S.

758. Goldmann D.A. (2000) Transmission of viral respiratory infections in the home. *Pediatric Infectious Diseases Journal* 19(10 Suppl), S97–S102.

759. El-Sahly H.M., Atmar R.L., Glezen W.P. & Greenberg S.B. (2000) Spectrum of clinical illness in hospitalized patients with "common cold" virus infections. *Clinical Infectious Diseases* 31(1), 96–100.

760. Pierres-Surer N., Beby-Defaux A., Bourgoin A., Venot C., Berthier M., Grollier G., Oriot D. & Agius G. (1998) Rhinovirus infections in hospitalized children: a 3-year study. *Archives of Pediatrics* 5(1), 9–14. [Abstract. Article in French]

761. Pitkaranta A. & Hayden F.G. (1998) Rhinoviruses: important respiratory pathogens. *Annals of Medicine* 30(6), 529–537.

762. Rakes G.P., Arruda E., Ingram J.M., Hoover G.E., Zambrano J.C., Hayden F.G., Platts-Mills T.A. & Heymann P.W. (1999) Rhinovirus and respiratory syncytial virus in wheezing children requiring emergency care. IgE and eosinophil analyses. *American Journal of Respiratory Critical Care Medicine* 159(3), 785–790.

763. Walker T.A., Khurana S. & Tilden S.J. (1994) Viral respiratory infections. *Pediatric Clinics of North America* 41(6), 1365–1381.

764. Turner R.B. (1997) Epidemiology, pathogenesis, and treatment of the common cold. *Annals of Allergy, Asthma, Immunology* 78(6), 531–539.

765. Hendley J.O. (1999) Clinical virology of rhinoviruses. *Advances in Virus Research* 54, 453–466.

766. Nahmias A., Yolken R. & Keyserling H. (1985) Rapid diagnosis of viral infections: a new challenge for the pediatrician. *Advances in Pediatrics* 32, 507–525.

767. Kasa R.M. (1983) Vitamin C: from scurvy to the common cold. *American Journal of Medical Technology* 49(1), 23–26.

768. Hemila H. (1996) Vitamin C supplementation and common cold symptoms: problems with inaccurate reviews. *Nutrition* 12(11–12), 804–809. [Abstract]

769. Fireman P. (1993) Pathophysiology and pharmacotherapy of common upper respiratory diseases. *Pharmacotherapy* 13(6Pt 2), 101S;143S.

770. Luks D. & Anderson M.R. (1996) Antihistamines and the common cold: a review and critique of the literature. *Journal of General Internal Medicine* 11(4), 240.

771. Smith M.B. & Feldman W. (1993) Over the counter cold medications: a critical review of clinical trials between 1950 and 1991. *Journal of the American Medical Association* 269(17), 2258.

772. Murray S. & Brewerton T. (1993) Abuse of over-the-counter dextromethorphan by teenagers. *South Medical Journal* 86(10), 1151–1153.

773. Eccles R. (1996) Codeine, cough and upper respiratory infection. *Pulmonary Pharmacology* 9(5–6), 293–297.

774. English J.A. & Bauman K.A. (1997) Evidence-based management of upper respiratory infection in a family practice teaching clinic. *Family Medicine* 29(1), 38.

775. Mainous A.G. III, Hueston W.J. & Clark J.R. (1996) Antibiotics and upper respiratory infection: do some folks think there is a cure for the common cold? *Journal of Family Practice* 42(4), 357.

776. Houglum J.E. (1983) Interferon: mechanisms of action and clinical value. *Clinical Pharmacology* 2(1), 20–28.

777. Seidenberg J. (1989) Antihistamines in pediatrics. *Monatsschrift Kinderheilkunde* 137(1), 54–56. [Abstract. Article in German]

778. Saroea H.G. (1993) Common colds. Causes, potential cures, and treatment. *Canadian Family Physician* 39, 2215–2216; 2219–2220.

779. Isaacson G. (1996) Sinusitis in childhood. *Pediatric Clinics of North America* 436, 1297.

780. Crome M.A., Dickinson J.A. & Reid A.L. (1983) The use of antibiotics in upper respiratory tract infection. *Australian Family Physician* 12(8), 585–587.

781. Zhu S., Wang N., Wang D., Wang M., Tong K., Xu H., Wang J., Li Q., Peng J. & Wang J. (1998) A clinical investigation on massage for prevention and treatment of recurrent respiratory tract infection in children. *Journal of Traditional Chinese Medicine* 18(4), 285–291.

782. Hu J. (2000) Acupuncture treatment of common cold. *Journal of Traditional Chinese Medicine* 20(3), 227–230.

783. Xu J. (1989) Influence of acupuncture on human nasal mucociliary transport. *Zhonghua Er Bi Yan Hou Ke Za Zhi* 24(2), 90–91, 127. [Article in Chinese]

784. Yu S., Cao J. & Yu Z. (1993) Acupuncture treatment of chronic rhinitis in 75 cases. *Journal of Traditional Chinese Medicine* 13(2), 103–105.

785. Oskolkova M.K., Podgalo D.A., Briazgunov I.P., Lukina O.F. & Meshcheriakov L.P. (1980) Acupuncture and electropuncture in the overall therapy of diseases in children. *Pediatriia* (3), 53–56. [Article in Russian]

786. Long X., Chang Q. & Shou Q. (2001) Clinical observation on 46 cases of infantile repeated respiratory tract infection treated by mild-moxibustion over acupoints on back. *Journal of Traditional Chinese Medicine* 21(1), 23–26.

787. Davies A., Lewith G., Goddard J. & Howarth P. (1998) The effect of acupuncture on nonallergic rhinitis: a controlled pilot study. *Alternative Therapy and Health Medicine* 4(1), 70–74.

788. Takeuchi H., Jawad M.S. & Eccles R. (1999) The effects of nasal massage of the "yingxiang" acupuncture point on nasal airway resistance and sensation of nasal airflow in patients with nasal congestion associated with acute upper respiratory tract infection. *American Journal of Rhinology* 13(2), 77–79.

789. Pothman R. & Yeh H.L. (1982) The effects of treatment with antibiotics, laser and acupuncture upon chronic maxillary sinusitis in children. *American Journal of Chinese Medicine* 10(1–4), 55–58.

790. Lindert K.A. & Shortliffe L.M. (1999) Evaluation and management of pediatric urinary tract infections. *Urology Clinics of North America* 26(4), 719–728, viii.

791. Lettgen B. (1993) Urinary tract infections in childhood. Old and new aspect. *Klinische Padiatrie* 205(5), 325–331. [Abstract. Article in German]

792. Ey J.L., Aldous M.B., Duncan B. & Williams R.L. (1994) Office laboratory procedures, economics of practice, patient and parent education, and urinary tract infection. *Current Opinions in Pediatrics* 6(6), 717–728.

793. Jadresic L., Cartwright K., Cowie N., Witcombe B. & Stevens D. (1993) Investigation of urinary tract infection in childhood. *British Medical Journal* 307(6907), 761–764.

794. Weir M. & Brien J. (2000) Adolescent urinary tract infections. *Adolescent Medicine* 11(2), 293–313.

795. Feld L.G. (1991) Urinary tract infections in childhood: definition, pathogenesis, diagnosis, and management. *Pharmacotherapy* 11(4), 326–335.

796. Jodal U. (1987) The natural history of bacteriuria in childhood. *Infectious Diseases Clinics of North America* 1(4), 713–729.

797. Watson A.R. (1994) Urinary tract infection in early childhood. *Journal of Antimicrobial Chemotherapy* 34 Suppl A, 53–60.

798. Linshaw M.A. (1999) Controversies in childhood urinary tract infections. *World Journal of Urology* 17(6), 383–395.

799. Downs S.M. (1999) Technical report: urinary tract infections in febrile infants and young children. The Urinary Tract Subcommittee of the American Academy of Pediatrics Committee on Quality Improvement. *Pediatrics* 103(4), e54.

800. Roberts K.B. (2000) The AAP practice parameter on urinary tract infections in febrile infants and young children. American Academy of Pediatrics. *American Family Physician* 62(8), 1815–1822.

801. Misselwitz J. & Handrick W. (1991) Urinary tract infection in childhood—an overview. Therapy. *Kinderarztliche Praxis* 59(3), 64–67. [Abstract. Article in German]

802. Arant B.S. Jr. (1991) Vesicoureteric reflux and renal injury. *American Journal of Kidney Disease* 17(5), 491–511.

803. Smellie J.M., Poulton A. & Prescod N.P. (1994) Retrospective study of children with renal scarring associated with reflux and urinary infection. *British Medical Journal* 308(6938), 1193–1196.

804. Aune A., Alraek T., LiHua H. & Baerheim A. (1998) Acupuncture in the prophylaxis of recurrent lower urinary tract infection in adult women. *Scandinavian Journal of Primary Health Care* 16(1), 37–39.

Appendix
Acupuncture
Meridians

TABLE A.1	Standard international nomenclature for the 14 meridians		
		Alphabetic code	
Name or meridian		**Agreed**	**Former**
Lung		LU	Lu, P
Large Intestine		LI	CO, Co, IC
Stomach		ST	S, St, E, M
Spleen		SP	Sp, LP
Heart		HT	H, C, Ht, He
Small Intestine		SI	Si, IT
Bladder		BL	B, Bi, UB
Kidney		KI	Ki, R, Rn
Pericardium		PC	P, Pe, HC
Triple Energizer		TE	T, TW, SJ, 3H, TB
Gallbladder		GB	G, VB, VF
Liver		LR	Liv, LV, H
Governor Vessel		GV	Du, Du Go, Gv, TM
Conception Vessel		CV	Co, Cv, J, REN, Ren

The meridians are illustrated in Figures A.1 to A.14.

The major acupuncture points are shown in Figures A.15 to A.31.

FIGURE A.1 *The Lung meridian.*

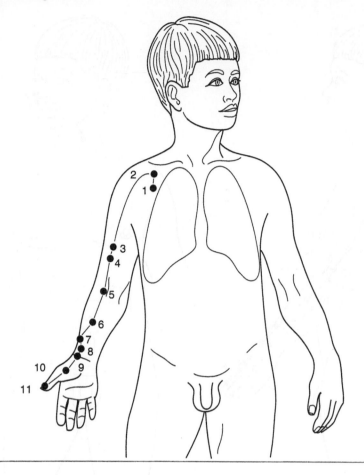

FIGURE A.2   *The Large Intestine meridian.*

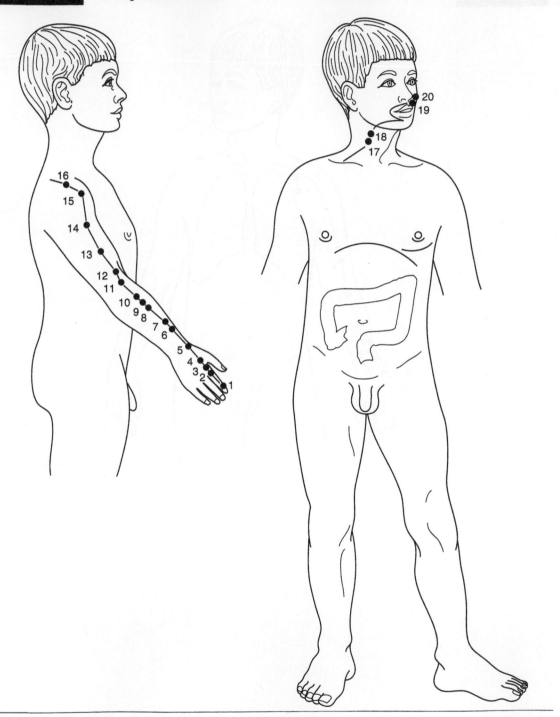

FIGURE A.3   *The Stomach meridian.*

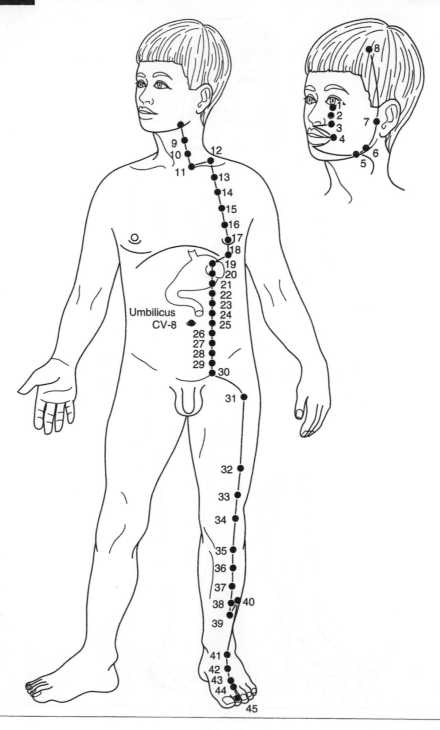

FIGURE A.4　*The Spleen meridian.*

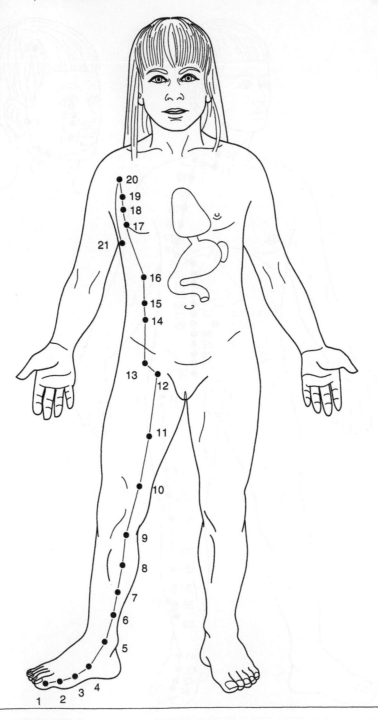

FIGURE A.5   *The Heart meridian.*

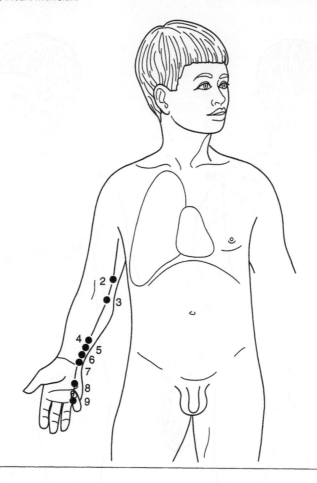

FIGURE A.6   *The Small Intestine meridian.*

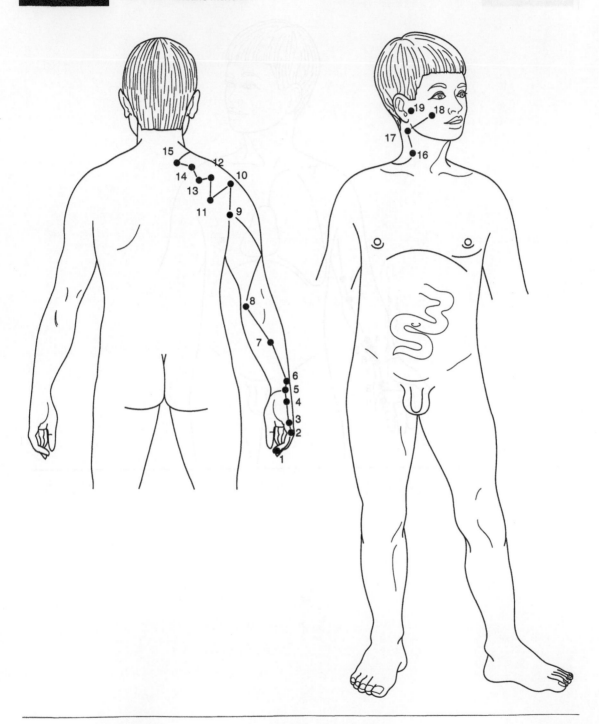

FIGURE A.7   *The Bladder meridian.*

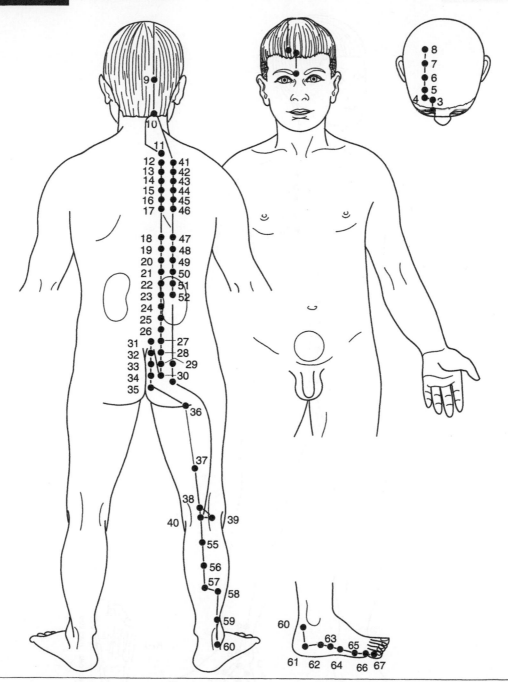

FIGURE A.8 *The Kidney meridian.*

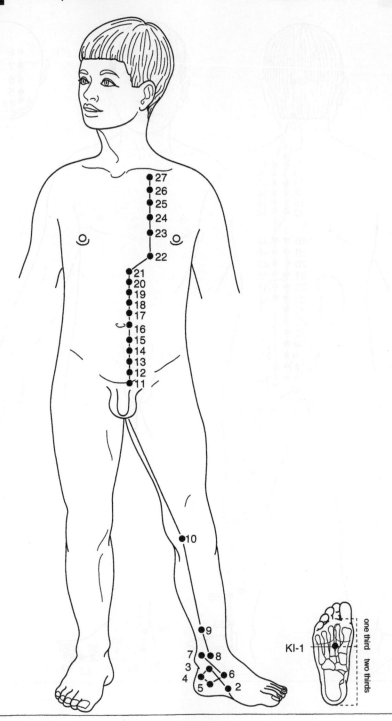

FIGURE A.9 *The Pericardium meridian.*

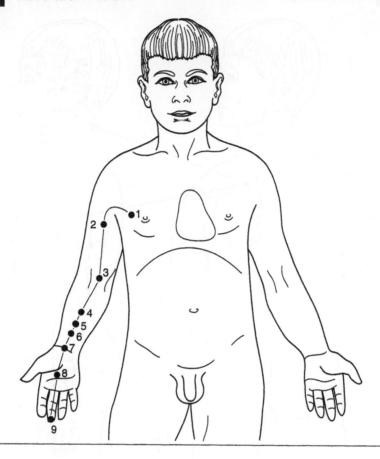

FIGURE A.10   *The Triple Energizer meridian.*

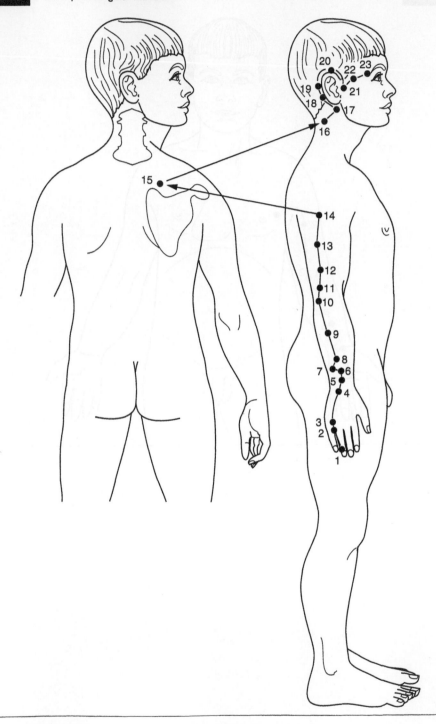

FIGURE A.11   *The Gallbladder meridian.*

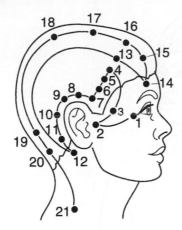
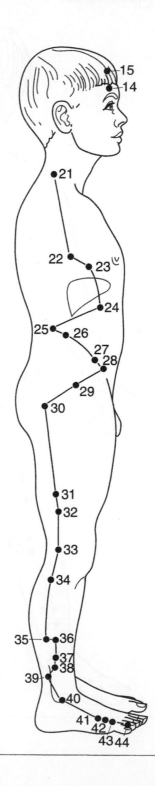

FIGURE A.12   *The Liver meridian.*

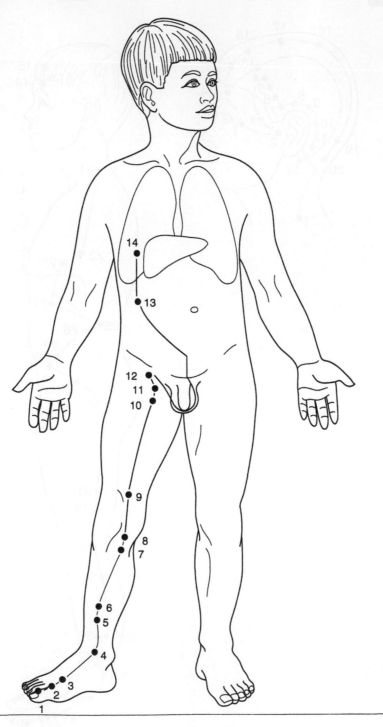

FIGURE A.13   *The Governor Vessel meridian.*

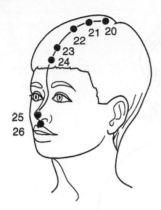
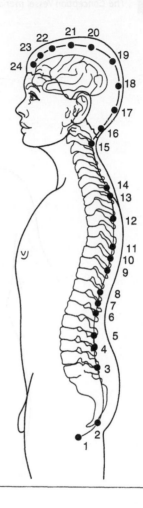

The Conception Vessel meridian.

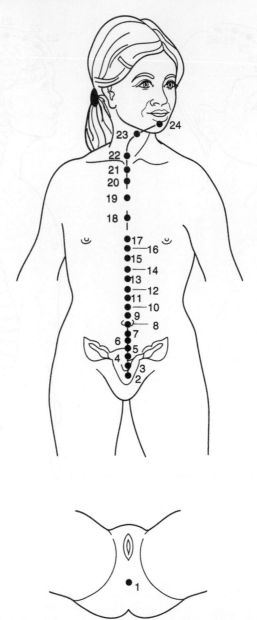

FIGURE A.15   *Major points of the upper abdomen.*

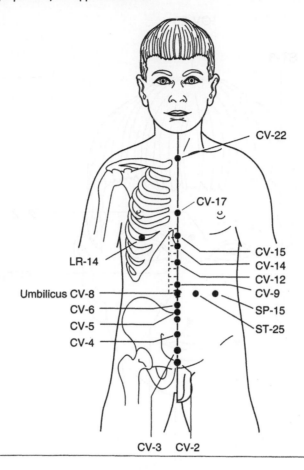

Major points of the face.

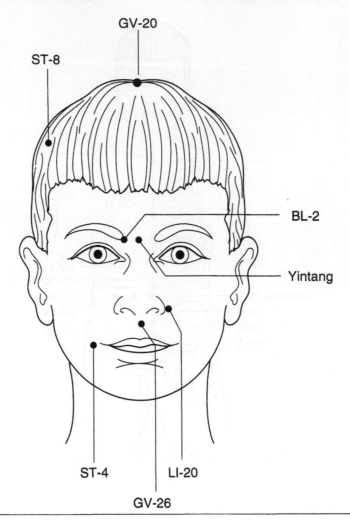

FIGURE A.17   *Major Governor Vessel and Bladder points.*

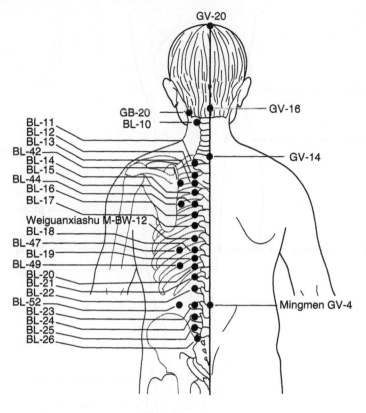

BL-42	Door of Corporeal Soul	BL-13	Lung Shu
BL-44	Hall of Shen	BL-15	Heart Shu
BL-47	Gate of Ethereal Soul	BL-18	Liver Shu
BL-49	House of Thought	BL-20	Spleen Shu
BL-52	Residence of Will	BL-23	Kidney Shu

FIGURE A.18   *Major points of the anterior lower leg.*

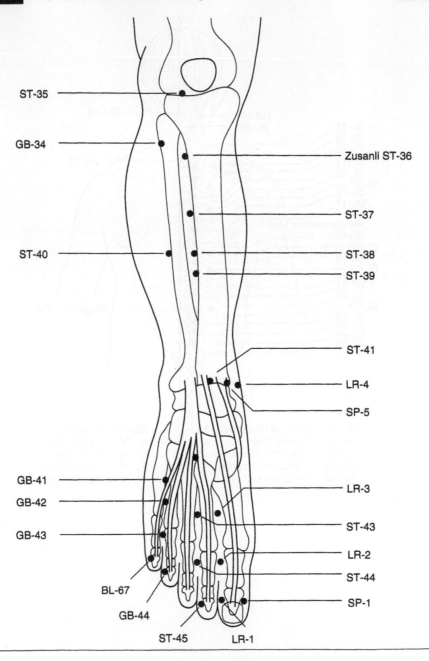

ST-35

GB-34

Zusanli ST-36

ST-37

ST-40

ST-38

ST-39

ST-41

LR-4

SP-5

GB-41

LR-3

GB-42

GB-43

ST-43

LR-2

ST-44

BL-67

SP-1

GB-44

ST-45   LR-1

FIGURE A.19   *Major points of the medial lower leg.*

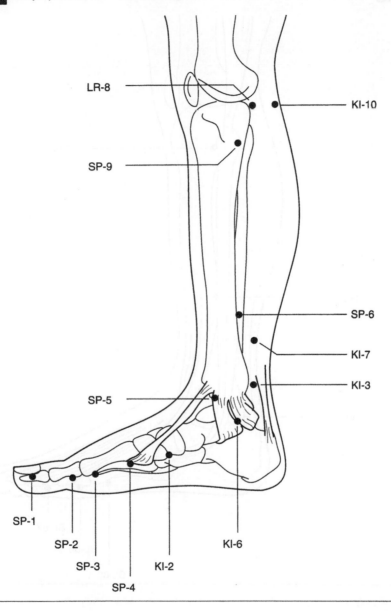

FIGURE A.20   *Major points of the lateral lower leg.*

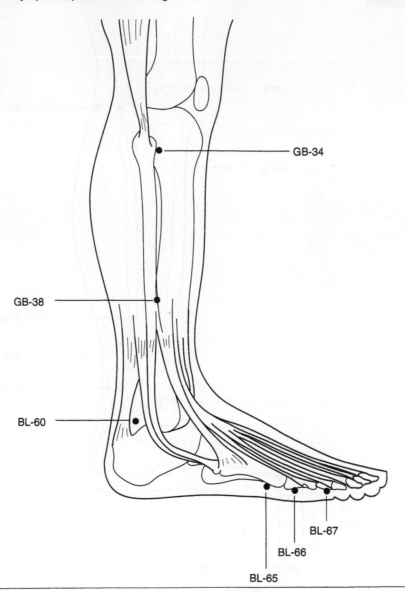

GB-34

GB-38

BL-60

BL-67

BL-66

BL-65

FIGURE A.21   *Weizhong point BL-40 on the leg.*

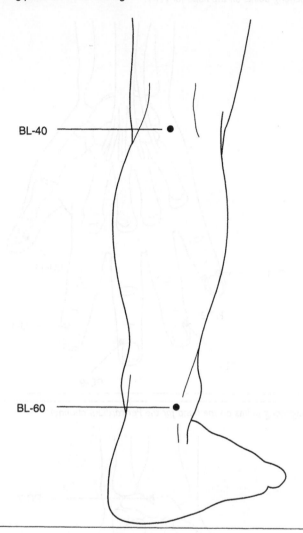

FIGURE A.22 *Shaochong points on the hand for HT-9.*

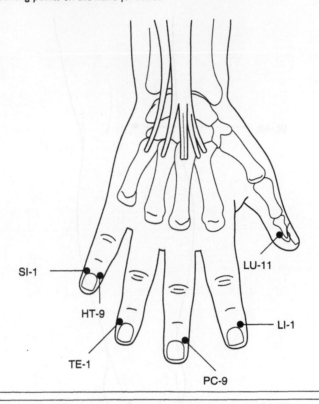

FIGURE A.23 *Zhongchong points on the hand for the Pericardium channel.*

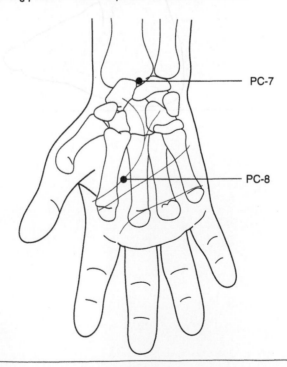

| FIGURE A.24 | Lingdao points HT-4 on the hand. |

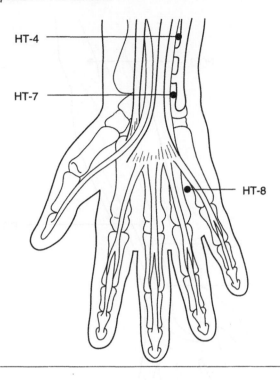

| FIGURE A.25 | Yangxi LI-5 points on the hand. |

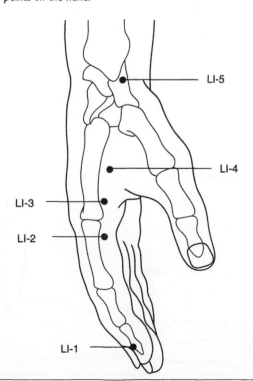

FIGURE A.26 Ximen points PC-4 on the arm and hand.

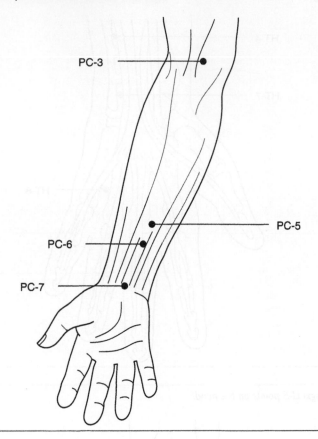

FIGURE A.27 Pianli points LI-6 on the arm.

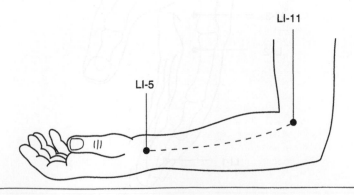

FIGURE A.28   *Shaohai HT-3 point.*

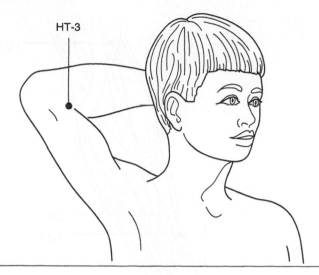

HT-3

FIGURE A.29   *Waiguan Triple Energizer points on the arm and hand.*

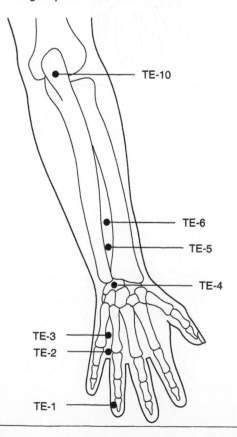

TE-10

TE-6

TE-5

TE-4

TE-3

TE-2

TE-1

FIGURE A.30 *Kongzui Lung points on the arm.*

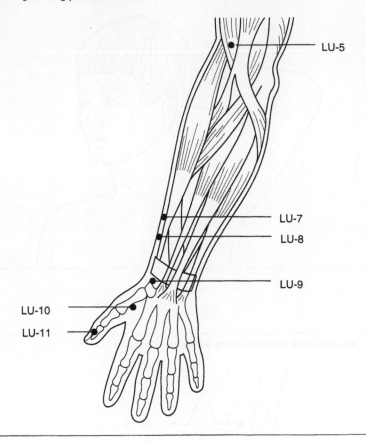

FIGURE A.31   *Zhizheng Small Intestine points on the arm and hand.*

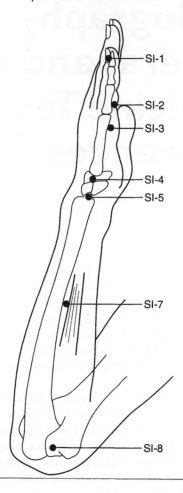

Bibliography of General and Chinese Medicine Texts and References

Bass, J.W. (1996) A review of rationale and advantages of various mixtures of benzathine penicillin G. *Pediatrics* 97(6 pt2), 960–963.

Beinfield, H. & Korngold, E. (1991) *Between Heaven and Earth, A Guide to Chinese Medicine*. New York, Balantine Books.

Bensky, D. & Gamble, A. (1993) Translated and compiled, *Materia Medica, Chinese Herbal Medicine*. Seattle, Eastland Press.

Cao, J. *et al.* (1990) *Essentials of Traditional Chinese Pediatrics*. Beijing, Foreign Language Press.

Chang, C.C. (1981) *Shang Han Lun: Wellspring of Chinese Medicine*, edited by Hong-Yen Hsu and William G. Peacher. Long Beach, Keats Publishing.

Chang, C.C. (1991) *Shang Han Lun* (in Chinese). Beijing, Beijing Press.

China Zhenjiuology, a series of video teaching tapes produced by "hundreds of renowned professors and specialists" from numerous Chinese Medical Colleges, coproduction by Chinese Medical Audio-Video Organization and Meditalent Enterprises Ltd.

Dahn, K.A., Glode, M.P. & Chan, K.H. (2000) Periodic fever and pharyngitis in young children: a new disease for the otolaryngologist? *Archives of Otolaryngology Head and Neck Surgery* 126(9), 1146–1149.

Deadman, P. & Al-Khafaji, M. (1988) *A Manual of Acupuncture*. Hove, Journal of Chinese Medicine Publications.

Diagnosis and Treatment of Gynecology and Pediatrics, in *China Zhenjiuology, A Series of Teaching Videotapes*, coproduced by Chinese Medical Audio-Video Organization and Meditalent Enterprises Ltd.

Ellis, E., Wiseman, N. & Boss, K. (1991) *Fundamentals of Chinese Acupuncture*, revised edition. Brookline, Paradigm Publications.

English-Chinese Encyclopedia of Practical Traditional Chinese Medicine. Beijing, Higher Education Press, volumes 1–14.

Flaws, B. (1997) *A Handbook of TCM Pediatrics, A Practitioner's Guide to the Care and Treatment of Common Childhood Diseases*. Denver, Blue Poppy Press.

Gunsberger, M. (1973) Acupuncture in the treatment of sore throat symptomatology. *American Journal of Chinese Medicine* 1(2), 337–340.

Helms, J. (1995) *Acupuncture Energetics, A Clinical Approach for Physicians*. Berkeley, Medical Acupuncture Publishers.

Hudson, D.E. (1997) Preliminary study to measure laser light and LED penetration through tissue. Respond Systems (Brand Ford, CT) Technical Report, 1–4.

Loo, M. (1999) Alternative therapies in children. In Spencer *et al.* (ed.) *Complementary/Alternative Medicine, An Evidence-Based Approach*. St Louis, Mosby.

Loo, M. Personal observations at TCM children's ward, Xinhua Hospital, Shanghai, China, 1999.

Lowrey, G.H. (1974) *Growth and Development of Children*. Chicago, Yearbook Medical Publishers.

Maciocia, G. (1994) *The Practice of Chinese Medicine, The Treatment of Diseases with Acupuncture and Chinese Herbs*. London, Churchill Livingstone.

Maciocia, G. (1995) *Tongue Diagnosis in Chinese Medicine*. Seattle, Eastland Press.

Maciocia, G. (1989) *The Foundations of Chinese Medicine, A Comprehensive Text for Acupuncturists and Herbalists*. London, Churchill Livingstone.

Matsumoto, K. & Birch, S. (1983) *Five Elements and Ten Stems, Nan Ching Theory, Diagnostics and Practice*. Brookline, Paradigm Publications.

Mussat, M. *Acupuncture Energetic Lectures*, part of video film library for UCLA acupuncture course.

Nei Ching, The Yellow Emperor's Classic of Internal Medicine, translated by Ilza Veith. Berkeley, University of California Press, 1949.

Nelson W.E. *et al.* (1996) *Nelson's Textbook of Pediatrics*, 15th edition. Philadelphia, W.B. Saunders Co.

Ni, M., & McNease, C. (1987) *The Tao of Nutrition*. Santa Monica, Seven Star Communications.

O'Connor, J. & Bensky, D. (eds) (1981) *Acupuncture, A Comprehensive Text*. Seattle, Eastland Press.

Oleson, T. (1996) *Auriculotherapy Manual: Chinese and Western Systems of Ear Acupuncture*. Los Angeles, Health Care Alternatives.

Raquena, Y. (1986) *Terrains and Pathology in Acupuncture, Volume One: Correlations with Diathetic Medicine*. Brookline, Paradigm Publications.

Reid, D. (1995) *The Complete Book of Chinese Health and Healing, Guarding the Three Treasures*. Boston, Shambhala.

Roy, C.C., Silverman, A. & Alagille, D. (1995) *Pediatric Clinical Gastroenterology*. New York, Mosby.

Ruppert, S.D. (1996) Differential diagnosis of common causes of pediatric pharyngitis. *Nurse Practitioner* 21(4), 38–42, 44, 47–48.

Schechter, N.L. (1995) Common pain problems in the general pediatric setting. *Pediatric Annals* 24(3), 139, 143–146.

Scott, J. (1991) *Acupuncture in the Treatment of Children*. London, Eastland Press.

Thomas, M., Del Mar, C. & Glasziou, P. (2000) How effective are treatments other than antibiotics for acute sore throat? *British Journal of General Practice* 50(459), 817–820.

Treatise on Febrile Diseases Caused by Cold with 500 Cases. Beijing, New World Press, 1993.

Index

Note: Page numbers in italics refer to figures and tables.

Printed and bound by CPI Group (UK) Ltd, Croydon, CR0 4YY

03/10/2024

01040366-0015